Children's Head Injury:
who cares?

This book is dedicated to the Children's Head Injury Trust

Children's Head Injury:
who cares?

David A. Johnson, David Uttley and Maria A. Wyke

Taylor & Francis
London • New York • Philadelphia

UK   Taylor & Francis Ltd., 4 John St., London WC1N 2ET

USA   Taylor & Francis Inc., 1900 Frost Road., Suite 101, Bristol, PA 19007

First published in 1989

British Library Cataloguing in Publication Data is available on request

ISBN 0–85066–846–8
ISBN 0–85066–846–X (pbk.)

Typeset in 11/13 Bembo by
Chapterhouse, The Cloisters, Formby L37 3PX

Printed in Great Britain by BPCC Wheatons Ltd, Exeter

Contents

List of figures

List of tables

Foreword

As a mother who has experienced the trauma of a son's horrific accident, his period of unconsciousness and rehabilitation, I am pleased to offer a foreword to this timely volume.

Its title is somewhat rhetorical, as I am sure that we all care about the health and welfare of our children who are suddenly placed at life's risk. Yet, the parent of a head-injured child often feels utterly alone in facing a prolonged and stressful ordeal; where neither the health care nor educational services seem interested in the longer term recovery of the child, nor have little to offer in the way of a comprehensive service for head injury victims. From the great number and variety of professionals attending the meeting in March 1988, I feel sure that many of them are sufficiently concerned to improve the care of these children.

It is abundantly clear that we must urgently fund research into the many questions raised by the contributing authors. I hope that this volume will serve to encourage enquiry and focus attention on this much neglected and needy population.

Anne Glennconner
London 1988

Preface

This volume presents the proceedings of 'Head Injured Children: who cares?'; a meeting held in London on 18 March 1988, organised by Atkinson Morley's Hospital and HEADWAY. The numbers attending from a wide diversity of professional disciplines far exceeded our expectations, and a common report was the feeling of isolation in working with head-injured children, and the desperate need for more information on how best to help.

Our thanks go to the contributors to this volume, who largely represent interested clinicians working closely with head-injured children. The range of subjects covered is far from exhaustive and there are many topics, such as epilepsy and cognitive development, which have been omitted either because of time or space. This volume is not intended as a comprehensive textbook as, indeed, it will be clear to the reader that there is relatively little scientific research material published which is specifically concerned with head injury in children. This small book represents a collective interest in the neglected morbidity of head-injured children, and a call for greater attention to be paid to the problems faced by the head-injured child in health, education and development.

HEADWAY, the National Head Injuries Association, backed the March meeting financially. As a small token of our thanks to HEADWAY, therefore, we are pleased to donate the royalties from sales of this book. We were surprised to find a total lack of interest and concern from the many pharmaceutical companies approached for help in staging this meeting, who failed to acknowledge the potential for neuropsychophar-macological research with this population, in order to improve outcome.

As a result of the interest shown in this venture, the CHILDREN'S HEAD INJURY TRUST has been established. Its general aims are to foster research and education into children's head injury, in association with other interested groups such as the National Children's Bureau, Child Accident Prevention Trust and HEADWAY. Further information concerning the CHILDREN'S HEAD INJURY

TRUST may be obtained by writing to the Chairman, Children's Head Injury Trust, Atkinson Morley's Hospital, Copse Hill, London SW20 0NE.

DAJ, DU, MAW,
London 1988

Acknowledgments

We are indebted to Sarah Bain and Ann Butt for their secretarial skills and help in completing this work.

Introduction: Why Should We Care?

The mention of injury to the head or brain strikes a note of apprehension in most people. Similarly, reports of any injury or debilitating tragedy to children arouse widespread sympathy and feelings of indignation that the young should suffer in any way. For the head-injured child, however, such public sympathy appears to be rather short lived, despite persisting and long-term difficulties stemming from the injuries. Head injury is never an all-or-nothing phenomenon, irrespective of the cause; rather, it is a matter of degree, producing relative changes in brain structure and function. As is evident from the contributions to this volume, the notion of greater plasticity and recovery of children who suffer head injury is not generally supported.

There is little age differentiation in the published reports on children's head injury: a paediatric population may range from birth to 19 years of age (Ward and Alberico, 1987). This has generated much confusion, especially in relation to evaluating outcome. Age demarcates stages or periods of development which reflect the underlying neurological substrate, although age alone is not a sufficient index (Jeffrey, 1980). Consequently, head-injured children as a population may reasonably be expected to show quite different, within-group responses to trauma, relative to their stage of development (e.g., Luerssen, Klauber and Marshall, 1988). Much of the early literature, especially neurosurgical and psychological, implies that the younger child is less vulnerable and shows a greater recovery from head injury than those who are older. There have been extensive methodological criticisms of such work, however, which suggest that given adequate evaluations, particularly of cognitive function, the young head-injured child does not show a preferential recovery rate. Relatively greater impairment appears in children younger than 8 years at the time of injury, but there has been a general failure to institute longitudinal studies of infants and toddlers with sufficiently sensitive outcome measures, and parallel neuroradiological confirmation. It appears that younger children may also be more vulnerable to a wide range of secondary factors, including nutrition and environmental stimulation.

Head injury to the child occurs in the context of development and incomplete neurological maturation. Consequently, the general concepts of critical periods and vulnerability are most pertinent to the younger child sustaining head-injury. It remains speculative as to what extent normal development proceeds after head injury but, given the greater vulnerability of immature neurones to insult and their tendency for more rapid degeneration, it seems reasonable that normal maturation must be at high risk in terms of either the sequence or rate of development, or both. Neither should we assume that recovery will show continual improvement indefinitely or at least until the child 'grows up'. As indicated throughout this volume, aberrant development may result from secondary factors in the recovery process, or subsequent atrophy of damaged tissue. Secondary neural degeneration in the head-injured child, for example, has not been widely reported (see Lange-Cosak *et al.*, 1979; Cullum and Bigler, Wider, Schlesner, 1985; Jellinger, 1983; Mortimer and Pirozzolo, 1985), but this often arises even in the presence of relatively good physical ability and appearance. The CNS (Central Nervous System) possesses a finite adaptive capacity to withstand the effects of any cerebral insult. Head injury reduces that capacity and, with increasing severity of trauma and subsequent atrophy, the remaining capacity of the CNS to adapt to any further neurological insult becomes relatively limited. With a decline in capacity, new signs and symptoms may appear as critical thresholds are reached. Consequently, reasonable measures should be taken to prevent any additional cerebral insult to the now more vulnerable head-injured child. As brain development results from complex interactions between genetic and environmental factors, it seems reasonable to suggest that the young head-injured child may be in greater need of early rehabilitation than his adult counterpart. It is suggested that investigation of specific neurotrophic agents may yield major contributions to recovery; for example, nerve growth factor and cholinergic functions in the basal forebrain (Korsching, 1986; Stein, 1981; Goffinet and Everard, 1986; Lauder and Krebs, 1978). There is undoubtedly a limited time in which any measures designed to limit neurological damage in the child can be effective. Rehabilitation should aim to manage effectively those avoidable complications of more severe trauma, such as inadequate nutrition, joint contractures and poor posturing. Moreover, rehabilitation must aim to facilitate as normal a pattern of development as possible, hence the need for follow-ups throughout the period of the child's remaining development (Kaiser, Rudeberg, Frankhauser *et al.*, 1986). Similarly, we must develop inter-disciplinary rehabilitation facilities specifically for the head-injured child, incorporating neurological, educational and social factors. Rehabilitation must become more scientifically based and practised in a coherent and neurologically meaningful way, rather than the haphazard, inconsistent guesswork which characterizes rehabilitation in this country.

When someone is injured it is assumed by both public and doctors that the best treatment is provided, based on sound knowledge of the pathophysiological response to trauma (Yates, 1988). Recent reports challenge this complacency and propose the concept of an integrated response to trauma, with expert care from road-side to rehabilitation (Cummins, 1987). The system of such care would be of far greater practical importance than any of its constituent parts. At present, most people working with head-injured children are a rather disparate group of interested specialists who either fail to consider each other's contributions, or are forced to work in isolation. We must either enact the otherwise mythical concept of an inter-disciplinary team approach to trauma care or dispel it once and for all. Removal of disciplinary barriers may open new scientific frontiers and clinical working relationships, creating a forum from which research may help to solve innumerable practical problems for the head-injured child and family (Miner and Wagner, 1986; Klivington, 1986; Rapin, 1986). Working from centres of excellence, neuro-trauma specialists could devote some of their time to injury prevention (Handel and Perales, 1986), increasing the awareness and education of public and other professionals alike. By such approaches, one may reasonably hope to improve community adoption of both preventative measures and of head-injured individuals, many of whom are typically maligned and, as a result, bear painful stigmata for many years.

In order to proceed further with research and practice in the area of children's head injury, it is crucial that we adopt a unified approach with greater methodological rigour. This requires clearly defined variables, carefully delineated sub-groups by mechanism and agent of trauma, extent and location of injury, maturity at time of injury, time since injury, general health and nutritional status; as well as a longer term follow-up with appropriate measures. Reliance upon singular testing procedures, whether the Glasgow Outcome Scale, or general IQ, has lead us, probably more than anything else, into perpetuating the dichotomous notion of 'recovery of function — no recovery' for age and brain damage relationships (Johnson and Almli, 1978). Similarly, we should examine carefully for the effects produced by mild head injuries in the child, particularly those cumulative effects produced by successive injury over many years. Pre-morbid factors may also require greater consideration, as some experimental studies suggest the importance of both physical (i.e., nutritional) and social (i.e., parental handling) factors prior to the injury, in determining outcome. There is seemingly little point in merely perpetuating the random fact gathering which has characterized so much clinical research and has lead to a gross misconception of the immature CNS and its ability to withstand the deleterious effects produced by various mechanisms of head-injury. How much of the good outcome reported for head-injured children is nothing but wishful thinking on our part, or the confusion of recovery with further development?

Trauma to the brain exerts perhaps the highest toll among all injuries, simply because it may dramatically alter the quality of future life for its survivors and their families (Shapiro, 1985; Lezak, 1988b; Waaland and Kreutzer, 1988). Nonetheless, we as a society continually fail to see the full implications of disability resulting from head injury in childhood (Haas, Cope and Hall, 1987) including increased educational support, lost or diminished careers, poor social and emotional adjustment, and later demands on mental health services.

Accidental head injury is not inevitable; many causes are preventable, given adequate attention to pedestrian safety and playground construction, for example (Bendixson, 1976; Handel and Perales, 1986; Atkins, Turner, Duthie *et al.*, 1988). Yet we continue to accept the carnage resulting from road traffic accidents, fail to implement comprehensive legislation for seat belt restraints, and fail to offer adequate protection from non-accidental injuries. Attention to such factors may help to reduce the probability of an increasingly disabled young population. In the absence of any effective treatments for the consequences of head injury, such preventative measures are urgently needed and may prove substantially cheaper than the increasing demands for continuing care as the true morbidity of this population is recognized. As Yates (1988) recently stated, an expenditure of 2 per cent of medical research budgets on trauma research seems insufficient, when more years of productive life are lost through injury, than through either cancer or cardiovascular disease (p. 1420).

It is hoped that readers of this volume will ponder the issues raised by the contributors and subsequently take positive action to instigate research and service development for this sadly neglected population.

Chapter 1

Mechanisms of trauma

B. A. Bell and Juliet Britton

Introduction

Head injury in children is common and one out of every ten children will sustain a significant head injury (Bruce, Schut and Sutton, 1985). It accounts for over 150,000 attendances per annum of children aged 14 years or under at casualty departments in the United Kingdom. About a third of these injuries occur at home, whilst playing or during a sporting activity. Falls account for about 15 per cent of the injuries, and around 10 per cent occur as a result of road accidents. Injuries at school and assaults make up approximately 5 per cent each (Strang, MacMillan and Jennett, 1978). Half of all the deaths each year in children aged under 15 years occur from head injury; with the death rate per 100,000 ranging from around seven in children aged from 0 to 4 years, to around ten in children aged from 5 to 9 years, and to about nineteen in children aged from 10 to 14 years (Klauber, Barrett-Connor, Marshall *et al.*, 1981).

Neonatal injuries

Head injuries at birth can result from the normal forces of labour and delivery, and steady pressure of the head against the pelvic prominence can produce a depressed 'table tennis ball' fracture and traumatic subarachnoid haemorrhage. Obstetric instrumentation can also cause head injury, particularly the misapplication of forceps, which can produce fractures of the skull vault and even the skull base. Traction injury to the spinal cord at the cervico-medullary junction, and to the brachial plexus may also follow a traumatic delivery.

Primary mechanisms of brain injury

Four differing mechanisms of injury can affect the brain, alone or in combination, to produce immediate tissue injury and dysfunction after a head injury.

Penetrating injury

The head may be struck by a sharp object, or the child may fall onto objects as diverse as an upturned 13 amp plug or a billiard cue. The penetrating object pierces the scalp and produces a depressed fracture of the skull, and may traverse the dura and enter the brain. The brain injury is normally localized, the child usually remains conscious, and the neurological signs will reflect the focal nature of any brain damage, e.g. a limb paresis if the appropriate area of the pre-central motor strip is penetrated.

Crushing injury

The head may be compressed between a moving and a stationary surface, such as by a mechanically operated door or by falling masonry. Inbending and fracture of the skull vault may be associated with basal skull fractures, whilst transient dislocation of structures such as the petrous ridges can damage the cranial nerves and brain stem.

Acceleration and deceleration injuries

This is the most common mechanism of head injury, occurring in the majority of road traffic accidents and falls. Rapid deceleration of the skull, as a vehicle is forced to an abrupt halt during an accident, will damage the brain as it moves against the inner surface of the skull by virtue of the brain's own momentum. Traumatic subarachnoid haemorrhage commonly results, with occasional frontal (Figure 1.1a) and temporal intracerebral contusions and, following falls, occipital contusions.

The internal elements of the brain are of differing densities and will decelerate at different rates, leading to shearing stresses within the substance of the brain. Fibre tracts in the brain stem and the junction between grey and white matter are particularly susceptible to damage. Free edges of dura such as the tentorial notch and the falx cerebri can create areas of focal damage in the midbrain and corpus callosum (Figure 1.1b).

The posterior cerebral arteries may also be compressed by the tentorium or the anterior cerebral arteries by the falx, leading to infarction of the brain supplied by these vessels. Linear forces are exacerbated by any rotational element which tends to produce

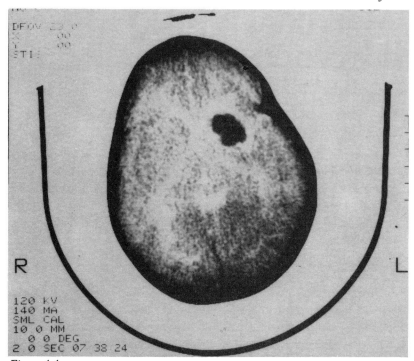

Figure 1.1a

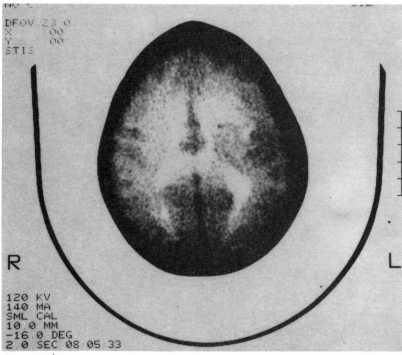

Figure 1.1b

lacerations across the brain and to tear cerebral vessels, creating acute intracerebral haematomas. The hypothalamus and pituitary stalk, and the olfactory nerves traversing the cribriform plate to reach the olfactory bulb, are particularly vulnerable to this mechanism of injury.

Child abuse

Most severe head injuries in children under 1 year of age are the result of child abuse (McClelland, Rekate, Kaufman *et al.*, 1980). Some 10 per cent of all traumatic injuries under 5 years of age will have a non-accidental cause. Head injury is the leading cause of death in child abuse, and of the 5 per cent of abused children who die, the mortality of the cranial component of the injury approaches 30 per cent. Half of the abused children with a head injury suffer permanent neurological and intellectual impairment (McClelland, Rekate, Kaufman *et al.*, 1980). The initial 'shaken baby syndrome' (Caffey, 1972) consisted of retinal haemorrhages, subdural haemorrhage, and subarachnoid haemorrhage, without visible signs of external trauma to the skull vault or scalp. The injuries are therefore usually ascribed to a whiplash-type injury (Caffey, 1974). Duhaime and her colleagues (Duhaime, Gennarelli, Thibault, *et al.* 1987) have recently suggested that there is commonly evidence of external trauma and the severity of the injuries is secondary to rapid deceleration and impact injury to the skull vault rather than simple shaking. Recurrent trauma is common (Figure 1.2), and the child may present with increasing head size and be found to have chronic subdural haematomas or hydrocephalus.

Figure 1.2

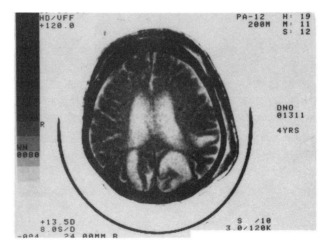

The presence of chronic subdural haematomas in an infant carries a high index of suspicion of non-accidental injury.

Figure 1.3

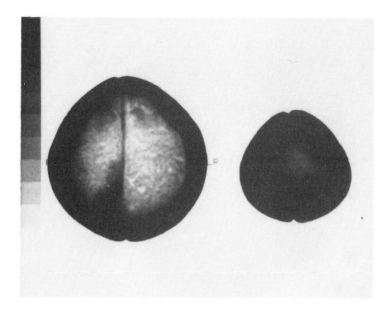

Features which may be identified on computed tomography (CT) scans in more acute presentations include acute subdural haematomas, which may be small and parafalcine (Figure 1.3), chronic subdural haematomas (Figure 1.4a), subarachnoid blood, intracerebral haematomas secondary to shear injuries, diffuse oedema — the mechanism of which is uncertain (Figure 1.4b), and arterial and venous infarction.

Arterial infarction is secondary to damage to the anterior or posterior cerebral arteries (Figure 1.2) where they run against the falx or tentorium. Shearing of the bridging parafalcine veins due to rotational forces may also cause bleeding within the falx and result in venous infarction. Indirect damage to the brain can also occur, and may be due to anoxia, possibly following compression of the neck or chest. Follow-up CT Scans are of importance in survivors of child abuse to detect enlarging subdural collections (Figure 1.5) or developing hydrocephalus.

Focal or diffuse atrophy can also be identified, commonly resulting from the diffuse oedema or more focal contusions and infarcts seen in the acute phase.

Figure 1.4a

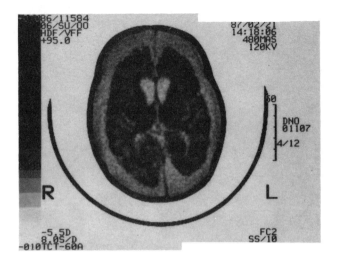

Figure 1.4b

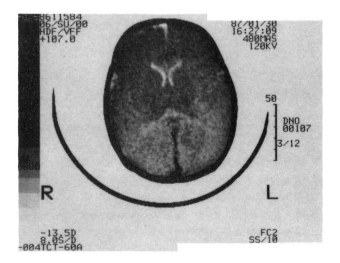

Figure 1.5a

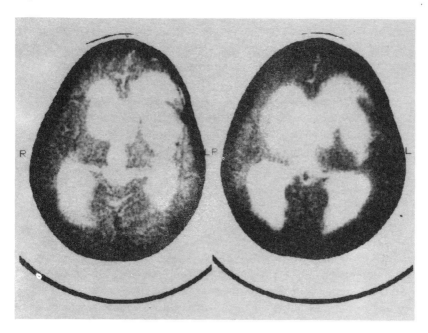

Figure 1.5b

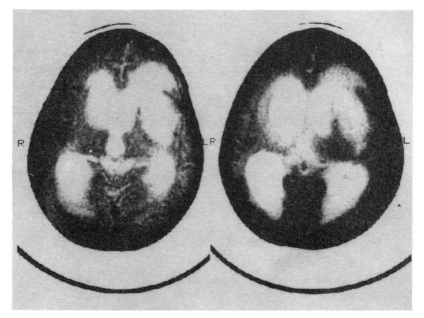

Missile injury:

The damage caused by a missile is proportional to its kinetic energy which is directly proportional to its mass and the square of its velocity. Thus a rifle bullet, which travels five times faster than a bullet from a pistol, will do twenty-five times as much damage to the brain. A low velocity bullet tends to leave an exit wound little bigger than the bullet itself, but the flight of a rifle bullet is rendered unstable during passage through the brain and leads to extensive fracturing and scalp damage at the site of exit from the skull. Children in deep coma after a missile injury rarely survive, and those that are conscious can rapidly deteriorate from brain swelling. Those remaining conscious will recover like any other penetrating head injury but with a high late post-traumatic epilepsy rate of about 45 per cent at 5 years (Jennett and Teasdale, 1981).

Structural brain injury

Computed tomography (CT) and now magnetic resonance imaging (MRI) have allowed the structural brain damage after head injury to be more accurately delineated during life. All unconscious children, and those with persistent vomiting, abnormal neurological signs, or a depressed skull fracture should have a CT scan.

Intracranial haematomas

Brain contusions (Figure 1.1b) are found in approximately 16 per cent of childhood head injuries, about half the incidence of 33 per cent found in adults (Zimmerman and Bilaniuk, 1981). Intracerebral haematoma (Figure 1.1a) is not common in children, with the incidence being approximately one-third of the 10 per cent incidence in adults. Extradural haematomas are also uncommon, affecting between 2 and 3 per cent of children under the age of 15 admitted after a head injury (Choux, Grisoli and Pergaut, 1975; Hendrick, Harwood-Nash and Hudson, 1964). Similarly acute subdural haematomas occur only a quarter as often as in adults (Zimmerman and Bilaniuk, 1981), but when they do occur they are highly likely to have been caused by child abuse.

Secondary mechanisms of brain damage

These secondary insults result from the brain's response to the initial impact, or from superadded infection.

Infection

Meningitis and intracerebral abscess can follow any injury where the integrity of the dura is breached, either directly in a penetrating injury with a depressed vault fracture, or indirectly in a basal skull fracture with a secondary dural tear. A dural tear is clinically manifest by a CSF leak, either from a scalp wound, or as rhinorrhoea or otorrhoea.

Diffuse cerebral swelling

This was proposed by Bruce and colleagues (Bruce, Alavi, Bilaniuk, *et al.* 1981) as a specific response to injury virtually confined to children. Bruce identified it in approximately 40 per cent of severely injured children who were in coma, and in over 20 per cent who were conscious. The authors suggested that in children who die from head injury, diffuse cerebral swelling manifest by obliteration of the intracranial CSF spaces and venous congestion is the most common autopsy finding (Lindenberg, Rischer and Durlacher, 1955). The swollen brain was thought to have normal Hounsfield numbers, implying that cerebral oedema was not the cause of the diffuse swelling, and increased cerebral blood volume was proposed as the aetiology. The definition of diffuse cerebral swelling was imprecise, and the concept was not accepted unequivocally. Later generation CT scanners have revealed that the swollen brain is not radiologically normal, showing impaired grey-white matter definition, and lowered density consistent with oedema that would not have been detected on the first and second generation CT scanners used by Bruce prior to 1981.

Hydrocephalus

Communicating hydrocephalus may develop following haemorrhage into the subarachnoid space (Figure 1.5).

Skull injury

Skull fractures are common in head injury in infants and young children and, despite being extensive on plain X-ray films, are only rarely associated with disturbance of consciousness and intracranial lesions. Unless the skull sutures are split, or the child has abnormal neurological signs, or is persistently vomiting, skull fracture without depression is not by itself an indication for a CT scan. An uncommon complication of skull fracture, when there is laceration of the dura and contusion of the underlying brain, is the 'growing skull fracture'. This usually follows an injury in which the level of consciousness is significantly altered, with an associated leptomeningeal cyst (Ito, Miwa and Onodra, 1977), and 90 per cent of growing fractures occur in children under three years of age.

Clinical evaluation

Seizures in the first hour following head injury in children are common, and rarely require medication. The incidence of late seizures in such children is below 1 per cent. Pallor, vomiting, and tachycardia are all very common following concussive injury in a child and, unlike adults, hypotension can be due to head injury in a small child. In children under one year of age, an extradural haematoma associated with a large skull fracture may leak through the fracture to the sub-galeal space, producing a combined extradural and sub-galeal haematoma that contains a significant proportion of the infant's blood volume. An infant with shunted hydrocephalus may also accumulate a large quantity of intracranial blood without elevating intracranial pressure, and thus become shocked.

Glasgow Coma Scale

In children under the age of two years the Glasgow Coma Scale (Jennett and Teasdale, 1981) is difficult to apply, and the verbal response may be scored by giving the child a value of five if there is any vocalization at all, and of zero if no crying is obtained. The motor component of the scale is applicable after the first few months of life, with the exception of the response to command, and is useful even on its own as the most powerful predictor of ultimate outcome of all three components of the scale in both children and adults. Despite the drawbacks of the application of the Glasgow Coma Scale to young children, it remains a good index of the depth of coma. The absence of a thoroughly evaluated alternative underlies the continuing value of this Scale in children. (See, for example, Simpson and Reilly 1982; Raimondi, Choux and Di Rocco, 1986).

Management

A child with an impaired conscious level following a head injury should have shock and hypoxia excluded as contributory causes. If arterial oxygen tension is low despite a clear airway and oxygen administration, the trachea should be intubated following pre-oxygenation with a bag and mask during which pressure on the cricoid cartilage prevents aspiration, and air entering the stomach. Thiopentone and muscle relaxants then allow endotracheal intubation without raising intracranial pressure further, and intermittent positive pressure ventilation should be adjusted to give a normal arterial oxygen tension (pO_2) and an arterial carbon dioxide tension (pCO_2) of between 25 and 30 mmHG. The child should leave the resuscitation room with a stable arterial pO_2 and systemic blood pressure, and management is then determined by CT scan findings. Surgical intervention is most commonly required for depressed skull fracture, the bone fragments being replaced after elevation, and with antibiotic cover if the fracture was compound. Extradural haematomas are promptly evacuated, as in adults, but a craniotomy is always used in preference to a craniectomy. Surgery for cerebral contusions and intracerebral haematomas should be avoided as far as possible, outcome being better with conservative management (Bruce, Schut and Sutton, 1985). Subdural haematomas are also best managed conservatively. The pia-arachnoid is easily stripped from the underlying cortex when the infant's brain is handled surgically, and extensive areas of brain ischaemia may be produced as the result of surgical intervention. The management of children with raised intracranial pressure aims to maintain the pressure below 20 mmHg, and therapy comprises elevation of the head to 30 degrees, hyperventilation to give an arterial carbon dioxide tension of 25 mmHg, diuretics, phenobarbitone, and finally mannitol.

Conclusion

Head injuries in children are common and there are four primary mechanisms underlying the brain damage in severe injuries. About a third of the injuries occur at home, and most severe head injuries in children under one year of age are the result of child abuse. Management of a child with an impaired conscious level following a head injury should initially treat shock and hypoxia and, following resuscitation, the child should be transferred to a neurosurgical unit with facilities for paediatric patients.

Chapter 2

Limits to cerebral plasticity

Robert Goodman

Introduction

Anyone who has looked after ill children will know that they often seem to bounce back very quickly after infections, broken bones or operations. Convalescent children are to be seen pedalling furiously around the paediatric ward at a stage when their adult counterparts would hardly have ventured out of their sick beds. Children's extraordinary capacity for physical recovery encourages both parents and professionals to hope that psychological recovery will be equally good, with little or no permanent aftermath. Sadly, however, this optimism is all too often ill founded after severe head injuries in childhood. We owe it to the children involved to face up to the limitations in the healing process. In the terrible days, weeks and months immediately after a severe head injury, optimism is essential for parents and professionals alike. In the longer term, however, children are not well served by the sort of blind optimism that goes on assuming that time will heal all. If head injuries result in lasting cognitive and behavioural deficits, these need to be recognized sooner rather than later — otherwise the child may be exposed to excessive demands, and the need for remedial help may not be appreciated.

This chapter begins by considering the individual's capacity to recover from brain injury, and then examines some of the limits to this recovery process. Recovery and its limitations are considered at two related levels: at the psychological level of which skills are acquired or re-acquired, and to what degree; and at the neurological level of how the brain reorganizes itself during the recovery process.

Recovery from brain injury

Severe brain injury can be followed by a striking degree of functional recovery, both in humans and experimental animals (see Finger and Stein, 1982). Brain-injured children and adults can regain lost abilities, whilst brain-injured children can also go on to acquire abilities that would normally have depended on the integrity of the damaged parts of their brains. Cerebral plasticity refers to the brain's capacity to reorganize itself after injury — a process that may facilitate recovery.

Lost abilities can be regained by restitution, in which the original means for achieving a particular end is fully or partly recovered, or by substitution, in which an alternative means is used to achieve the same end. To put this another way, restitution involves the brain reorganizing itself after injury in order to be able to achieve the same goals in the same way, while substitution involves the acquisition of a variety of alternative strategies for achieving the same goals in novel ways. Both restitution and substitution can vary in their degree of adequacy, and one is not necessarily better than the other. The remainder of this chapter is concerned with the brain's capacity for restitution, but this exclusive focus should not suggest that substitution is unimportant. On the contrary, substitution is of great practical and theoretical importance, particularly for anyone involved in rehabilitation.

Excellent recovery from early injury: three examples

To illustrate cerebral plasticity at its best, three examples have been chosen of excellent restitution of function after extensive but early brain injury. Two examples are drawn from animal experiments, and the third from clinical observations.

The first example concerns the recovery of vision in cats after bilateral damage to the visual cortex, involving cortical areas 17, 18 and 19 (Spear, 1979). If this damage is acquired when the cat is already an adult, the result is a severe deficit in a variety of visual abilities, including form and pattern discrimination. The loss of vision is not total, however, and the cat has some residual ability to distinguish between different forms and patterns. This residual ability depends principally on the integrity of the lateral suprasylvian (LS) cortex — a region that is not normally essential for this sort of discrimination. As time goes on, the cats recover some of their former ability to discriminate between different forms and patterns, with the LS cortex playing a central role in this recovery. If the LS cortex is subsequently damaged, the recovered abilities are lost again. Recovery from adult-acquired damage appears to be based on the cat learning how to make progressively more use of the surviving visual input, rather than on any fundamental reorganization of neuronal connections.

When the same sort of damage to the visual cortex is sustained not by an adult cat but by a newborn kitten, the recovery of visual abilities is much more complete. Few if any deficits remain by the time the kitten has grown up. Once again, the recovery of form and pattern discrimination depends mainly on the LS cortex. In this instance, however, a major neuronal reorganization occurs within the LS cortex, resulting in a pattern of neuronal connections which closely resembles that of the lost visual cortex.

A near-perfect recovery of function occurs, apparently as a result of the greater cerebral plasticity of the young brain.

The second example of excellent recovery after early damage involves the effect of bilateral prefrontal damage on delayed-response learning in monkeys (Goldman-Rakic, Isseroff, Schwartz *et al.*, 1983). In a typical delayed-response task, the monkey observes food being hidden in one of two foodwells, after which both wells are briefly hidden by a screen. Delayed-response learning is judged by the monkey's subsequent success at retrieving food from the correct well. The dorsolateral portion of the prefrontal cortex is essential for delayed-response learning in adult monkeys, but plays little or no role in delayed-response learning in young monkeys. If the dorsolateral cortex of an adult monkey is damaged bilaterally, the result is a permanent impairment on delayed-response tasks. When comparable damage is acquired in infancy, no deficit is evident initially because the dorsolateral cortex seems to play little or no role at this stage in life, but a permanent deficit in delayed-response learning becomes apparent when the monkey reaches adulthood. By contrast, when dorsolateral damage occurs prenatally, little or no deficit on delayed-response tasks is present when that monkey reaches adulthood. The capacity for long-term recovery after prenatal damage may be due to extensive reorganizations in the pattern of neuronal connections within the frontal lobes.

The final example of a particularly good recovery of function after early damage is drawn from a case report of a young boy who lost most of the left side of his brain (Smith and Sugar, 1975). The boy was first noted to have a right hemiplegia — that is, weakness and stiffness of his right arm and right leg — at five months of age, reflecting damage to the left cerebral hemisphere that was probably sustained at, or before, birth. Epileptic seizures began just before he was 4 years old, and became so frequent and uncontrollable that a left-sided hemispherectomy operation was performed at the age of 5 and a half years, with nearly all of the damaged left hemisphere being removed. Subsequent progress was remarkably good: the hemiplegia was no worse, seizures ceased entirely, and he was subsequently able to attend a normal school, play in the school band, complete a university degree, and find employment as an industrial executive. At the age of 26, he had an IQ of 116, with above-average scores on both verbal and nonverbal tests. Although this outcome was exceptional and does not reflect the serious problems that can be associated with hemispherectomy (see Goodman, 1986), the case is instructive. As a rule, the two cerebral hemispheres of the human brain show clear specialization of function, with language functions depending mainly on the left hemisphere, and with visuospatial and some musical functions subserved mainly by the right hemisphere (see Corballis, 1983; Gordon, 1983). When hemispherectomy follows unilateral damage sustained in late childhood or adult life, the individual is left with persisting deficits in the functions that were dependent on that hemisphere (Smith, 1972; Patterson, Vargha-Khadem and Polkey 1989). In the case described by Smith and Sugar (1975), by contrast, early damage to, and then removal of, the left hemisphere did not result in any subsequent deficit of language function. Indeed, the remaining right hemisphere was able to support above-average verbal abilities. Furthermore, this relatively unusual lateralization of language to the right hemisphere was not obtained at the cost of a loss of other abilities. In response to early damage to the left hemisphere, the right hemisphere was able to take over left-hemisphere language functions without apparently sacrificing its own right-hemisphere visuospatial and musical functions. Since this remarkable degree of recovery is not seen after comparable later damage, it presumably reflects the greater cerebral plasticity of the young brain.

What sort of reorganization of the nervous system might contribute to the extraordinary capacity for recovery from early brain damage that has been illustrated by the preceding three examples? Before turning to the neural mechanisms that are thought to underlie cerebral plasticity, it is worth taking several steps back to review the main features of normal brain development.

Normal brain development

From a functional point of view, it is the pattern of connections between neurones that is of central importance. A disconnected neurone is of no value, and a misconnected neurone may be worse than useless. On the other hand, the loss of millions of neurones can have little or no detrimental effect, provided the overall pattern of interconnections remains intact, e.g. clinical symptoms of Parkinson's disease do not generally appear until about 80 per cent of the zona compacta of the substantia nigra has degenerated (Marsden, 1987).

How does the brain's intricate pattern of interconnected neurones come into being? Used as we are to assembly lines and industrial production, the first stages of brain development come as no surprise: the components are manufactured, moved into position and then joined up — or to put it another way, cell division in the germinal layers produces neurones that subsequently migrate to their definitive position and form multiple axonal and dendritic connections (Ebels, 1980; Geschwind and Galaburda, 1985). Multiplication and migration are largely completed by the time a child is born (Geschwind and Galaburda, 1985), while the formation of connections starts before birth and continues at a high rate during infancy (Schade and van Groenigen, 1961). If brain development were like the production of a computer, the finished product would be ready once all the components were in place and connected. In fact, brain development proceeds rather differently, with a lengthy phase of fine-tuning by selective loss of cells and connections. In brain development, as in the development of practically all biological systems (Glucksman, 1951) there is a mixture of additive and subtractive processes. If additive processes are akin to industrial production, with a series of parts being added until the final product is complete, then subtractive processes are akin to sculpting a statue from a block of stone, with bits of stone being chipped away until the finished statue is shaped. As a first approximation, additive processes largely determine the broad outline of brain organization, while subtractive processes contribute to subsequent fine-tuning (Cowan, Fawcett, O'Leary *et al.*, 1984; Janowsky and Finlay, 1986). In most neuronal systems, roughly half of the original neurones die off during a well-defined period that is characteristic of each neuronal population. This selective cell death may eliminate neurones that have formed erroneous connections, as well as helping to match the size of each neuronal population to the size of its target field. Selective elimination of some of the axon collaterals of an individual neurone can increase the specificity of that neurone's connections. Fine-tuning by selective loss probably continues throughout childhood. In the human frontal cortex, for example, synaptic density reaches a peak in the second year of life and then progressively declines until late adolescence, presumably as a result of selective loss (Huttenlocher, 1979). It is worth emphasizing that head injuries in childhood generally occur in the midst of these subtractive processes, but at a time when the additive processes are complete or nearly complete.

Neuronal responses to brain injury

After this brief review of normal brain development, it is now possible to return to considering the brain's response to injury. Dead neurones cannot be replaced after the prenatal proliferative phase, but there is now abundant evidence from animal experiments that surviving neurones can form new synaptic connections in response to brain injury, particularly when the injury occurs early in life (Finger and Stein, 1982).

When an axon is transected by brain injury the distal portion dies, but the proximal portion may form growth cones and regenerate new terminals. This regenerative sprouting can result in the formation of appropriate new connections close to the site of injury (Kromer, Bjorklund and Stenevi, 1981). Successful axonal regeneration over longer distances is probably hampered because brain injury disrupts tissue alignment and vascularization, and also leads to the production of glial and connective-tissue barriers (Finger and Stein, 1982). In addition to initiating regenerative sprouting, brain injury can also initiate collateral sprouting: when the injury destroys some of the axons innervating an area, the remaining axons may produce side-branches (collateral sprouts) that reoccupy the vacated synaptic sites.

The neuronal response to brain injury depends, in part, on the age at injury (van Hof, 1981; Finger and Stein, 1982). Both regenerative and collateral sprouting occur more readily in young animals than in adult animals. In addition, if the brain is damaged before or during the stage of selective axonal loss, the accidental losses of some axonal collaterals can potentially be counterbalanced by a reduction in the normal losses of other axonal collaterals (Janowsky and Finlay, 1986). Finally, if the brain is injured at a very early stage, before the developing axons have reached their normal destination, some of the growing axons can eventually reach alternative destinations instead. As a result of these and other differences, early brain damage is more likely to elicit the production of anomalous connections, i.e. neuronal connections that are either absent or inconspicuous in a normal brain. Early brain-damage elicits more regeneration and remodelling, and so the young brain is said to show greater cerebral plasticity or neuroplasticity.

Although this section has focused primarily on structural reorganization after brain injury, it is worth noting that important functional changes in neuronal transmission can occur in the absence of structural changes. Recovery from brain injury may involve the reactivation of latent synapses (Wall, 1977) as well as the creation of new synapses.

Neuroplasticity may potentially be enhanced by a variety of chemical factors, including Nerve Growth Factor (NGF) (Bjorklund and Stenevi, 1972) and noradrenaline (Kasamatsu, Pettigrew and Ary, 1979). Stein, Palatucci, Kahn, *et al.*, (1988) have recently proposed that trophic factors released by foetal brain-tissue transplants account for the beneficial effects of these transplants on the behavioural recovery of brain-damaged experimental animals. Perhaps some of the age-related decline in neuroplasticity is due to a progressive decline in the brain's capacity to produce neurotrophic factors in response to injury.

In some studies, the degree of functional recovery after a brain injury has been correlated with the neuronal responses to that injury (Schneider, 1979; Spear, 1979). These correlational studies have demonstrated that the immature organism's greater cerebral plasticity may be adaptive, but it is not invariably so. The anomalous connections formed after brain injury can restore normal functions, but they can also lead to maladaptive responses if the anomalous connections are between the 'wrong' sites. Schneider's (1979) studies in hamsters provide a particularly clear illustration of this principle. If the midbrain tectum is lesioned at birth, redirected growth of the optic tract leads to the formation of anomalous connections. In some instances, these anomalous connections result in the sparing of visually elicited turning responses that are lost after comparable lesions in adulthood. In other instances, however, the anomalous connections lead to a maladaptive turning responses, e.g. persistently turning the wrong way as a result of anomalous retinal projections to the wrong side of the midbrain. These misdirected movements can be abolished by surgical division of the relevant anomalous pathways.

Limits to recovery related to timing and location of damage

Having considered examples of excellent recovery from early brain injury, and having reviewed some of the neural processes that may contribute to this recovery, it is now appropriate to turn to the limitations of the recovery process. Since the timing and location of the brain injury impose important limitations on the completeness of recovery, these factors will be considered first.

When damage affects both sides of the brain symmetrically, recovery of the functions normally served by that part of the brain may be poor unless the damage was sustained around the time of birth or even before. This limitation is suggested, for example, by the way in which monkeys make good long-term recoveries from dorsolateral prefrontal lesions if these lesions are sustained prenatally, but not if they are sustained in infancy (see Goldman-Rakic, Isseroff, Schwartz *et al.*, 1983). Perhaps in this instance a limit arises because the extensive neuronal reorganization needed to circumvent bilaterally symmetrical damage cannot take place if the additive processes of axonal and dendritic growth are largely completed. Since most childhood head injuries occur long after birth, and since closed head injuries commonly produce bilaterally symmetrical damage, the implications for head-injured children are not encouraging. For example, if both frontal lobes are damaged in middle childhood, there is little reason to suppose that brain reorganization can effectively reconstruct frontal-type cortex elsewhere.

Good recovery of function is more likely when the damage is limited to one side of the brain, and when the function under consideration is normally lateralized to just one hemisphere — even if the function is normally lateralized to the hemisphere that has been injured. Language acquisition provides a good example (Goodman, 1987). In most individuals, language skills depend principally on the left hemisphere (see Bradshaw and Nettleton, 1983; Springer and Deutsch, 1985). If the left hemisphere is damaged very early in life, however, the individual with an intact right hemisphere can still acquire language that is normal or nearly normal (Smith and Sugar, 1975; Dennis and Whittaker, 1977; Woods and Carey, 1979; Vargha-Khadem, O'Gorman and Watters, 1985). When the left hemisphere is damaged in somewhat older children, persistent language deficits are more likely, though these too may be relatively subtle (Woods and Carey, 1979). After puberty, the capacity for left-to-right transfer is still present in some individuals (see Kinsbourne, 1971), but is generally less dramatic than after early brain damage. It would seem, then, that as brain development progresses, the right hemisphere generally becomes less able to take over the skills that are normally lateralized to the left hemisphere. Conversely, the left hemisphere becomes progressively less able to take over right-hemisphere functions (Woods, 1980). It is tempting to speculate that a developing hemisphere can only take over the other hemisphere's functions if the pattern of selective axonal loss can still be modified (Janowsky and Finlay, 1986) — this would explain why the capacity for left-to-right or right-to-left transfer progressively diminishes during childhood as the phase of selective loss moves towards completion.

Another factor influencing the degree of recovery from brain injury is whether the injury occurs suddenly or gradually. In general, when brain damage occurs gradually, as a result of a slowly expanding lesion or a succession of small injuries, the degree of recovery is greater than when the same amount of damage has occurred suddenly (Finger and Stein, 1982). Thus recovery from damage to one hemisphere due to an open head injury may well be less complete than recovery from comparable brain damage due to a slowly expanding abscess or benign tumour.

Why are limitations in recovery overlooked?

Given the previous considerations, it seems likely that cerebral plasticity will be most evident when brain injury has occurred very early in life, has affected just one hemisphere, and has come on gradually. Severe head injuries in childhood frequently fulfil none of these criteria. In view of this, total recoveries may turn out to be the exception rather than the rule. If this is true, it is probable that residual deficits often go unrecognized. Why should this happen? Incorrigible optimism or low expectations may play some part, as may a tendency for parents and professionals to deny the existence of residual deficits in order to protect themselves from their own feelings of despair and powerlessness. In addition, there are three aspects of the residual deficits that may make them genuinely easy to miss. First, the deficits may be subtle in nature; secondly, the deficits may only become apparent as the child grows older. Finally, deficits in the capacity for new learning may be much more pronounced that deficits in existing skills. These three issues will be considered in turn.

Deficits may be subtle

In many instances, subtle but important deficits are apparent to the people who know the child best, although they may not be able to pinpoint exactly what is amiss. As these deficits are subtle, they may not be recognized on superficial acquaintance in a doctor's surgery, or from ordinary psychological testing. Children who have sustained very early unilateral damage are generally thought to make particularly good recoveries, and yet even in these children it is possible to detect persistent language and 'frontal lobe' deficits provided appropriately sophisticated tests are employed (Vargha-Khadem, O'Gorman and Watters, 1985; Vargha-Kardhem, personal communication). If this is so after early unilateral damage, it is likely that similar or more marked deficits also occur after later-onset head injuries causing bilateral damage. It would be wrong to assume that a deficit that only shows up on sophisticated testing is necessarily unimportant. In the child's everyday world, social or school failure could result from relatively subtle and hard-to-pin-down deficits in language, attention, memory or social responsiveness, to name but four key areas.

Deficits may worsen with time

Some of the deficits acquired after head injury resolve with the passage of time. Unfortunately, other deficits may actually worsen. To put this another way, head-injured children may grow out of some problems but grow into others. This possibility is suggested by the studies of brain-damaged monkeys described earlier (see Goldman-Rakic, Isseroff, Schwartz *et al.*, 1983). After bilateral dorsolateral damage sustained in infancy, the monkeys initially seemed to be doing well, with no disturbance of delayed-response learning (which does not depend on the dorsolateral cortex of the frontal lobe until later in life). As they grew up, however, deficits in delayed-response tasks did become apparent as the monkeys reached an age when the dorsolateral cortex was necessary for the performance of these tasks. This late emergence of a previously silent deficit is sometimes referred to as a 'sleeper' effect. Similar effects may occur after childhood brain injury. In humans, the prefrontal cortex is a late-maturing part of the brain, as judged, for example, by its rate of dendritic maturation as compared with the primary visual cortex (Schade and van Groenigen, 1961; Takashima, Chan, Becker *et al.*, 1980). Consequently, when severe head injury in early or middle childhood results in bilateral prefrontal damage, some frontal lobe deficits may initially be relatively mild because the damaged cortex had not yet acquired many functions. The deficits may later become more apparent as the individual reaches an age when the damaged cortex would have played an important role. For example, in a longitudinal study of head-injured children, there was no major increase in conduct problems until four or five years after the head injury, Black, Blumer, Wellner *et al.*, (1971). This late rise in conduct problems may reflect the emergence of 'sleeper' effects, though it is equally possible that the rise is simply a consequence of the children moving towards or into adolescence.

Deficits may particularly affect new learning

Another reason that residual deficits may escape detection is that, as Hebb (1942) pointed out, brain injury may disrupt the capacity for new learning more than the capacity to retain existing skills. Since we generally expect a child's current academic standard to be a good guide to that child's ability to make further academic progress, a disproportionate impairment in new learning may well baffle parents and professionals alike. Thus, if a 10 year old child sustains a severe head injury, and if that child retains enough previously learned skills to be able to read at an 8 year old level, we typically expect his or her reading level to go on increasing rather like that of a normal 8 year old. This expectation may be ill-founded. Perhaps the child's capacity for new learning is more akin to that of an average 6 year old or even 4 year old. If so, it is not difficult to see that the child will have difficulty making further progress. Intellectual stagnation, with little or no change in a child's mental age over the course of four or more years, has been noted in some children with severe epilepsy (Corbett, Besag, Goodman *et al.*, unpublished observations). Somewhat similar cases of developmental stagnation have been reported in the very different context of disintegrative psychosis of childhood (Hill and Rosenbloom, 1986). These examples illustrate the way in which brain disorders in childhood can have a far more devastating effect on the acquisition of new abilities than on the retention of existing ones. There is a danger that the resultant learning disorders will unfairly be attributed to insufficient motivation on the part of the child, or to broader psychosocial problems.

Misconnections: A disadvantage of cerebral plasticity?

As described earlier, animal experiments suggest that the young brain's greater capacity to form new connections after injury is something of a mixed blessing. In some instances, the new connections enhance recovery. In other instances, however, the new connections are misconnections, and these misconnections interfere with recovery. Little is known about misconnections after childhood brain injury, though their existence is suggested by the occurrence of patchy hyperaesthesia and abnormally persistent mirror movements in brain-injured children (Schneider, 1979). Speculatively, misconnections in childhood might contribute to a variety of educational and behavioural problems. Widespread misconnections would channel irrelevant information between regions of the brain that would not normally be connected, and this might well interfere with the normal functioning of each region. Most of us have experienced how difficult it is to follow a complex argument at a noisy party, or how hard it is to pass on a telephone message on a crossed line. These difficulties may be analogous to the sorts of problems that could face an individual trying to make sense of the world against the background of noise generated by widespread misconnections. It is not hard to imagine that a poor signal-to-noise ratio would impair concentration and the regulation of activity, interfere with problem solving and disrupt the acquisition of new knowledge. In other words, widespread misconnections could plausibly lead to poor concentration, hyperactivity, learning problems and lowered IQ.

Although focal brain injury in childhood is less likely to produce a specific psychological deficit (such as a lasting aphasia) than comparable injury sustained in adulthood, childhood injury is more likely to result in general intellectual and scholastic impairment (Rutter, 1984; Rutter, Chadwick and Shaffer, 1984). Is this general impairment the result of crowding too many specific functions into too little remaining brain? The case report of Smith and Sugar (1975) suggests that this is not so. As described above, a boy who has lost practically half of his brain grew up without specific psychological deficits, and with superior intelligence and academic abilities.

Although we cannot know what this boy might have achieved with an intact brain, the case does suggest that the intellectual and scholastic impairments that commonly follow early localized brain damage cannot simply be attributed to crowding too much into the remaining brain. Instead, it seems possible that the advantages of greater cerebral plasticity after early brain injury, in terms of better recovery of specific abilities such as language or vision, are often although not invariably offset by the disadvantages of this greater plasticity, in terms of intellectual and academic impairments due to misconnections. If so, it will be essential to study whether possible therapeutic interventions, such as the administration of neurotrophic factors intended to enhance the formation of valuable new connections, also increase the formation of disruptive misconnections. This is clearly an important area for future research.

Conclusion

Hans–Lukas Teuber stated: 'If I'm going to have brain damage, I'd best have it early rather than late' (quoted in Finger and Stein, 1982). Although there is clearly some truth in this view, it is an oversimplification. The benefits of cerebral plasticity are sometimes exaggerated, with residual deficits being missed because of their subtlety, late onset, or disproportionate impact on new learning. In addition, greater cerebral plasticity may have potential disadvantages, with widespread misconnections resulting in a variety of intellectual, educational and behavioural difficulties.

Chapter 3

Early recovery: can we help?

David A. Johnson

'One hopes for extensive recovery after long periods of recuperation and physical therapy, but there is very little done to manipulate the recovery process directly' (Stein, 1981, p. 424).

Introduction

The increasing recognition and importance attached to rehabilitation after head injury is evidenced by the burgeoning journal and textbook literature. Yet, as Stein's observation suggests, we have been somewhat tardy in our attempts to achieve the best possible outcome for our adult head-injured patients. The situation for head-injured children, however, is much worse and significant for the paucity of accurate information and knowledge. This appears in the presence of the substantial literature on recovery in animals which, not only highlights the misconceptions surrounding the myth of early recovery after brain injury (Isaacson, 1975) but, offers practical frameworks within which to improve the head-injured child's recovery. This apparent inactivity may reflect the rigidity of our thinking and our lack of intellectual conscience. For example, Zuccarello, Facco, Zamperi et al., (1985) concluded that 'Clinical experience indicates that children recover from head injury better than adults and these impressions receive support from the clinical studies of Cedermark (1942) and Akerlund (1959)'. Regrettably this is typical of statements founded on assumptions based on inadequate knowledge and insufficient examination.

The process of active rehabilitation typically begins only several months after injury, when the patient has passed through the early, critical stages of recovery. In the period immediately after injury all attention is naturally focused on the patient's survival. As life is secured, however, a waiting game generally ensues; let's wait and see how well and how quickly he recovers without further specific and aggressive medical intervention. Any treatment at this stage is predominantly physical and essentially passive in nature, such as chest physiotherapy, but still innumerable and potentially avoidable clinical problems persist, such as heterotopic ossification, inadequate nutrition, badly splintered limbs, swallowing disorders, poor communication, and unduly anxious parents, all of which complicate progress in later rehabilitation. That rehabilitation for head-injured children is, with one or two exceptions, non-existent in this country is undoubtedly due to ubiquitous, unreliable and invalid statements such as 'he will make an excellent recovery, as most young brains do'. This apparently remarkable potential for recovery may indeed be attributable to a lower threshold at which neurophysiological dysfunction of a reversible nature would produce overt symptoms without significant structural damage (Molnar and Perrin, 1983). It may simply represent ignorance and misinformation on our part, a lack of awareness and attention to the neurobehavioural sources of problems. This may be compounded by our inability to predict the sequelae of neurological dysfunction when it is not thrust in front of our eyes.

Outcome studies are few in this area and generally subject to criticisms of population heterogeneity, inappropriate outcome measures, relatively short follow-up period, or simply small numbers (e.g., Gaidolfi and Vignolo, 1980). If children die from their head injury, they do so early (Berger, Pitts, Lovely *et al.*, 1985) and, for the survivors, aggressive and early rehabilitation could make a substantial difference to length of hospital stay, return to school, family dynamics, the child's independence and ultimate outcome. A major question is which approach would produce optimal recovery: working simply to restore general health, on the assumption that this will automatically help spontaneous recovery, which is simply playing the waiting game once the child is medically stable; or protecting the individual from stimulation so that the injured CNS is not overloaded in its reduced capacity; or using individually tailored programmes of stimulation and rehabilitation (Rosenzweig, 1980). It is this latter approach which may offer the greatest potential but, in order to progress clinically in this area, we must look to the results of animal experimentation. The caveat being that there is no directly comparable animal model of diffuse, traumatic brain injury detailing longtitudinal recovery. Experimental reviews (e.g., Stein, Rosen and Butters, 1974, Finger, 1978, Almli and Finger, 1984) highlight the primary necessity of disregarding the heterogenous population of 'head-injured children' and paying more critical attention to delineation of actual brain state, differentiation of primary and secondary effects, time since injury and maturational stage. In our attempts to treat some condition or difficulty, one must have at least a basic understanding of the actual bases of the problem, in order to apply the principles of rehabilitation and consider the possibilities for alternative explanations or solutions. 'It is important at least to be conversant with the other side of the coin . . . the challenges of recovery of function and rehabilitation . . . the techniques and resources of research with animal models' (Rosenzweig 1980, p. 163). Regrettably, this is seldom the case for those dealing with head-injured children.

Cerebral concussion from head injury causes a diminished level of brain activity, relative to the severity of biomechanical forces involved (Ommaya and Gennarelli, 1974, Gennarelli and Thibault, 1985). This principally involves disruption or damage to the extensive neocortico-thalamo-reticular pathways, as well as any focal lesions. In addition to structural damage, the brain's normally tight coupling between neuronal activity, oxidative metabolism and blood flow is seriously disrupted and, although autoregulation may still be present, it may not be normal (Rosner, 1987). It is the potentially reversible dysfunctions which, when accurately evaluated, may give crucial indications for treatment. The essential feature of unconsciousness is a reduction in behavioural responsiveness to external stimulation and inner needs (Tsubokawa, 1987). Unable to interact with his surroundings, the child's sensation may operate only at the barest level of survival. The assessment of coma, by grading the degree of decline in observable responses to external stimulation (e.g., Glasgow Coma Scale GCS) is not yet standardized with children. This may not, however, correlate necessarily with a reduction in general levels of brain activity, as desynchronised EEG may occur in coma for example. Although normal cognition and emotion require a level of arousal and information processing not attainable in the severely-injured brain, coma may involve a more active process than previously supposed, with responses occurring at subclinical levels (Engel, 1980). Clinical recovery or deterioration may parallel changes in heart rate, EEG, or neurochemical activity (Evans 1978; van Woerkom, Minderhoud, Gottschal, *et al.*, 1982; Johnson, Richards, Roethig-Johnston, 1988). As Teuber so often reported, the CNS is never passive but operates upon its own inputs, emitting a continuous activity which is affected in surprisingly similar manner by deprivation and by defects.

As the primary pathological focus in coma-producing head injury, the brainstem is also the integral axis from which normal mental development and behaviour evolve. Information processing within brainstem sensory nuclei and the adjacent reticular formation may indeed be one of the most critical and relevant areas for investigation in head-injured children. In addition to any primary injury, for example, the brainstem vestibular, auditory and other sensory relay nuclei may be particularly vulnerable to secondary insult (e.g., Buchwald, 1975) and subsequent degeneration. Brainstem pathology may significantly disturb the normal encoding of information into appropriate neuronal firing patterns, thus rendering it of limited meaning for memory (Teuber, 1975) and higher cortical activities. Without such patterned input to higher cortical centres, via the specific sensory pathway, the remaining portion of the CNS may be incapable of supporting normal behaviour.

The hypothesized pathological basis of head injury may cause substantial disruption to the 3-dimensional or stereomorphophysiological nature of the CNS (J. Moore, 1980). The phylogenetically newer components are particularly vulnerable, perhaps because of their greater metabolic demands, less established vascularization, anatomical proneness and high dependence upon lower systems. Disruption of this basic dichotomy of dependence is clinically apparent at all stages after injury, when lower functions are released from cortical regulatory inhibition and lose their ability to create the necessary foundations for normal learning and higher level function. This notion of dependency appears at all levels of recovery and includes structural dependency on morphological integrity, metabolic dependency on physiological events during information processing, and informational dependence on processing of coherent information. As recovery proceeds, the previously dependent subcortical and neocortical centres expend extra energy, albeit from a reduced capacity system, to interpret a multitude of deficient and aberrant signals.

Head injury resulting in a period of altered consciousness may produce relative degrees of sensory deprivation (SD). This essentially represents any change in the internal or external environment that deprives the organism of normal and necessary stimuli. This may include the intensive care unit, general wards, use of sedative drugs, confinement to bed and lack of movement. The need for stimulation is inherent in normal adaptive behaviour (Suedfeld, 1979), and progressive SD in otherwise healthy adults may cause widespread changes in brain activity. Most organisms will seek stimulation that has been in short supply, in order to redress the balance; the importance of maintaining sensory equilibrium has been emphasized by studies on SD and the sensory inadequacies of short-term hospitalization. Confined to the sterile, impoverished environment of intensive care or the busy recovery ward, the head-injured child is unable to change this situation. He will be unable to cope with primary survival needs to seek and select the appropriate nutrition, temperature levels, or sensory stimulation. Consequently, the effects of reduced sensory input are likely to be of much greater significance than that experienced by normal or other hospitalized patients (Barrie-Shevlin, 1987). Furthermore, emerging from unconsciousness or SD, into a more stimulating environment may create a substantial stress upon the child, which interferes with previously learned or organized processes and may cause inappropriate behaviour. For example, an initial hypersensitivity after SD may lead to avoidance of ordinary levels of light, sound, interpersonal contact and an irrational fear of space and novel environments which, in severe cases, may easily result in withdrawal or disturbed behaviour. In a model of emergence-stress (Fuller, 1967), excessive arousal in an organism exposed to a myriad of unfamiliar stimuli is assumed to produce overload in neural systems underlying many forms of behaviour. The notion of overstimulating a recovering child, therefore, would seem to be more applicable to the usual routine of keeping him on a busy or noisy ward, rather than in a quiet and distraction-free environment and working intensively on a one-to-one basis. A traumatic state of SD, however, does not end abruptly as the child regains consciousness. It is likely to persist to varying degrees throughout recovery and over a period of many years in the more severely injured child. If the child has limb disabilities, or becomes increasingly withdrawn, their relative inactivity and isolation creates a degree of SD which may continue long after injury, resulting in morphological, behavioural and emotional changes which operate in a vicious circle. The neurological effects of SD may be similar to those of muscles deprived of their normal functions, with a gradual loss of tone, function, and eventual atrophy after prolonged disuse. When structural damage and degeneration are compounded with sensory and nutritional deprivation, the head-injured child's prognosis must be correspondingly poor. Experimental evidence for both types of loss (Rosenzweig, 1980) appears from focal occipital lesions accompanying reduced weight and DNA in the remainder of the cortex (Will, Rosenzweig, Bennett *et al.*, 1977), and disuse atrophy resulting from stimulus deprivation enhancing deterioration. Many deficits after head injury may be partly due to secondary neuronal loss (Buchwald, 1975; Jellinger, 1983), depending upon the maturational status of the damaged region and its interrelated areas. In the prefrontal cortex for example, different components mature at different rates: subcortical before cortical, and orbital (sulcal) before dorsal convexity (medial) cortex (Nonneman, Corwin, Sahley *et al.* 1984), with immature structures being more susceptible to degeneration. Unless the region or structure concerned has developed a mature pattern of connections with functionally related brain areas, then the effects of insult may not become apparent for some years (see Goodman, this volume). Development is not simply a matter of overt behaviour, but also of physiological change and growth. Consequently, if the CNS is damaged, or its ontogenetic development disrupted by head-injury, then behaviour, in its broadest sense, must change. Loss of functional integrity simply means that the functional responsibilities of an injured area, such as the prefrontal cortex, are changed in relation to all other areas. We have yet to undertake longitudinal studies of secondary and progressive deterioration following head injury in children but it is of critical importance, to the theory and practice of early rehabilitation and clinical management decisions, to consider the situation at least as parallel to that of the head-injured adult (Strich, 1956).

CNS morphology interacts with the uses to which it is put so, when visual, auditory and tactile senses are deprived during early growth or recovery, their sensory fields and cortical projections are left in an underdeveloped or underused condition. With experimental eyelid closure in animals, for example, passage of light is not prevented but is non-patterned and correspondingly poor in information (Bondy and Morelo, 1971). Interference with visual input may cause vascular deficits, which extend to widespread secondarily innervated areas within the cerebral hemispheres, implicating a further risk of impaired metabolism and function outwith the damaged area (Reivich, Gur and Alavi, 1983). Reviewing the evidence, Layton, Corrick and Toga (1978), concluded that changes in the normal sensory environment may lead to physiological and behavioural abnormalities despite structural integrity. These effects may be reversible in cases of transient deprivation, but continuing absence of meaningful sensory input may permanently restrict optimal brain development, perhaps due to prolonged cerebro-vascular insufficiency, or changes in the concentration of putative neurotransmitters, and the orderly maturation of the biochemical system (Walker, Kelley and Riesen *etal.*, 1975).

As neural activity changes, a complex system responds, involving blood flow, biochemical events and electrical changes. A relationship between changes in functional activity of the brain and alterations in cerebral metabolism has been documented for many years (e.g., Roy and Sherrington, 1890; Risberg, 1986). Depression of cerebral activity due to concussion (Williams and Denny-Brown, 1941) has been shown to be associated with lowered cerebral blood flow and metabolism (Reivich, Gur and Alavi, 1983). Social isolation in rats may reduce prefrontal dopamine (DA) activity and potentiates the response of mesocortico-prefrontal DA neurons to somatic stressors, (Kraemer, 1985). Conversely, environmental enrichment helps to reverse behavioural and physiological deficits in rats with neonatal neurotoxic lesions of brain catecholaminergic (CA) systems. The situation is probably more complex in the socially developed primate, as cortical CA concentration and synthesis rate is higher than in rodents. One should recall Layton, Corrick and Toga's (1978), reservations, however, that whilst the extent of behavioural and perceptual recovery after experimental deprivation has been considerable, a corresponding degree of physiological recovery has not been reported.

Bases for intervention

The environment is clearly a major determinant of the organization and function of the CNS in higher mammals. The development of intricate neural structures, complex perceptual organization and behavioural precision, all depend upon its demands (Riesen, 1975, Renner and Rosenzweig, 1987). Early experience derived from specific types of environmental stimulation may be critical for the development and maintenance of appropriate and well-coordinated responses and general neuropsychological development. The environment's considerable influence over the inherent adaptability of the CNS offers the potential to influence recovery significantly, either adversely or beneficially. There is ' ... overwhelming evidence that CNS neurons may undergo structural and or biochemical changes according to use or specific experience, as a consequence of normal synapse replacement, or in response to injury' (Marshall, 1984, p. 278). In general terms plasticity refers to this adaptability, the CNS's potential to modify its structural organization to environmental changes, a fundamental property of the developing organism.

Early deprivation of sensorimotor experience, particularly during critical development, has been blamed for a considerable proportion of mental retardation and social inadequacy in man (Fuller, 1967). Intact neurochemical, physiological and behavioural mechanisms are axiomatic to adequate environmental interaction (Kraemer, 1985), supporting the improvement and elaboration of specialized skills in normal development and recovery after brain injury. Primary neurological systems, such as the reticulolimbic, can be stimulated in such a way that the effects of sensory deprivation may be ameliorated. The behavioural and neural deficits following deprivation during certain developmental stages in cats (Chow and Stewart, 1972), for example, are diminished by forced usage strategies. There is general agreement that raising animals in enriched environmental conditions (EC) results in positive structural and biochemical changes within the CNS which, in turn, contribute to improved learning and cerebral development (Ferchmin, Bennett and Rosenzweig, 1975). There are, however, some conflicting reports, (see review by Rose, 1988), and difficulties in making methodological comparisons (Renner and Rosenzweig, 1987). Reviewing the effects of environmental manipulation on recovery, Greenough and Fass De Voogd (1976), report that brain-lesioned rats placed in an enriched condition (EC) do as well on maze learning as normal rats, an effect which may occur irrespective of age (Altschuler, 1976). Greatest recovery was demonstrated by rats with intact brains and EC, whilst lesioned rats in an impoverished environment (IC) performed most poorly (Schwarz, 1964). The rate and amount of functional recovery have been reported to improve with EC, yielding significant changes in RNA:DNA ratios, cholinergic activity, increased dendritic growth, a doubling of synaptic density, increased cortical glial cells and cortical weight unrelated to body weight. The fact is that EC promoted behavioural recovery implies increased metabolic activity, a mechanism which may partially compensate for the impaired brain growth observed with lesioned animals. The often substantial differences between IC and EC subjects are enhanced further among lesioned rather than control subjects, perhaps because of increased sensitivity to environmental effects, reflecting a biochemical adaptability to injury (LeVere, 1988). Alternatively, methodological limitations suggest that the task performance of brain-injured subjects is less affected by ceiling or floor effects.

It has been suggested that beneficial environmental manipulation may exert a non-specific arousing function, in turn suggesting further possibilities for neuropharmacological intervention. Unfortunately, not all kinds of CNS activation may be equally efficient with regard to recovery (e.g. Harrell, Rawbson and Balagura, 1974), particularly of cognitive function, and the quality of arousal may be a critical factor. The evidence is contradictory on the effects of co-administering CNS stimulant drugs with EC. Renner and Rosenzweig, (1987), metamphetamine to augment the effects of EC in normal rats, but concluded that this combination did not produce the desired results, perhaps because of drug specificity on behaviour. Renner and Rosenzweig (1987) report earlier work using (inetamphetamine to augument) A recent clinical report of co-administering amphetamine with physical therapy to adult stroke patients, apparently yielded facilitated recovery of motor function (Crisotomo, Duncan, Propst *et al.*, 1988). Outwith the consideration that this study was conducted for only a few days, it unfortunately administered vitamins as a placebo control which may have altered neurotransmitter activity and hence behaviour.

Environmental enrichment appears a powerful tool for aiding functional recovery. Its effectiveness is most likely to be attributable to an optimal quantitative and qualitative increase in the level of activation, the nature of which would not be produced by passive sensory stimulation, irrespective of age (Held and Hein, 1963; Bland and Cooper, 1970). The few negative findings appear to be concerned with specific sensory capabilities known to be dependent upon rather limited regions of the brain. Finger (1978) reported that rearing under EC did not improve tactile stimulation performance after extensive one-stage somatosensory cortex ablation. If the neural damage prevents processing the sensory information required for that particular problem, then EC may have no beneficial effect in specific sensory tasks. The impact of a stimulating and complex environment may further depend upon the extent to which skills can be generalized across situations (Greenough, Fass and De Voogd, 1976). The beneficial effects of EC may be in terms of a general adaptive capacity (Finger, 1978), resulting in improved task performances, such as maze learning, which can be solved by various strategies.

One clinical application of these general experimental findings has been with infant stimulation programmes. The only apparent study purporting to show that early infant stimulation had no effect (Piper and Pless, 1980) was unfortunately conducted over a short time and did not consider development as a dynamic process whereby beneficial or adverse effects may not be immediately apparent, factors of clear importance to the growing child with head injury. In contrast, early and short periods of stimulation using a variety of visual, audio-visual, audio-vestibular and physical stimulation, with added instructions to parents, is reported to result in a slowing of developmental decline and improved psychosocial performance (Sharov and Shlomo, 1986; Williams, Williams and Dial, 1986). The results obtained in the between-group comparisons are not always statistically different in these studies, but the behavioural measures appear relatively insensitive. Such programmes appear to be effective on some level but, in order to confirm and extend this efficacy, the underlying physiological or anatomical substrates must be delineated (Ferry, 1986).

This line of evidence highlights the potential benefits of EC, at least for the immature and lesioned CNS (Finger and Stein, 1982; Will and Eclancher, 1984). A logical extension of this work attempting to provide clinical EC, is the controversial and highly emotive area of coma stimulation. Claims for and against coma stimulation are made on ethical or moral grounds, on individual case reports, or unselective press reports (e.g. Miller, 1985); for example, the child who is reported to wake up suddenly from coma in response to hearing a tape from his favourite pop star. There appear to have been no adequately controlled studies in this potentially important field, and there are numerous methodological problems in those few reports available, limiting the potential importance of their findings. Proponents of coma stimulation programmes stress the importance of treating every aspect of the patient, extending care beyond routine physical maintenance (Freeman, 1987). The approach of Le Winn (1980) aims to stimulate all five sensory modalities with simple but intense stimuli, thereby arousing severely head-injured patients from coma and improving their chances of recovery. Subsequently, Le Winn and Dimancescu (1978) reported that sixteen stimulated coma patients all survived and made good therapeutic progress compared to fourteen unstimulated patients, of whom eleven died. A recent report (Quine, Pierce and Lyle, 1988) refers to a small subgroup of children, aged 1 to 18 years, receiving a form of coma stimulation programme, but their findings do not indicate any further details on the effects of such interventions. Some authors (e.g., Yanko, 1985) maintain that early recovery is not considered the time to introduce novel stimulation because of the patient's processing impairments, suggesting instead that they respond much better to familiar stimuli. This appears to neglect the arousing properties of stimulus-novelty and salience, however, and there may be no difference in responsiveness to stimulus familiarity in the early recovery period. Moreover, sensory stimulation should not reasonably cause adverse effects upon intracracranial pressure, contrary to some suggestions (e.g., Yanko, 1985).

The principal aim of stimulation programmes with head-injured children is to effect significant changes in central arousal-activation systems, which have become traumatically disordered. As the experimental and clinical reports suggest, physiological and behavioural abnormalities may exist in the presence of structural integrity. These circulatory, metabolic and functional depressions may occur in areas remote to the localized injury (Stirling-Meyer, Hata and Imai, 1987) but states of diaschisis may be reversible by specific intervention (Laurence and Stein, 1978). As there are different thresholds of arousal it is important to have some indices of activity within the various physiological systems when working with stimulation approaches. Neurophysiological and biochemical measures may be sufficiently sensitive and accurate to allow therapeutic and predictive implications to be derived from the data (Oken and Chiappa, 1985). The importance of incorporating EEG and other physiological measures during recovery is widely acknowledged (Johnson and Lubin, 1967; Evans, 1978), particularly as disruption in the regulatory control of physiological responses during cortical processing may persist. EEG changes during and after sensory motor stimulation (Weber, 1984) and may be regarded as signs of cortical and autonomic reactions to sensory input (Pfurtscheller, Schwarz and List, 1986). The close relationship between EEG and heart rate suggests that stimulation of the brainstem activating system results in nonspecific, indirect arousal-activation. Heart rate activity may be taken as indices of primay or secondary injury (Evans, 1979), as well as retention of stimulus discrimination by the patient's response to stimulation (Le Fever, 1986). This would seem consistent with the suggestion that, in later stages of recovery, changes in heart rate accompany adjustments in cortical activity during attentional processes (Levine, 1976; Brouwer, 1985). Not surprisingly, there may be some relation between good outcome and stimulus-induced EEG alteration, with poor outcome indicated by loss of reactivity to external stimuli. This is difficult to differentiate if simply using behavioural measurements, however. The possible metabolic response to stimulation is suggested by Reivich, Gur and Alavi (1983), who demonstrated alterations in local cerebral glucose metabolism during auditory, tactile, visual and cognitive stimulation.

The notion that neurological recovery may be facilitated by neuropharmacological manipulation is not new (Ward, 1950; Gualtieri, 1987). Unfortunately, however, there are few reports of its application with adults in the acute stage (Di Rocco, Maira, Meglio *et al.*, 1974; Minderhoud, van Woerkom and van Weerden, 1976) and, apparently, none solely concerned with head-injured children. The modulation of effects produced by experience, via hormones, neuropeptides, and non-specific neurotransmitters has recently assumed renewed importance as in the study of sleep and learning, for example. The long term influences of neurones are the metabolic activity of their target cells. Loss of trophic or nourishing influences from damaged neurones after brain injury could lead to disorganized post-synaptic cellular metabolism (see Goodman, this volume), and reduced synaptic transmission in the affected cells. This may be reversible by exogenous nerve growth factor (NGF), for example, a complex protein with powerful neurotrophic effects (Stein, 1981; Gage and Varon, 1988). In addition to those changes caused directly by the injury, environmental changes may cause further, secondary alterations in neurotransmitter activity (Kraemer, 1985; Panksepp, 1986). Catecholamines (CA) and the indoleamine serotonin (5-hydroxytryptamine, 5-HT) are those principally investigated, with the greatest changes reported in noradrenaline (NA) and 5-HT activity in unconscious patients, at varying times after injury, from day one through to six months (Vecht, van Woerkom, and Teelken, 1976; van Woerkom, Teelken and Minderhoud, 1977; Clifton, Ziegler and Grossman, 1981; Ikeda and Nakazawa; 1984, Hamill, Woolf, McDonald *et al.*, 1987). There is, however, no report of the long term outcome of these head-injured patients in relation to neurochemical status but, after subarachnoid haemorrhage, poor clinical outcome has been related to increased adrenaline and NA levels (Peerless and Griffiths, 1975). Increased 5-HT activity has been correlated with abnormal oculocephalic and oculovestibular responses (OVR) in the acute recovery stage after head injury (Maccario, Backman and Korein, 1972). OVR's may indicate the level of brainstem dysfunction in coma (Plum and Posner, 1982), correlating with level of conscious response, clinical improvement (Maccario, Backman and Korein, 1972, Minderhoud, van Woerkom and van Weerden, 1976), and outcome prediction (van Woerkom, van Weerden and Minderhoud, 1984). The finding of a rapid phase of nystagmus invariably related to improvement in consciousness (Poulsen and Zilstroff, 1972) raises questions of possible relationships between neurological state and condition of the central vestibular pathways (Yules, Krebs and Gault, 1966). The presence of a

Paradoxical Caloric Response (PCR) implies that the brainstem is largely, not necessarily wholly, suffering from a functional disturbance; i.e. the structures are not irrevocably damaged but may be in a state akin to shock. Abnormal OVR's have in turn been related to poor neuropsychological function at long term follow up in severely head-injured adults (Levin, Grossman, Rose, *et al.*, 1979) and so, may have some predictive value for treatment and outcome. If such dysfunction has a neurochemical basis then specific neuropharmacological intervention may facilitate 'unblocking' (Luria, 1963) or disinhibition of the traumatically disordered regions of the brain.

Important advances in this area were made by the Groningen researchers (e.g., Minderhoud, Huizenga and van Woerkom, 1982). Critical variables were found to be initial GCS, time of intervention, and presence of a PCR. Of sixteen patients studied, ten had an accelerated phase of recovery which suggested a neurological condition partly determined by reversible lesions, but in which too few exogenous and endogenous stimuli could be effectively utilized. Those patients with poor GCS long after the accident did not show any improvement with neurotransmitter replacement, suggesting predominantly irreversible lesions. Failure to detect differences in outcome may largely be due to insensitive outcome measures, notably the Glasgow Outcome Scale (GOS: Jennett and Teasdale, 1981). Physostigmine, a cholinesterase inhibitor, has an activating effect upon the brainstem reticular formation and may improve the caloric response of patients with disturbed consciousness. Nystagmus patterns characterized by saccadic oscillations associated with the quick phase of caloric nystagmus were reported in nine vegetative severely head-injured patients, five of whom were under 12 years of age (van Woerkom, van Weerden and Minderhoud, 1984). The children showed high incidence of saccadic oscillations, but their initial clinical picture was not worse than that of adults. Among the practical considerations for extraocular eye muscles are their crucial roles in visual scanning, tracking and fixation, and in the fine saccadic movements used in reading, writing, painting, or performing other fine visuomotor skills. Early examination of the oculovestibular system for improvement potential may, therefore, be of substantial benefit to the child's long term outcome.

The important anatomical and functional relationships between the vestibular, reticular and thalamocortical systems are well documented. Located proximally to the reticular system are the vestibular nuclei, vestibular system pathways and other structures involved with eye movements and balance. The midbrain reticular formation, diffuse thalamic system, cerebral cortex and cerebellum have modulating influences upon nystagmus and the EEG during vestibular stimulation. Within these same regions are located major neuronal groups and pathways for neurotransmitters involved in arousal, sleep, and eye movements. Particularly important are acetylcholine (ACh.), 5-HT and the CA's, which may exert significant effects upon the brainstem reticular system and vestibular nuclei (R.Y. Moore, 1980), and all of which are likely to be major considerations in delineating substrates of recovery and areas for intervention (e.g., Bogdanovitch, Bazarevitch and Kirillov, 1975).

There appear to be no published reports of vestibular stimulation with head-injured children at any stage of recovery. The available sources of evidence include animal experiments and clinical studies with non-trauma groups which variously report using a water caloric, optokinetic, rhythmic movement, or acceleration stimulus. Vestibular nuclei may be activated not only by the end organ, but also strongly and reliably by proprioceptive stimulation to the limb and neck afferents, and to moving visual fields which cause optokinetic nystagmus. Optokinetic vestibular stimulation in animals increases thalamic activity (Buttner and Henn, 1976) and in cortical Areas 2 and 3 (Parietal region) (Buttner, Buettner and Henn, 1981). Vestibular stimulation by calorics in neurologically intact adults may result in significantly increased regional cerebral blood flow in the cerebral cortex, notably the contralateral superior temporal region which may reflect a primary corticovestibular projection area (Roland and Friberg, 1983; Friberg, Olsen, Roland *et al.*, 1985). An extraordinary plasticity of vestibular function is present during the formative years of childhood, with a rapid decrement in vestibular reactivity in development which parallels the decrement in rapid eye movement sleep (REMS) (Ornitz, 1983). Important modifications of central vestibular mechanisms may rapidly occur during the first few years of life, therefore, and continue at a slower pace throughout childhood, playing a pervasive role in general maturation. As vestibular mechanisms follow a maturational sequence they, in turn, may be manipulated to influence maturation. Normal infants during their first year typically produce a large variety of rhythmical, stereotyped movements, such as waving, banging, rubbing, licking, and bouncing, which appear as developmental profiles. They seem dependent upon the maturation of proper neuromuscular pathways, and age at onset correlates with rate of motor development (Fisher-Thompson and Thelen, 1986). The reinforcement characteristics of vestibular stimulation have been extended to autistic, retarded and multiply handicapped children (Sandler and McLain, 1987), indicating its potency over other reinforcers such as food, praise, or sensory stimulation. This is consistent with observations that movement is an integral part of play throughout early and late childhood, and the rapid acceleration, movement and deceleration create a central component of vestibular stimulation. Institutionalized and non-ambulatory children, for example, experience an environment which is particularly barren of vestibular input. Their inability to obtain appropriate movement stimulation through their own efforts may make vestibular stimulation especially important. Improved sensorimotor skills are reported following vestibular stimulation with normal and preterm infants, Down's Syndrome, cerebral palsy, general developmental delay and multiply handicapped children. Abnormal OVRs have also been reported in some hyperactive children (HAC) who present with disorders of physiological arousal, attention, and motor control, and who subsequently benefit from vestibular stimulation. Improvements in motor and visuomotor functions, learning ability, and general behaviour of HAC (Bhatara, Clark, Arnold *et al.*, 1981), suggest that vestibular function may be selectively facilitated, in parallel with neurophysiological (Satterfield, 1976) and cerebral blood flow changes. There is no indication that rotational stimulation precipitates epileptic seizures, or that caloric stimulation of the semicircular canal facilitates abnormal EEG activity (Barac, 1967; Kantner, Clark, Atkinson *et al.*, 1982). The head-injured and HA child may have similar deficits in arousal-activation-control (see Taylor, this volume). Given that vestibular stimulation may result in altered levels of activity in cerebral, autonomic and behavioural systems, it seems reasonable to suggest that it may similarly affect the head-injured child. It seems likely, therefore, that a decisive role may be the interaction between the vestibular nuclei and surrounding reticular formation with its multiple reciprocal connections. Complex interactions are evident within the oculovestibular system and the conceptual system of arousal-activation, even when one confines the analysis to input from three sources, vestibular, visual, and eye movements. The effects can only be conjectured when the afferent input from other sensory systems, such as hearing, is added. Reports on vestibular therapies have important methodological inadequacies and the feasibility of this type of stimulation for all populations is clearly questionable. Not all children show physical tolerance of vestibular stimulation, and there may be age levels for its effectiveness (Ornitz, 1983). There is, however, theoretical and clinical potential in pursuing trials during early recovery from head injury, although it is emphasized that no such evaluations have been reported with head-injured children and clinical trials should proceed with caution.

Concluding Remarks

The high incidence of paediatric head injury and the increasing morbidity in such a young population demands that clinical neuroscience at all levels carefully discard traditional medical prejudice. We must refute unsubstantiated claims, for instance, that children recover from head injury better than adults, with scientifically acceptable evidence. This requires that we urgently pursue research leading to an understanding of the immature brain's response to head injury, its initial and potential recuperative capacities, and the effective remediation of trauma's debilitating effects. We know so little about head injury in children that it is vital we 'we look upon each patient as a research model capable of relaying valuable data concerning loss and recovery of function' (NIMH, 1984, page 17). The true extent of marked disabilities may only become evident in the later stages of recovery from head injury, when greater demands on the child are made, or when developmental stages are brought into play for the first time. Attempts at prosthetic remediation are likely to be of limited benefit at this relatively late stage and, considering the potential benefits of early, intense and individually tailored rehabilitation, it is no longer acceptable for the health service to pay lip service to the glaring inadequacies of clinical management and yet play the wait-and-see game, merely trusting the myth of full and spontaneous recovery in the young brain. Is it necessary, asks J. Moore (1980), that we have floods of public case histories before we are willing to open up the intellectual barriers of our minds and recognize the fascinating potentials that are available within the nervous system for stimulating and enhancing the recovery process through multiple therapeutic techniques? We should at least prepare the ground for optimal recovery, guiding and enhancing the child's potential as soon as possible, establishing greater continuity in care throughout recovery, and improving communication between hospitals and carers. To evaluate both the theoretical and more popular claims for helping early recovery, it is essential that appropriate and valid measures of functioning are taken in experimentally controlled designs. Many such ideas are otherwise wasted, losing innumerable hours of staff and patient time in fruitless data collection and inefficient patient care. The widespread, well intentioned, but unscientific and consequently unproven use of stimulation programmes with little or no theoretical background can only delay the discovery of effective treatment by systematic search. If this proves unattainable, then stimulation programmes can cease beclouding a stark reality that may call for greater prevention and fewer prosthetic palliatives. Human studies are, of course, more problematic than animal research and it is often difficult to bridge the gap between the two (Weiskrantz, 1977; Warren and Kolb, 1978), but it is possible that the factors which enhance or retard recovery in rats, cats and monkeys may play a similar role in man. Although the animal literature in this field is far from exhaustive, especially regarding the effects of brain injury coupled with the normal development of the target behaviour (Johnson and Almli, 1978), there are some experimental principles (J. Moore, 1980; Finger and Stein, 1982) which offer general guidelines for treatment approaches:

1   Sensory deprivation may be preventable by starting active rehabilitation as soon as possible after injury. The reticulolimbic system is one of the most important systems to activate with therapeutic techniques, because it has multiple efferent and afferent connections with all other systems of the central nervous system. It readily reacts to changes and acts as a stimulator of other neural systems. The effects of a critical amount of cell damage in the initial processing stages of sensory input, distorting that information into redundant noise, may be more disabling than complete loss of function within a sensory system. Tailoring therapy programmes to individuals is of great importance.

2   Any stimulation should be intense and varied for the duration of hospitalization, especially when the child is bedridden. The intensity of stimulation required to produce a response should not in any way be underestimated. Compare the intensity of a painful stimulus required to

elicit a motor response, for example, with that of talking to the patient in a quiet sickroom voice, gently calming the troubled brow. Placing objects simply in the line of vision (Yanko, 1985), on the locker or above the bed is unlikely to be of any use because of acute visual, perceptual or attentional disturbances. Highly stimulating material, such as holographic paper or sound effects tape, may be of greater help initially than family photographs or the ubiquitous pop music radio playing in the background. The child adjusts to the intensity and quality of stimulation with frequent repetitions over time. His adaptation signals progress, whilst habituation to the stimuli used should be avoided at all stages.

3   Passive experience of a stimulating environment may be necessary at the very beginning of treatment but, it is not sufficient and active participation must occur as soon as possible. The nervous system learns by doing, and optimal learning is facilitated by multiple use of senses. Combining verbal and physical guidance to obtain responses is an effective interim procedure, particularly with recalcitrant patients.

4   Facilitation and inhibition are fundamental physiological properties of the nervous system normally held in a complex balance which, following brain injury, may be considerably disturbed and require a clear external structure to guide behaviour.

5   *The pattern of recovery typically* follows the developmental sequence, that is subcortical integration of function preceding cortical. Neocortical components are usually the most vulnerable to trauma and are the last to recover, if at all. The majority of normal functioning is integrated automatically at subcortical levels, but this may not occur for the younger head-injured child who must exert greater conscious effort and control in many aspects of behaviour which would otherwise be automatic or habitual. Cortical overdrive can be a powerful inhibitor of skill, in that too much conscious effort usually causes unnecessary tensions resulting in a reduction of performance, which is tedious and exhausting for all concerned. Individual stimulation programmes should begin with the conception of simple intense stimuli in the early stages of recovery, aiming to rouse and stimulate basic functions, which then lead to more complex demands and activities as the head-injured child progresses. The younger the organism is at the time of injury, the greater the chance that the old systems are still dominant, or less differentiated and, therefore, can aid in the recovery function (Johnson and Almli, 1978; J. Moore, 1980).

6   The rate of rehabilitation should be related to the child's needs, and not dictated by how many patients the therapist must see. The process is typically long and tedious before any measures of progress are demonstrated. It is not known if and when recovery stops, particularly in the still-

developing organism. Major gains are clearly made early and then the child appears to reach a plateau, but further changes may continue for some time, albeit more slowly. Unfortunately, the therapeutic input often falls far short of maximizing the child's early potential. It is the extra effort required in this apparently last phase which can bridge the crucial gap between sitting back and doing nothing, or returning successfully to education.

7   Relatives and carers are potentially an invaluable source of help in the child's recovery. They can increase the total period of stimulation, facilitate consistency and generalization. They may also derive some benefit themselves from helping, increasing their understanding and acceptance of the patient's acute disabilities, and assisting in planning realistic long-term goals (Quine, Pierce and Lyle, 1988).

8   Experimental evidence suggests that the outcome of brain injury may be largely dependent on the social and physical environment in which the subject was living either before or after the CNS injury (Will, 1981) and this factor needs investigation in order to evaluate its contribution to clinical recovery potential. Physical (e.g., nutritional) and experiential variables have largely been ignored, with greater attention focusing on the broad dichotomy of recovery – no recovery (Johnson and Almli, 1978). Any programme of extra stimulation should accord with the general treatment plan and not be detrimental to other patients, hence the creation of sections within units for head-injured patients would be advantageous.

The experimental reports suggest that, with infants and pre-schoolers at least, environmental enrichment is a primary requisite of which parents, educational and hospital staff alike should be aware. If, by determining the conditions under which hypotheses are correct, we may begin to delineate the structural and metabolic changes which occur following traumatic brain injury at various ages in childhood and adolescence, then we shall be in a substantially more advantageous position to design and implement effective and rational rehabilitation. If stimulation of any form leads to improvement, does this really reflect true recovery of function, or simply an additive effect superimposed upon that caused by the lesion? Rosenzweig concludes that ' . . . at the least . . . even damaged brains can benefit from experience and that their full capacity cannot be determined without training and or enriched experience' (1980, p. 142). Even though brain-injured rats appear to learn less well than intact controls, they nevertheless benefit from exposure to a complex environment. The caveat here is that if the critical minimal neural substrate is not available, then no amount of therapy is going to produce any functional recovery. The definition of recovery is an important variable. If the EC animals show a return to more normal levels of performance, they could be said to show 'recovery' from the effects of a lesion in a complex environment. This may not amount to restitution of function as such, rather the elaboration of a new set of strategies to replace those lost by injury. On the basis of his earlier work, Rose (1988) suggests that the post-operative environment may stimulate compensation for loss in one sensory modality by increased use of others, which cannot be construed as recovery *per se*.

It is imperative, therefore, that recovery, adaptation, and further development are differentiated as far as possible. The apparent paradox between recovery assessed physiologically (i.e., permanent abnormal change) and behaviourally (i.e., apparently good outcome) is probably more a reflection of the greater discriminative power of physiological measurement. This discrepancy characterizes the head-injured child and thus argues strongly for a combined approach examining both physiology and behavior in recovery of function, since conclusions about recovery on one level cannot be generalized to another.

The head-injured child presents many challenges and opportunities for understanding the complex interactions of a malfunctioning system, one that is trying to recuperate and reorganize itself in relation to what was once a normal and integrated organism, and yet continue its ontogenetic programme of development (see, Greenough, 1975, Kaiser, Rudeberg, Frankenhauser *et al.*, 1986). Longtitudinal research with this population will help to redress our dependence on comparing adult-child head injury and delineate the time course of neurological and behavioural change (Johnson and Almli, 1978). In so doing, we shall be forced to avoid testing the child in an adult world, and design appropriate procedures for the disabled but developing child, identifying their capacity rather than simply task success or failure. Whilst the young child head-injury and the adult patient may share similar mechanisms and severity of injury, they have clearly not shared equivalent interaction or experience with their environments. The likelihood is, therefore, that normal development is disrupted in the young head-injured child, implying a greater need for stimulation or enrichment in their hospital, school and home, covering not only cognition, but also nutrition and social factors. The practical impact of treatment-induced changes in brain and behaviour after head injury would be very considerable indeed, particularly in terms of earlier and faster progress through formal rehabilitation, and the social significance of a relatively more abled population. In their present form, these ideas for early intervention may turn out to be ineffective at worst but, with sufficient methodological rigour, they may provide early benefits, improve coping abilities, and maximize outcome. The alternative is a life for the child and family which is increasingly dominated by handicap, dependence, despair and isolation.

Chapter 4

Rational drug interventions

Peter Eames

Introduction

There is no published data that bears directly on drug treatments of disorders related to head injury in children. This in part reflects the relatively small numbers involved, and the fact that few rehabilitation centres have concerned themselves in any specific way with this population. Studies of pharmacological interventions in adults with acquired brain injury are still very limited (Gualtieri, 1988), though the field is expanding rapidly. It is already apparent that some drug treatments can be of help in a number of areas, which may be common to both head-injured children and adults, including attention, memory, learning and social behaviour. Fundamental research, however, is still desparately needed. This chapter will consider the theoretical and practical issues involved in drug treatment of head-injured patients, in the hope of provoking further attention to possible applications in children.

General considerations

Pharmacology is the science concerned with the nature and mode of drug effects. Therapeutics concerns the use of drugs in clinical conditions. Clearly, pharmacology should be the main basic of therapeutics, but the teaching of these subjects tends to happen at different stages in medical training and, as a result, their relationship is often loosened. Most commonly, pharmacology is taught preclinically as a basic science in a coherent course. Subsequently, therapeutics is invariably taught piecemeal, as different disorders are encountered during clinical training. Unless clinical teachers actively encourage students to relate treatments to their previously acquired knowledge of pharmacology, this science becomes relegated to the past, along with botany and inorganic chemistry. Indeed, in ordinary medical practice the commonest basis for drug prescription is an almost automatic disorder-drug association, rather than the logical development of a therapeutic solution from pharmacological knowledge. An example may clarify this point. An outbreak of apparent hysteria, involving bizarre head, face and neck movements, was reported in an overseas armed forces community which acted as a base for desert training. It transpired that all of the patients had been admitted to the medical centre with acute diarrhoea and vomiting, and the so-called hysteria was in fact a series of acute dystonic reactions to the drug Stemetil (prochlorperazine). This had been prescribed in an almost reflex fashion, the learned automatic disorder-drug association being 'Nausea and Vomiting — PING! — prescribe Stemetil'. In discussion, it transpired that the medical officers involved did not know that Stemetil is a phenothiazine and, therefore, capable of provoking dystonic reactions. The real catch, however, was that the stores officer had taken in supplies of 25 mg tablets, instead of the usual 5 mg, and the drug was being prescribed at 'Stemetil one tablet three times a day'. As a result, the patients were receiving a dose appropriate in the treatment of severe psychiatric disorder, but five times the usual dose for nausea and vomiting.

The great majority of treatments in medicine, both effective and irrelevant, are empirical. This means that a drug has been found to be effective and, in the best instances, the finding has been upheld after careful study using double blind controlled conditions. It also implies that there is little knowledge of how the effect is achieved. Ideally, of course, all drug treatments should simply redress some specific pathophysiological abnormality which underlies the clinical abnormality. This ideal of rational drug intervention however, can be achieved only when some clear pathophysiological disturbance is known to be the cause of the clinical condition, and this is a rare occurrence. Perhaps the best example involving the central nervous system (CNS) is the use of L-dopa in the treatment of Parkinson's disease, although even this is not as straightforward as it might seem. As far as the target symptom or disorder is concerned, the empirical approach generally works quite well, but two particular problems are associated with it. First, automatic disorder-drug associations tend to be made so quickly that important aspects of the whole context may be overlooked. For example, it requires a significant degree of self-discipline to remember to enquire about a previous history of asthma before prescribing propranolol for migraine prophylaxis. Secondly, the process tends to focus attention on a desired effect of the drug, so that additional effects may be overlooked. The common expression used to describe these is 'side effects', but this is a term which is in itself misleading. In normal circumstances any drug has a range of effects; in the treatment of a particular symptom or condition, some particular effect is desired, but the others will occur nevertheless, and there is nothing truly 'side' about them. As an illustration, the drug orphenadrine is marketed by one pharmaceutical company for the treatment of Parkinsonian disorders, but by another as a skeletal muscle relaxant. In the promotional material neither company mentions the other's use or indeed action, and these omissions result from a marketing agreement between the companies. Which is the side effect?

Context can be very important in predicting drug effects. For head-injured children, a feature of obvious importance is age. For some drugs, different effects can be expected in children from those seen in adults, though probably the most important difference in most cases relates to dosage. Some drugs are metabolized quite differently in two age groups. An example where this can mislead is the anticonvulsant carbamazepine, for which the different balances between its two major catabolic pathways require that much the same dose levels be used in children as in adults. A much greater distortion of standard drug effects is produced by severe diffuse head injury, which presents an extremely complex, though nonetheless broadly predictable special context. For example, whilst the use of prochlorperazine for the treatment of nausea and vomiting presents few problems when the appropriate dose is used in otherwise normal subjects, in the head-injured individual it may have two adverse effects; first, it is epileptogenic, and this is of particular importance to the head-injured since they already carry an increased risk of epilepsy and the onset of post-traumatic epilepsy is known to have very serious effects on educational and occupational outcomes, as well as on the general quality of life. Second, even quite low doses of prochlorperazine may produce extrapyramidal movement disorders in head-injured patients. This example highlights the fact that potential adverse effects are most easily overlooked when drugs are prescribed for symptomatic disorders unrelated to the primary problem; for example, trivial viral symptoms in a person recovering from a severe head injury.

The obvious solution is for all physicians dealing with the head-injured is to develop the habit of thinking pharmacologically, but it must not be imagined that this is easily achieved. Only in the last decade has the whole range of problems resulting from severe head injury begun to be appreciated. Even now it is rare, at least in England, for the condition to be treated in special units wholly devoted to it. The much wider development of 'categorical' head injury rehabilitation units in the United States has not been attended by consistent or committed medical interest in many cases. As a result, little is yet known about specific aspects of drug treatments in the head-injured generally, and virtually nothing is known about the special problems of head-injured children. Inevitably, most problems are approached by comparison with superficially similar ones in other pathological states, and trying out the appropriate drug treatment. This sort of approach is inadequate in many ways. More creative thinking is needed, based on actual knowledge of the brain disorders caused by head injury. A major impediment to this is the ingrained attitude, particularly prevalent in academic centres, which effectively demands that a drug treatment be already described in the literature before it can be considered proper to use it. On closer inspection, it is apparent that this attitude stems from rules which apply more to therapeutics than to pharmacology. Ironically it seems much more likely that what is needed is creative *pharmacological* thinking.

Pharmacology and head injury

There is a rapidly expanding literature on drug treatments for head injury disorders. (See reviews in the Journal of Head Trauma Rehabilitation, 1987, Gualtieri, 1988.) The bulk of this literature however, consists of reports of studies of very small groups, or of single cases, the motivation for which can be seen to come from traditional drug treatments of conditions other than head injury. It is distressing to see how often the conclusions of these studies lead to recommendations which clearly ignore potential adverse effects which are predictable from current knowledge of the drugs and of head injury disorders. For example, Mysiw and Jackson, (1987) state that tricyclic antidepressants may diminish agressive behaviours and 'are rapidly gaining recognition as having a major impact on the rehabilitation course of the TBI (traumatic brain injury) patient'. No mention is made of the considerable and well established risk of provoking epilepsy (Markowitz and Brown, 1987; Hayes and Kristoff, 1986) and, in fact, their confident statement is based on a single study of one patient, by their own group (Jackson, Corrigan and Arnett, 1985), and a further study not then published. The latter subsequently reported twenty patients with agitation (out of a total of fifty-eight patients treated for head injury) of whom thirteen showed 'dramatic decrease in agitation' one week after starting treatment with amitryptiline (Mysiw, Jackson and Corrigan, 1988). The proportion of patients who responded to the drug, however, dropped dramatically with decreasing degree of confusion, inviting the alternative interpretation that their agitation resolved spontaneously as post-traumatic confusion cleared. Given that these drugs increase the risk of epilepsy by only a few per cent, it is not surprising that this problem did not make itself apparent in their study. If, however, their recommendation were to be followed by physicians around the world, one could confidently predict, on the basis of the extensive literature on antidepressants, a significant increase in the number of individuals developing post-traumatic epilepsy. In his review, Gualtieri (1988) mentions that one particular antidepressant, maprotiline, 'is known to lower seizure threshold . . . and is therefore probably contraindicated in TBI patients'. He also states 'one advantage of amitriptyline is that it is the tricyclic antidepressant least likely to lower seizure threshold', but the study he quotes in support of this (Clifford, Rutherford, Hicks *et al.*, 1985) is in fact a study of the effects of drugs locally applied to specific sites in animal preparations, and the findings are quite different from those in man which, in fact, show this drug to be the antidepressant most likely to provoke epilepsy. Very similar considerations apply to the small literature, frequently overinflated by reviewers, claiming beneficial effects from neuroleptic (antipsychotic) drugs on behavioural disorders after head injury. Cardenas (1987) quotes three studies (with eighteen, twelve, and eleven patients respectively) and one report containing a few case examples. She notes that most of the studies have flawed methodological designs, yet concludes that it is a fact that antipsychotic medications can alleviate symptoms following brain injury. In her review of adverse effects she does not even mention the possible provocation of epilepsy, and recommends diphenhydramine for treatment of neuroleptic-induced extra-pyramidal disorders in the elderly, despite that fact that even the American Physicians Desk Reference Book warns of the significant epileptogenic actions of this drug.

An even more ominous point is that all antidepressant and neuroleptic drugs have more or less marked anticholinergic activity, which is known to have deleterious effects on cognition. A few of the published head injury studies claim useful effects on behaviour without cognitive deterioration, but these claims turn out to be based on screening procedures that assess well established and static intellectual functions, rather than the often subtle kinds of cognitive disorder, such as attention and learning, that characterize the head-injured, and are particularly sensitive to the effects of these drugs.

Similarly, there is a growing literature on the use of stimulant drugs for behavioural and attentional disorders after head injury. Close scrutiny, however, reveals that the claims are built upon alleged similarities between these patients and children with Attention Deficit Disorder, coupled with just three published studies, one well-designed (Evans, Gualtieri and Patterson, 1987), the others 'open' case reports (Weinstein and Wells, 1981; Lipper and Tuchman, 1976). Each of these three studies concerns just one patient.

Seeking rational therapies

If rational drug treatments are desirable, then they must be sought. The obvious way to proceed is to identify as far as possible the individual deficits which contribute to functional disorders, to achieve an understanding of pathophysiological causes of the deficits, and then attempt to correct them in as direct and physiological a way as possible. This is the essence of the use of L-dopa in Parkinson's Disease, for example. It may be helpful at this stage to point out a distinction between two forms of drug effects. A naturally occurring biological agent which influences the biochemical or biophysical processes in which it is ordinarily involved may be said to be acting 'physiologically'. A substance not usually incorporated in, or produced by, natural processes may nevertheless alter metabolism. The commonest reason is probably that the substance (drug) has a part of its molecular structure which closely resembles, or is identical to, the structure of the physiological agent. Thus, the drug may be used to produce a physiological effect, but often the affinity of the drug for the natural system may be different, so that higher concentrations may be required. More troublesome is the possibility that some other part of the molecular structure may resemble another natural agent sufficiently closely to provoke additional effects, perhaps completely unrelated to the desired effect, some of which may be actively deleterious. Drugs which act in this way are said to be 'pharmacological' agents. Sometimes the same substance may have both kinds of effects. For example, cortisone in certain doses may simply replace a deficiency, as in Addison's Disease (adrenal insufficiency), whilst in much higher doses it may have a pharmacological action in suppressing the natural processes of inflammation.

In trying to establish rational drug treatments it is of course essential to study the effectiveness of any interventions only in controlled conditions. Regrettably, purely physiological ways of intervening are unlikely to be possible very often. The next level of intervention is to try to manipulate the pathophysioloigcal state with pharmacological agents (drugs), as opposed to physiological ones like L-dopa. This will bring new problems in the form of additional effects of the drugs, which may have nuisance value, or may be frankly deleterious. Most of these effects will be predictable from knowledge, however, and may even be correctable. For example, the arrival of the dopamine D2 blocker, sulpiride, makes it possible to prevent the psychotogenic effects of the D1 and D2 dopamine agonist bromocriptine, without significantly reducing its positive effects on the extrapyramidal motor systems. Some adverse effects of drugs are, however, completely unpredictable and come to light, not from pharmacological studies, but from the clinical trials which form the basis of therapeutics. Zimelidine was one of the most promising of the new wave of antidepressant drugs with a relatively pure effect on 5-HT, until it had to be withdrawn because it was found to induce a serious clinical neurological syndrome. A new anticonvulsant, zonisamide, which was very promising in clinical trials, had to be withdrawn because of an alarmingly high incidence of renal stones.

Aims of treatment

A further conceptual distinction for clarification concerns the targets of drug interventions. Most information currently available is about the use of various drugs in the treatment of the effects of head injury. An equally or, perhaps, more legitimate concern is whether drug treatments may be able to influence the rate or extent of recovery processes themselves. Feeney's group have published results from a number of studies on this topic, (Sutton *et al.*, 1987) and other sources are mentioned below. Clearly, preventive measures are more 'rational' than treatments of established deficits which might have been prevented, and it seems important to encourage research into this aspect.

In view of the multidisciplinary audience, a brief review of the basic functioning of the neurone is offered, together with the ways in which it may be disordered, or manipulated. Working from this basis, existing 'rational drug treatments' will be discussed, and some of the possibilities for future developments in the management of severe head injury, both restorative and preventive, will be considered.

The Neurone

Figure 4.1: Simplified Neuronal Mechanism

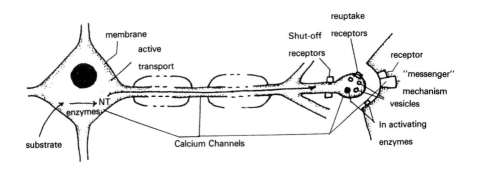

The diagrammatic representation of a neurone (Figure 4.1) is designed to highlight aspects of function which can be manipulated either physiologically or pharmacologically. There are three distinct aspects of functioning which need to be considered, namely membrane stability, conduction of the electrical impulse, and the control and effects of neurotransmitter chemicals. The electrical stability of the nerve cell membrane and particularly that of the cell body, is the first requirement for effective nerve action. Two factors known to be important to this stability are the physical shape of the cell body, which may be distorted by local mechanical interferences such as scar tissue, and the composition of the extracellular fluid, which may be disturbed in metabolic disorders. The commonest effect of the former is unexpected, environmentally irrelevant electrical discharge, which of course produces epilepsy. Metabolic disturbance, on the other hand, may cause either hypoexcitability or irritable discharge.

If the action potential is not conducted smoothly and at the expected velocity, the integration of the activity of groups of cells is likely to be disturbed. Moreover, both the conduction process and the release of neurotransmitter depend upon the proper functioning of specialized channels through the membrane for the transport of calcium ions, which may be disturbed by a wide range of metabolic disorders. There is a large literature on this complex topic, but a helpful simplified summary is available in Greenberg (1986). [For further reading on these topics, see Cooper, Bloom and Roth 1986; Iversen and Iversen, 1981]. At a much simpler level, conduction depends on the acid-base balance of the extracellular fluid and on temperature, and these agents have greater effect on neurones with defective myelination.

Neurotransmitter chemicals are, in most cases, elaborated in the cell body from chemical substrates which enter the cell, with specific enzymes and co-factors required for the transformation. The neurotransmitter molecules are then transported down the axon, by means of specific transport mechanisms, ultimately being stored in microvesicles in the nerve terminals. The quantity of neurotransmitter in each vesicle is fairly constant. Storage is not permanent and, perhaps as a result of gradual leakage from the vesicle, the neurotransmitter substance is eventually inactivated by a variety of enzymes within the terminal or, if not so inactivated, may re-enter a vesicle. The arrival of an action potential at the terminal causes a usually standard number of vesicles and, therefore, a standard quantity of neurotransmitter to be released from the terminal into the synaptic cleft. Transmitter molecules may then attach themselves to specific receptors on the post-synaptic cell membrane, thus causing changes in its permeability or, in the activity of 'second messenger' mechanisms. In either event, there is a change in membrane excitability, and each presynaptic action potential thus changes the probability that an action potential will be generated in the post-synaptic neurone. Some neurotransmitters increase this probability (i.e., stimulate the cell) whilst others reduce it (i.e., inhibit the cell). Again the effect is not permanent, and neurotransmitter molecules detach themselves from the receptor, move back into the cleft where they are either inactivated by specific enzymes, or are taken up into the presynaptic terminal through specific re-uptake channels. Finally, in order to allow self-regulation of the terminal, there are receptors on the terminal itself which, when activated by the arrival of neurotransmitter molecules, change the excitability of the last part of the axon so as to prevent the conduction of the action potential. All of these features probably apply to all of the different neurotransmitters. The classical neurotransmitters comprise acetylcholine, noradrenaline, dopamine, 5-hydroxytryptamine (5-HT), gamma-aminobutyric acid (GABA), glutamic acid, aspartic acid, and glycine; any one neurone contains only one of them. Indeed, it used to be thought that this rule was absolute but, in the last decade a new class of neurochemicals has been identified, which are peptides. It now appears that many neurones have parallel systems involving one 'classical' and one peptide transmitter. To complicate matters even further, there are two rather distinct ways in which neurones deliver their neurochemicals to post-synaptic receptors. The arrangement described so far involves a physically close connection, resulting in an effect on just one part of the membrane of one target cell. Some cells, or more properly, cell systems, however, release their chemicals into synaptic structures which are very extensive and in the form of lakes or interlacing channels, making them available to a wide range of post-synaptic cells at more or less the same time. There are even neurones which appear to release the neurochemical into the ventricular systems of the brain, thus achieving very widespread effects within a particular neurotransmitter system. This kind of effect is known as neuromodulation and, although some of the classical substances are sometimes delivered in this way, it is probably more typical of some of the neuropeptides.

It is important to understand that any of the neurochemicals may act in either a neurotransmitter or a neuromodulator fashion, depending on the microanatomy of the particular neuronal system. For any particular neurochemical, there are different kinds of receptors. They all respond to the same chemical, and the differences are probably related to structural differences between neurones in different functional systems, and perhaps to variations between neurotransmitter and neuromodulator functions. Their importance comes from the fact that it has proved possible to identify drugs which selectively affect a single type of receptor. For example, I have cited (above) the possibility of preventing the psychotic changes which can be produced by bromocriptine. This is a dopamine agonist, which is not very selective, and stimulates both the D1 and D2 types of dopamine receptor. Its typical use is to replace the missing dopamine stimulation of the nigrostriatal pathway in Parkinson's Disease. Sometimes the concomitant stimulation of the mesolimbic pathways is sustained (i.e. there is inadequate down-regulation — see below), and the patient becomes psychotic. This can be counteracted without undoing the helpful nigrostriatal effects by administering sulpiride, a drug which blocks only the D2 (mesolimbic) receptors. This is obviously a very complex arrangement, even though the preceding account is simplified. It is composed, however, of all those factors which can be affected by known drug actions.

Drug effects on the neurone

It is possible to interfere with neurotransmitter functioning by many different means. The simplest is to increase the concentration of the neurotransmitter substrate in the cell body. Large loading doses of substrate will force an increased rate of production of neurotransmitter, through the effect known as the Law of Mass Action, which is likely eventually to increase the quantity released by each action potential and, therefore, to increase the post-synaptic effect. On the other hand, production can be reduced by drugs which interfere with the enzyme involved in the transformation. Theoretically it should be possible to alter the rate of neurotransmitter transport down the axon. There are drugs which will deplete the nerve terminal of its neurotransmitter stores, thereby reducing its activity, (after a brief initial increase, of course). Receptors may be blocked by antagonist drugs, whose molecules will fit onto them but do not activate them or will activate but not detach themselves, or they may be activated by agonist drugs which act just like the neurotransmitter. Neurotransmitter action may be prolonged by blocking inactivating enzymes or, alternatively, by blocking re-uptake mechanisms. Drugs which selectively stimulate 'shut-off' receptors will, of course, inactivate the neurone. Alternatively, those which block these receptors will prevent auto-regulation and thus increase activity. It happens that these latter receptors are most commonly affected by very low doses of drugs which in higher doses may produce opposite effects by blocking post-synaptic or re-uptake receptors. This is a rather subtle example of the intuitively obvious fact that dosage is an important determinant of drug action. There are, however, other important determinants. All living systems have a natural tendency to resist imposed change (homeostasis) and the neurone is no exception. There are several mechanisms which serve to return the level of activity of the neurotransmitter system to its norm, of which the shut-off receptors are one example. Another is the propensity for new receptors to sprout when existing ones are blocked for any length of time. This particular mechanism undoubtedly makes for much confusion in the interpretation of drug effects in the intact animal, because the rate of and delay before sprouting vary between different kinds of neurone, and also depend on the duration of blockade by the drug in question. This general phenomenon is known as regulation, and sprouting is clearly an example of up-regulation. If a drug increases the availability of neurotransmitter in the synaptic cleft, by blocking inactivating enzymes for example, down-regulation may occur as a result of shrinkage of the number of receptors, as well as through stimulation of shut-off receptors. One important consequence of regulation is that the immediate effects of a drug on being first introduced may be quite different from effects which will appear if it is administered for a long period of time. The commonest example of this phenomenon is that almost any drug which affects the nervous system will produce sedation when first introduced, even though its main chronic effect may be to enhance alertness. Another important example is that almost all antidepressant drugs need to be administered for at least several days, at an adequate dose, before the antidepressant effect appears. A further aspect of regulation should be mentioned, which is particularly relevant to head injury. Regulation is a normal function, which operates fully only if the neurone is in a normal state. Using the example of Parkinson's Disease, once again, the nigrostriatal neurones are underfunctioning because of inadequate enzymatic transformation of L-dopa (the substrate) into dopamine. The cell would like to up-regulate, but it cannot do so. Large doses of L-dopa increase its concentration in the cell body, and thus increase the amount of dopamine formed, with the level of neuronal activity returned towards its norm. There is no cause here for down-regulation, since the change imposed by the interference is in the direction sought by the homeostatic mechanisms. After the initial recovery period, however, neurones in a traumatically injured brain are either too damaged to function at all, or they function normally, so regulation can be expected to occur. In thinking pharmacologically, therefore, regulation effects should be anticipated.

The effects of head injury

Brain disorders from head injury result from different causes at different stages. Neurones which are irreversibly damaged at the time of injury are obviously a constant factor. In the early stages of recovery, however, many cells are disturbed in their functioning, but may subsequently recover. Most nervous functions depend on activity in groups or systems of neurones, rather than on single cells, and there are almost certainly recovery processes which result from reorganizations of group action, to make up for cells which are permanently lost. Some recovery processes are thought to be maladaptive and introduce new disturbances of function later in recovery. Physical damage to the brain is healed through the formation of scar tissue which, as it shrinks with maturation, may distort remaining normal cells and render them electrically unstable. Other late developments, such as hydrocephalus, chronic haematoma or hygroma, may compress and distort parts of the brain, even to the point of renewed cell destruction. Of all these effects, however, the one which has most implications for drug treatments is undoubtedly the initial axonal damage associated with the concussive effect of closed head injury. It has now been demonstrated that diffuse axonal injury damages the axonal membrane, particularly at nodes of Ranvier, in such a way as to allow escape of intracellular calcium ions, and there is some evidence to suggest that this escape may be responsible for much of the permanent neuronal damage in this condition (Gennarelli, Adams and Graham, 1986). It is possible that prevention of the leakage in the very early period after injury may limit the damage. The fact that many axons are damaged permanently, however, has important implications for drug treatment. Extrapyramidal disorder again provides a particularly helpful example; it is possible to improve the dopaminergic activity of nigrostriatal cells in Parkinson's Disease by increasing the depressed rate of dopamine formation with high concentrations of L-dopa. If nigrostriatal function is deficient after head injury, however, it is because some of the neurones have been damaged, and most of the damage is to axons. Even if the cell bodies are functioning and can be induced in this way to increase their dopamine content, the neurotransmitter cannot be deployed, because it cannot be transported down the axon to a functioning terminal. The only fully rational way around the problem is to find another means of delivering dopamine to the post-synaptic receptors. This is the aim of surgical implantation of foetal or autologous adrenal dopaminergic neurones into a damaged striatum. This approach has not yet been attempted in head-injured subjects, whilst its effects in those with Parkinson's Disease are only just being assessed. The current solution is a second level one, mainly to use a dopamine agonist drug like bromocriptine. It is not yet known whether regulation occurs only in individual neurones, or whether grouped neurones can interact in this respect. If they could, then it might be possible to increase activity in the system even if a proportion of neurones were damaged beyond repair. For example, L-dopa would increase the activity of each functional cell, at least until the sum of activity in the system reach its norm, though beyond this, down-regulation mechanisms would prevent further increase. A further example concerns the rational approach in relation to epilepsy. Some forms of this condition appear to result from a relative insufficiency of GABA in nerve terminal vesicles. This can be overcome by blocking inactivating enzymes in the synaptic cleft with the drug sodium valproate, which has shown itself to be particularly effective in primary generalized epilepsy. Because this anticonvulsant produces so little deleterious effect on cognitive functions, it has been suggested as a suitable treatment for post-traumatic epilepsy. There are two rational arguments against this, however; firstly, epilepsy after head injury is nearly always of focal origin, resulting from localized cortical damage. There is no good reason to assume any inherent defect of GABA metabolism and any increase in the duration of GABA action is, therefore, likely to be reduced through down-regulation; secondly, any GABAergic neurones which have been damaged cannot have their function enhanced, since no GABA reaches the nerve terminals.

Current examples of rational treatments

Membrane stability

The main problem resulting from instability of cell body membranes after injury is, of course, the hyperexcitability and proneness to spontaneous discharge which underlie post-traumatic epilepsy. The anti-convulsant carbamazepine appears to exert its effects mainly through stabilization of abnormally excitable membranes, which makes it a very suitable drug for the treatment of this condition. Although there are other anti-convulsants which share this action, the absence of significant interference with cognitive functions through sedation makes it the drug of first choice, not only for frank epilepsy, but also for other conditions which are based on instability of neurone groups, in particular the various temporo-limbic syndromes. Electrolyte and protein disturbances are other potential causes of membrane instability. It is now well established that severe nutritional deficiencies can develop during coma after head injury and greater attention must be paid to the patient's nutritional status if the best outcome is to be achieved (Hadley, Graham, Harrington, *et al.*, 1986; Fruin, Taylor and Pettis, 1986).

Nerve conduction

It is sometimes possible to reverse the transient exacerbations of multiple sclerosis (MS) which occur in excessively hot weather, or in circumstances of acidosis, by manoeuvres which reduce body temperature, or by giving bicarbonates. The results in MS are not particularly impressive, and treatments have not apparently been tried in post-traumatic conditions, but they may perhaps find a place in the treatment repertoire and would at least be worth investigating. On the other hand, it is likely that there will soon be trials of treatment with gangliosides and calcium channel blockers in the very acute phase of severe head injury, in an attempt to reduce the degree of permanent axonal injury. Animal experiments have already been reported with gangliosides (see Karpiak, Li and Mahadik 1987).

Neurotransmitters

Most current attempts at rational drug intervention involve the manipulation of neurotransmitters. Tryptophan has been used effectively in the treatment of post-traumatic sleep disorders (Webb, 1981). L-dopa has been used in acute head injury management, but long-term outcome has not been assessed, so that effectiveness has not been demonstrated in a convincing way. Combinations of lecithin, an acetylcholine precursor, with anticholinesterases have been shown to improve memory in dementia, and have been used in post-traumatic cognitive deficits with promising results (Levin, Peters and Kalisky, 1986; McLean, Stanton, Cardenas *et al.,* 1987). Amphetamine and methylphenidate have produced improvements in attention and memory in one head injured subject (Evans, Gualtieri and Patterson 1987). Open studies of naltrexone, an opioid antagonist, have shown impressive effects in post-concussional symptoms (Tennant, 1987) and post-traumatic bulimia, excessive food-seeking behaviour (Childs, 1987). Preliminary experience with this drug in brain-injured patients with manipulative and dissociate disorders suggests that these are systematically reduced, while attention is improved (Eames, unpublished data). Successful treatment of akinetic mutism following surgical damage to the diencephalon has been reported with bromocriptine, a dopamine agonist, (Ross and Stewart, 1981). Fisher (1983) pointed out that the anergic, aspontaneous state which he calls abulia, is a lesser degree of this disorder. Although no studies in head injury are yet published, it has been found in a number of centres that abulic states, especially if associated with extrapyramidal motor disorders, often respond well to bromocriptine. Vasopressin is a peptide hormone which is secreted by the posterior pituitary gland and has effects on renal and uterine function. This has been known for decades but, more recently, it has been shown in animal studies to be released as a neuromodulator in the diencephalon, and to be involved in attention and memory, perhaps through an effect on arousal (Gash and Thomas, 1983; de Wied, 1983). Numerous human studies have been reported with conflicting results but, overall, it seems that a particular synthetic version, lysine-vasopressin, may sometimes have useful effects in post-traumatic disorders of learning and attention.

Future possibilities

The acute stage

Mention has already been made of the possibility of limiting axonal damage by trying to protect the axon against the effects of leakage. From animal models, a wide variety of substances are known to give some unspecified protection against neuronal damage, even if they are administered after the insult. These include the increasing range of so-called nootropic drugs derived from piracetam (Giurgea, 1973), codergocrine mesylate (Berga, Beckett and Roberts, 1986), opioid antagonists (Baskin and Hosobuchi, 1981), megavitamin therapy, glutamate antagonists (Kochhar, Zivin, Lyden *et al.*, 1988), and pyritinol (von Wild and Dolce, 1976), although few clinical studies in head injury are yet available (see Kitamura, 1981).

At the moment, much interest is being focused on the effects of severe head injury on neurotransmitter systems. From both animal and human work, there is evidence to suggest that all of the major neurotransmitters are discharged from neurones as a result of acute trauma (Sachs, 1957; Edvinsson, Owman, Rosengren *et al.*, 1971; Porta, Bareggi, and Collice 1975; Bareggi, Porta and Selenati 1975; Benedict and Loach, 1978; Hamill, Woolf, McDonald *et al.*, 1987). There are two distinct problems which may result; the large quantities of neurotransmitters diffusing freely through the extracellular fluid of the brain may have toxic effects wherever they meet appropriate receptors. Secondly, this neurotransmitter loss effectively depletes neurones of their stores, which will inevitably take time to replenish, and the nutritional deficiencies in coma may well delay this further. There are thus reasonable grounds for considering a treatment approach which at first sight appears contradictory. On the one hand, it may be advisable to try to protect receptors against the sudden excess of freely circulating neurotransmitters for a period of time which would be estimated on the basis of demonstrated patterns of the rise and fall of excesses in blood and cerebrospinal fluid. On the other hand, there may be a need to speed up the replenishment of stores of neurotransmitters by providing large amounts of their substrates. It must be remembered that the enzymatic transformations require various co-factors, particular vitamins, which may also need to be provided. For example, one proprietary preparation of tryptophan comes ready-mixed with pyridoxine and vitamin C, both necessary co-factors in the transformation to 5-HT. Improved outcome has been demonstrated in rats treated immediately after injury with anticholinergic agents (Hayes, Lyeth, Dixon *et al.*, 1985). Some concern about the application of such findings in human head injury arises from demonstrations of effectiveness of the pro-cholinergic actions of anticholinesterases (Luria, Naydin and Tsvetkova, 1969) in terminating coma, and improving cognition. It may well be, however, that both protection and repletion of neurotransmitter stores need to be provided concurrently, as early after injury as possible. The potential methods of achieving repletion of stores seem likely to involve the administration of large amounts of neurotransmitter substrates, although depleted action may, in the short term, be enhanced by the use of drugs which reduce the rate of breakdown by blocking inactivating enzymes. Because of the effects of regulation, only intact neurones can be manipulated in this way and any shortfall in activity resulting from loss of functioning neurones can be made up only through the use of direct stimulation of post-synaptic receptors with agonist drugs. It also seems apparent that this latter option will be available only for modulatory systems, since the administration of the drug by current methods makes it available only in a very diffused fashion and it cannot provide discrete, temporally appropriate stimulation.

Putting all of these possibilities together, it seems that there may be considerable benefit in giving the acutely head-injured patient a cocktail of neurotransmitter substrates (choline, L-dopa, tryptophan, glutamic acid), co-factors and high-energy nutrients, one or more of the metabolic protectors (glycosides, nootropic agents, and so on), and receptor blocking agents (perhaps scopolamine, phenoxybenzamine, propranolol, cyproheptadine or pizotifen, pimozide or sulpiride, and naltrexone). The problems with this idea are enormous; first, it must be demonstrated that each of the substrates is safe to give, and that their combination in appropriately large quantities does not give rise to metabolic interactions that are intrinsically dangerous, or that inactivate any of the constituents; secondly, the known potential hazards of the pharmacological agents, both individual and interactional, must be considered; thirdly, to satisfy the need to be sure of what is and is not necessary and useful, extensive trials of all possible combinations would have to be undertaken, studying not only the short term effects, but also ultimate outcome. Because of the great variation in outcome of patients with apparently similar states at the time of hospital admission, very large numbers of head injury victims would have to be included in any such studies. From a theoretical and pharmacological point of view, such a triple approach to the problem of traumatic neurotransmitter release seems likely to have much to offer, but practical application is probably a long way off.

Another area of great potential research interest involves the possibility of using in-dwelling micro-delivery systems, so that pharmacological or physiological agents can have their effects only at the desired sites. There is some animal work along these lines which is promising, but the techniques are likely to need considerable further development before they can be applied to the human brain.

The chronic stage

It is altogether more practicable to begin to apply the results of creative pharmacological thinking to functional problems which are apparent once consciousness is restored and the tempo of recovery has slowed to the point that deficits can be more easily characterized. There are several approaches which have already been tried, but need formal controlled study. The indentification of others will require more careful analysis of functional deficits than is commonly made in rehabilitation centres, as well as increasing knowledge of brain function and neuropharmacology, and improved methods of assessing outcome.

Chapter 5

Food for thought: a role for nutrition in recovery

John W.T. Dickerson, David A. Johnson and Anne Maclean

Introduction

The effects of injury upon the body's metabolism and the relationship to post-injury nutrition have been the subject of increasing research. When considering the effects of head trauma in children, however, our attention is also drawn to the effects of injury and nutrition on the brain. Unlike most other organs in the body, the brain has a single growth spurt with limited ability for regeneration. Before birth, brain growth and development are dependent upon the nutrition, health and well-being of the mother; after birth, these processes are subject to a number of environmental factors, including nutrient supply, hormonal balance and the sensory environment (Dickerson, Merat and Yusuf, 1982; Morgan and Winick, 1980). These interdependent variables may be altered after head injury and disturb complex relationships affecting the management of the head-injured child.

Developmental studies have usually focused on the effects of chronic protein energy malnutrition (PEM) on the brain, but it is now apparent that normal variations in nutrient availability may directly influence cerebral metabolism. Changes in blood chemistry which follow variations in the amounts of protein and carbohydrate consumed in each meal cause changes in cerebral neurotransmitters and may thus affect brain function. In this chapter we consider the current knowledge of these complex inter-relationships and their bearing on children recovering from head injury.

Brain development

The brain accounts for 13 per cent of body weight at birth, but just 2 per cent in the adult. In the newborn, cerebral oxygen consumption is low but rises rapidly with cerebral growth and maturation. Cerebral blood flow reaches a peak at different times in different regions, and is proportional to the speed of regional maturation; areas with high density of white matter show the highest blood flow at peak myelination; and blood flow is proportional to metabolic rate. By 6 years, the brain has achieved about 90 per cent of its adult size and by 12 years, a child has a head which is almost as large as his father's (Sinclair, 1978). Cerebral blood flow and oxygen consumption are maximal at 6 years of age (about 60 ml/min/brain) and represent over half the basal metabolic rate, which is higher than the 20–30 per cent in adults (Anderson, 1981).

The normal fuel for the brain, glucose, must be derived from the diet, since the brain contains negligible amounts of glycogen and neutral fat. During periods of starvation, the brain uses ketones for energy and this facility is more easily activated in babies than in adults. The growth spurt of the brain constitutes a critical, or vulnerable period when nutritional deficiencies are likely to have their greatest effect (Dobbing, 1968). The period of growth and development in man, however, is absolutely and relatively longer than in laboratory animals, so the brain remains sensitive to chronic PEM for longer and deficiencies may well affect further myelination, dendritic and synaptic growth. Moreover, since vitamins and minerals are involved in brain metabolism, selective deficiencies may affect the brain and its function at any age, irrespective of its effects on growth. Whether the effects of such deficiencies are reversible depends upon the severity and chronicity of the depletion. In rats, synthesis of the neurotransmitter serotonin (5-HT) is dependant on diet (Dickerson and Pao, 1975) and probably so at any age. The growing brain appears to have no special priority when dietary inadequacy occurs and is not spared at the expense of other tissues.

The limiting factors operating during growth may determine the level of cerebral function achieved, but the final result may depend upon the severity of the limitation and on the degree of environmental stimulation provided. The extent of dendritic arborization linking the neurones plays an essential role in brain function. An impoverished environment results in lower brain levels of acetylcholinesterase, for example (Rosenzweig, Bennett, Diamond *et al.*, 1969, 1972). In contrast, the effects of PEM in rats is reduced by increasing their population density (Bell, 1975). Long term active avoidance conditioning (Savaki and Levis, 1977) and early stimulation in nutritionally deprived pups (Morgan and Winick, 1980) cause an increase in dendritic growth. There is at least experimental evidence to suggest that the proper development of the brain is affected by both the plain of nutrition and by sensory stimulation. Furthermore, cortical control via the senses may be important to the head-injured child's nutritional status.

Control of appetite and oral feeding

A child normally plays an active role in structuring the environment so as to facilitate his own development; for example, a homeostatic drive may ensure constant checks of nutrient levels and their regulation by daily food intake (Riesen, 1975). In the rat, the hypothalamus plays a central role in feeding behaviours; the lateral hypothalamus, substantia inominata and inferior temporal visual cortex contain neurones which may selectively respond to either the taste or sight of food, or its physical attributes, such as shape, size, and orientation of the stimulus, whilst other food-related neuronal activity may depend upon the animal's motivational state (Rolls, 1985). Similarly, forebrain-hypothalamic inputs have important influences on appetitive behaviours; with projections to brainstem autonomic regions, for example, implicating the generation of autonomic responses to the sight of food. Such feeding information may be used for the initiation and control of feeding behaviour, involving prefrontal and supplementary motor cortical projections. The hypothalamus may have a central role in the presence of traumatic brain injury, in relation to the anterior pituitary and sympathetic pathway activity. The sympathetic and adrenocortical responses to injury correlate with injury severity and extent of metabolic and catabolic changes (Gadisseaux, Ward, Young *et al.*, 1984). The incidence of hypothalamic lesions and the extent of dysfunction after head injury in the child appears unreported.

The crucial role of appetite is to ensure that the blood contains adequate concentrations of all nutrients, including minerals and vitamins, from consuming a varied diet. Nutritional deficiencies may cause alterations in neurotransmitters such as amino acids, monoamines and peptides, which maintain normal cerebral function and behaviour. Meal composition may exert an effect by altering the availability of precursors, or the nutrients required as cofactors in metabolic pathways leading to neurotransmitter synthesis. 5-HT neurons, for example, may convey information about the metabolic consequences of changes in nutrition, growth and developmental processes, and reactions to stress. Similarly, cholinergic systems may regulate processes important to sleep, learning and memory (Panksepp, 1986).

Diet and neurotransmitters

Major neurotransmitters are manufactured from polypeptides and amino acids, obtained from dietary protein, which pass from the blood stream into brain cells by rate-limiting specific carrier systems distributed throughout the brain capilliaries. Amino acids also function as substrates for the synthesis of structural proteins and enzymes, and for the growth of dendrites. The dietary essential amino acids tryptophan, tyrosine, histidine, and threonine are precursors for 5-HT, catecholamines (CA), histamine and glycine respectively, whilst acetylcholine (ACh) requires choline. These neurotransmitter precursors cannot be synthesized in the brain. Moreover, the specific transport mechanisms by which they pass into the brain are regulated by diet, plasma concentration and the availability of co-factors. Almost all vitamins and minerals are necessary for normal neurological growth, operation and repair. Sodium and potassium are crucial to neuronal function, for regulation of electrical activity and nerve conduction; potassium may be depleted by diuretics, corticosteroids, antibiotics or inadequate dietary sources. Those vitamins needed for the production of neurotransmitters include vitamins C, B2, B6, folic acid and iron. Oligodendroglial cells produce myelin mainly from cholesterol and complex lipids supplied by dietary fat, but vitamin B12, a dietary essential, is involved in this process. Vitamin B6 is involved in myelin repair, the production of 5-HT and gamma-aminobutyric acid (GABA), and of non-essential amino acids by transamination. Vitamin C, found in high concentrations in the adrenal glands and brain, is crucial to norepinephrine (NE) and epinephrine (E) production, and conversion of folacin to the coenzyme tetrahydrofolic acid, important in the biosynthesis of amino and nucleic acids and in cell division. Some anti-convulsants, particularly phenytoin and phenobarbitone, increase the requirement for folate and, in the absence of adequate dietary intake, may cause a macrocytic anaemia. Drugs have this effect by stimulating the production of drug metabolizing enzymes which require folate as a co-factor (Labadarios, Obuwa, Lucas *et al.*, 1978). With dietary inadequacy of certain vitamins and minerals exacerbated by drug prophylaxis, normal brain function is clearly at risk.

Tryptophan, the precursor of 5-HT, is the least abundant of the essential amino acids in dietary protein; the body's store is relatively small and blood levels are sensitive to intake. Studies in rats have shown that single ingestion of a meal containing protein and carbohydrate modifies the blood levels of tryptophan, tyrosine and other large neutral amino acids (LNAA) (leucine, isoleucine, valine, and phenylalanine) which compete with the tryptophan for the same transport system into the brain (Young, 1986). Carbohydrate leads to secretion of insulin which increases the ratio of the concentration of tryptophan to the sum of the concentrations of the other competing amino acids, and this facilitates the passage of tryptophan into the brain (see Fernstrom and Wurtman, 1974), thus increasing the synthesis of 5-HT. In contrast, a protein-rich, low carbohydrate diet elevates the level of competing amino acids in the bloodstream. Plasma tryptophan levels may also change with a characteristic daily rhythm (Fernstrom, Wurtman, Hammarstram-Wiklund *et al.*, 1979), which may be of importance in the presence of disordered diurnal rhythms after severe head injury.

Dietary effects are equally important for plasma tyrosine and phenylalanine ratios, which influence brain catecholaminergic (CA) activity. Tyrosine is derived either from dietary proteins or from hepatic hydroxylation of phenylalanine. The ratio of plasma tyrosine to other NAA's controls brain tyrosine levels in rats and, in turn, influences the rate of DA (dopamine) and NE synthesis and release. Injections of tyrosine, which elevate brain tyrosine, or of tryptophan or leucine which lower brain tyrosine, may respectively increase or decrease the rate of hydroxylation of tyrosine to dopa. The ingestion of meals that modify plasma tyrosine ratios and brain tyrosine levels may have similar effects.

Administering choline to rats increases blood and brain choline, and brain ACh levels, and may be a major determinant of the rate of ACh synthesis and release

(Blusztajn and Wurtman, 1983). Clinical use of choline has followed, in conditions thought to involve inadequate central cholinergic function (Barbeau, Growdon and Wurtman, 1979). As suggested, both serotonergic and cholinergic neurons may act as sensors which inform other brain neurons about the general metabolic state. These signals may be integrated cortically and contribute to regulation of both neuroendocrine response and behaviour. The main source of choline is dietary, in the form of lecithin, but it is found in only small amounts in food. Lecithin increases peripheral and brain ACh levels in rats, and elevates serum choline levels in humans more effectively than choline chloride (Growdon, 1979), although the extent of brain ACh synthesis and release remains unclear, and clinical efficacy of administration has been variable.

How a particular meal affects precursor availability for net transmitter metabolism may depend on meal composition and the previous state of repletion of the neurones. Twenty-four hour food deprivation in rats leads to increased brain tryptophan, 5HT and 5-HIAA (5-hydroxyindoleacetic acid), and may be compounded by maternal-social deprivation to a greater extent in younger organisms (Curzon, 1985, Spear and Scalzo, 1985). Human controls given tryptophan show small increases in 5HT, but much greater increases in 5-HIAA, suggesting a large fraction of the 5HT is destroyed. Although modest deprivation may increase precursor availability, persistent deprivation must eventually deplete stores and increase the probability of suboptimal functioning.

Effects of trauma

As with other accidental injury, head injury creates physiological imbalances which exacerbate the condition both peripherally and centrally. Susceptibility to infection, which remains a major cause of death for those surviving the initial brain injury, may be related to the severe protein and caloric deficiencies after trauma, exacerbated by use of steroids, catheters, or surgical wound contamination (Gadisseaux, 1985). The acute response to infection and tissue injury is characterized by fever, neutrophilia, decreased albumin synthesis, changes in serum levels of iron, zinc and copper, and increased synthesis of acute-phase proteins such as C-reactive protein (Wannemacher, Dupont and Perarek, 1972) and may last for at least three weeks (Young, Ott, Beard *et al.*, 1988).

The metabolic hallmarks of serious injury are hypermetabolism, hypercatabolism, and glucose intolerance, which are related to injury severity.

Hypermetabolism

A greatly increased need for calories and energy arises mainly from synthetic and biochemical inefficiency. Increased breakdown of muscle proteins also occurs, which increases the supply of amino acids for gluconeogenesis and greatly accelerated synthesis of acute phase reactant proteins, those essential to immunologic defence, wound healing and the maintenance of vital organs. There is a concomitant increase in the need for B vitamins and the manufacture of some neurotransmitters induced by the hypermetabolic state. McClain, Twyman, Ott *et al.*, (1986) reported significantly altered zinc metabolism, with urinary excretion more than $7,000 \mu g$ per day, in severely head-injured adults, with implications for protein metabolism and cognitive function.

The autonomic status of severely head-injured patients is similar to that of surface burns patients, with hypertension, tachycardia, hyperthermia, and wasting of body mass, even when food intake seems to be adequate (Clifton and Robertson, 1986). Hypermetabolic intensity is related to a hyperadrenergic state, manifest as increased nutritional requirements and a hyperdynamic cardiovascular state with increased oxygen delivery to tissues (Clifton, Robertson, Grossman *et al.*, 1984). Serum and urinary catecholamine levels generally appear to increase in relation to injury severity (Clifton, Ziegler and Grossman, 1981), and are implicated as a major component in post-traumatic hypermetabolism, also as cofactors with steroids (Deutschmann, Konstantinides, Raup *et al.*, 1987). Hyperadrenergic states may arise from increased muscular tone, since paralysis and sedation may reduce Resting Metabolic Expenditure in some patients, suggesting activity level as a contributory factor (Fruin, Taylor and Pettis, 1986). Normovolaemia is of primary importance to early recovery, as volume depletion impairs the supply of oxygen and glucose to damaged organs and so increases the mortality rate. Similarly, as oxygen consumption increases in proportion to CA elevation, the combination of hypermetabolism and inadequate delivery of oxygen is destructive. As the patient's neurological and general stress condition improves, so the hypermetabolic process should resolve, although a history of other disease, or inadequate nutrition may hinder this early recovery.

Hypercatabolism

Severe hypercatabolism and massive nitrogen loss occurs in some head-injured patients, with increased tissue loss relative to the severity of brain injury (Rapp, Young, Twyman *et al.*, 1983). As indicated, some amino acids are used for protein synthesis, and others for gluconeogenesis. At least part of the excessive protein catabolism associated with head injury has been attributed to concomitant use of corticosteroids, but where steroids are excluded, nitrogen losses decline to amounts comparable to those for skeletal trauma.

The nutritional requirements of head-injured patients are correspondingly greater than normal, with every 1 gm of nitrogen loss representing 6.25 gms of protein loss, equivalent of almost 30 gms of muscle tissue. In the absence of adequate feeding, many patients with average metabolic changes will lose 15 gms of nitrogen a day, equivalent to some 90 gms of protein or about 400 gms of tissue, mainly skeletal muscle. Young, Ott, Norton *et al.*, (1985) reported that head-injured patients who received high levels of intravenous nutritional support nonetheless demonstrated increased energy expenditure and nitrogen loss. As suggested, the patient's activity level may be another determining factor of caloric expenditure (Deutschman, Konstantinides, Raup *et al.*, 1986).

Glucose intolerance

When the normal supply of glucose is limited during starvation, the CNS uses alternative sources. Ketone bodies are derived from a breakdown of body fat stores, and can supplement 60–70 per cent of cerebral energy requirements, although B-complex vitamins and minerals are still necessary as co-factors. Altered glucose metabolism is one of the most commonly noted metabolic abnormalities in critically ill patients. Hyperglycemia may be a function of increased hepatic glucose production rather than lowered glucose utilization. A relative insensitivity to both insulin and glucose may also arise. Insulin and growth hormone are the major anabolic hormones, which stimulate repair processes and promote energy storage as glycogen and fat and increase muscle repletion. When insulin is deficient large amounts of protein are converted into glucose and the patient becomes wasted.

The body's responses to trauma are an attempt to supply alternative substrates and energy under conditions of food deprivation and acute stress, when normal appetitive intake is impossible. Despite the apparent significance of this response to the patient's survival, protracted metabolic abnormalities will result in considerable muscle wasting; this cannot be regarded as a suitable condition in which the patient should undergo active and intensive rehabilitation. Neurons consume energy rapidly, have very limited glycogen storage, utilize few energy substrates, and are thus extremely vulnerable to energy depletion. Other nutrients most likely to suffer from this depletion are those not stored in the body in adequate quantities, such as vitamins C and B complex, which are also in greater demand during stress.

Adaptations to the acute stress of trauma, hypoxia-ischaemia or excitotoxic seizures, may be mediated by glucocorticoids secreted by the adrenal glands. It may be important to outcome that the principal steroid target is the hippocampus. Glucocorticoids may act catabolically to compromise the capacity of these neurons to survive co-incident metabolic insults (Sapolsky, 1987).

The metabolic response to head injury in the child and adolescent includes increased energy expenditure and decreased serum albumin levels similar to that observed in head-injured adults. Depletion of body reserves are much more critical in children, however, and more so in the infant, because of relatively smaller nutrient reserves. The proportion of energy needed for basal metabolism varies with the individual's weight. A 5 kg infant uses approximately 65 per cent of its basal metabolic energy for cerebral metabolism, whilst a 20 kg child uses 42 per cent and an adult uses about 25 per cent (Heird, Driscoll, Schullinger *et al.*, 1972). Weight loss of 1-2 per cent in a week may be significant and of major concern in hospitalized patients, because of a correlation with increased morbidity and mortality.

In addition to the general metabolic responses to trauma, areas of focal injury may cause specific and long-term changes in nutritional status and behaviour. Experimental data (Rolls, 1985) suggests that severe bitemporal damage in the monkey may result in both food and non-food items being placed in the mouth. Visual discriminative learning difficulties may lead to difficulty in forming correct associations between stimulus (food item) and reinforcement. Orbitofrontal injury may alter food preferences, with failure to control inappropriate feeding responses.

Treatment and recovery

Despite methodological restrictions, age and species constraints, these observations may have important applications in the care of head-injured children. Dietary intake must relate to the child's nutritional status, metabolic response to trauma and other factors, such as drugs, which influence neurotransmitter activity. Since loss of immunocompetence is observed during protein-energy malnutrition, early feeding may improve the metabolic changes after trauma, restore infection defence mechanisms, decrease susceptibility to infection and thus improve recovery. Despite the recognition of the metabolic response to injury with its increase in requirements and the potential for nutritional deficiency, few reports of early nutritional support appeared before 1980. Feeding was conventionally delayed until the return of adequate gastrointestinal (GI) function which, unfortunately, is often prolonged after coma-producing head injury. Enteral feeding may be delayed by increased gastric residues, prolonged paralytic ileus, abdominal distension, aspiration pneumonitis and diarrhoea.

The intensity of the hypermetabolic response may vary widely among head-injured patients, as it does among patients suffering from burns or multiple trauma, although there is inadequate data on less severe post-traumatic hypermetabolism. With severe head injury, the acute hypermetabolic response may be substantial, with Mean RME up to 150 per cent above baseline in some cases (Clifton and Robertson, 1986). Adequate protein and energy should be provided early, otherwise large cumulative negative nitrogen and energy balances occur at the expense of immuno-competence and survival (Clifton, Robertson and Contant, 1985; Twyman, Young and Ott, 1985).

It is a golden rule in clinical nutrition that patients should be fed via the gastro-intestinal tract whenever possible. Enteral feeding is recommended, therefore, as soon as normal GI function returns. Many seriously ill, obviously depleted patients may receive no nutritional support for up to ten days after injury, despite the fact that the probability of clinical nutritional deficiency is widely acknowledged. Indeed, those who care for such patients appear to take a positive decision to induce malnutrition, by their very inaction. Conversely, it is reasonable to suggest that early nutritional support could facilitate early recovery from severe head injury by providing energy and protein in order to control the catabolic phase, replace nitrogen loss, prevent muscle wasting and protein depletion, improving resistence to infection, and hastening wound healing (Gadisseaux, 1985), although the timing and mode of feeding may be critical factors. Some beneficial effects of early feeding after head injury have been reported; in a prospective study of young adult severely head-injured patients, Rapp, Young, Twyman *et al.*, (1983) compared enteral with Total Parenteral Nutrition (TPN) finding an improved survival rate at eighteen days, with TPN provided within forty-eight hours after admission. The authors concluded that ' . . . administration of TPN prevented early death and . . . (may) provide the opportunity for eventual neurological recovery . . . ', the basis of which was suggested to be an enhanced immunologic response to infection. In a recent study, Hadley, Graham, Harrington *et al.*, (1986) reported that severely head-injured adults given TPN within forty-eight hours and over fourteen days, had significantly greater than average daily nitrogen intakes and average nitrogen losses, than did enteral patients, but such changes do not necessarily benefit the patient. As with the majority of outcome studies in head injury, the absence of no-treatment controls and inadequate measurement of functional outcome appear to negate any unequivocal statements of the possible long term contribution of nutritional support; many otherwise significant improvements in clinical status may have been obscured by the use of global outcome categories. Nonetheless, the complications of acute parenteral feeding are well documented, whilst enteral feeding may be administered and tolerated within a few days in most severely injured patients.

There is increasing recognition of the value of nutritional care teams, yet the extent of nutritional support may vary greatly between hospitals; patients may be maintained only with intravenous fluids (glucose or saline without added amino acids, minerals or vitamins) until GI function returns but, in no sense is a patient being fed with such a programme, as 10 litres of 5 per cent dextrose are needed to provide 2000 kcal. Intolerance of enteral feeding in the first week after injury makes early TPN a reasonable alternative until GI function returns; although TPN given for less than four days is unlikely to be utilized maximally because of the time necessary to adapt to intravenous nutrition. Young, Ott, Rapp *et al.*, (1987) recommend that enteral feeding is not started until bowel sounds are active and gastric residual volumes are less than 100 ml/hour. At the start of enteral feeding it may be better to pass the fine bore (1-2 mm diameter) tube past the pyloric sphincter into the duodenum or jejunum, but this is not possible in all patients. A pump should be used with the tubes so that the flow can be maintained easily at the desired rate. Metoclopromide can be given to facilitate gastric emptying. Education of nurses in the management of patients being fed parenterally or enterally is vitally important and emphasises the advantages of having a clinical nurse specialist responsible for such feeding throughout the hospital. In such hospitals, parenteral and enteral feeds are not only used more economically, but the patients benefit from a reduction in the 'too little — too late syndrome' and in the incidence of infection.

If patients need to be fed intravenously, the solutions should be complete nutritionally with amino acids, energy substrates, vitamins and minerals; only two energy substrates, glucose and fat, need now be considered (Lee, 1988). Overload of either amino acids or energy, particularly glucose, should be avoided in the seriously ill. Patients fed parenterally should be monitored daily for their tolerance to enteral feeding, which is more physiological, safer and much less expensive. Protein seems to be the preferred fuel in severely head-injured patients fed enterally from ten days after injury; those given a high protein (2.2 g/kg/day) enteral feed had a mean cumulative nitrogen balance of + 9.2 g over a ten day period, compared with − 31.2 g in patients given a standard protein (1.5 g/kg/day) feed (Twyman, Young and Ott, 1985). This amount of protein may be combined with no more than 7.0 g/kg/day of dextrose and 2.5 g/kg/day of lipid (Young, Ott, Rapp *et al.*, 1987).

Metabolic complications of chronic drug treatments have been increasingly recognized, and include nutrient malabsorption, or inefficient use causing increased need for a nutrient (Dickerson, 1988a). Calcium abnormalities are associated with long term anticonvulsant therapy, with reports of osteomalacia in adults, and rickets in children particularly from phenytoin, phenobarbitone and primidone. Anticonvulsants may induce changes in liver metabolism, increasing requirements for vitamin D (Stamp, Flanagan, Richens *et al.*, 1978) and folic acid. In view of the apparent importance of folic acid in cerebral metabolism, its deficiency may be causally implicated in neuropsychiatric disorders in both epileptic and non-epileptic patients. Folic acid administration to children with folate depletion failed to show any effect on either seizure or behaviour (Bowe, Cornish and Dawson, 1971). The relationship between anticonvulsant drug levels, behaviour and cognitive performance of epileptic children attending a special school revealed psychomotor slowing, drowsiness, irritability, and distractibility (Trimble, Corbett and Donaldson, 1980). Children with lowered Performance IQ (Wechsler, 1974) had significantly higher mean phenytoin and primidone levels. Corbett and Trimble (1984), concluded that anticonvulsant-induced disorders of folic acid metabolism may be implicated in both cognitive deterioration and behaviour disorders in children. The over-reliance placed on relatively insensitive IQ measures has been criticized elsewhere.

Rehabilitation

As growing and developing organisms, children have different nutritional status and dietary requirements from adults. Their therapeutic management would be quite different for adequate maintenance of body mass, outwith the demands of growth and recovery (Wharton, 1978). Having survived the acute injury, the child faces the stressful stages of physical, cognitive and educational rehabilitation, during which optimal nutritional requirements may change, exacerbated by inadequate food intake. Moreover, such increased demands are made upon restricted physical resources. Patients are frequently underweight at this stage if nutritional support has not been initiated during intensive care. If the GI tract can be used, but an adequate amount of food cannot be consumed orally, enteral feeding via a nasogastric tube should be commenced. Oral feeding should be encouraged, however, so that the tube, which may cause discomfort and agitation, can be removed as soon as possible. Nurses should monitor the oral food intake carefully so that the tube is not removed until an adequate amount of food is consumed by mouth. As an interim measure, the oral intake may be supplemented by a liquid 'sip' feed. Nurses should be aware of changes in the patient's sense of smell, taste and hunger, which can be major factors in causing a suboptimal nutritional intake. As with cancer patients (Dickerson, 1988a), the ordinary hospital diet may be unacceptable and liaison with kitchen staff be necessary to provide a diet which the patient will eat. Patients with physical handicaps may have difficulty achieving an optimal intake because of problems in feeding themselves, or in sucking, biting, chewing or swallowing foods. Overeating may arise in the later stages of recovery; parents may be unwilling to restrict food intake in the recovering child, or simply be less strict in controlling his behaviour. Immobile children may have such small energy requirements that it is difficult to provide a balanced diet with a minimum energy value. The overweight child who is learning to walk will be restricted in movement, thus hampering early recovery and possibly setting the stage for social ridicule from peers. Overeating has shown a consistent increase at 2 year follow-up in some head-injured children (Rutter, Chadwick and Shaffer, 1984) although nutritional analyses were not undertaken. Parents should be given clear dietetic advice, therefore, when their child leaves hospital, and at regular follow up.

Pre-accident nutritional status may influence recovery in all head-injured children; suboptimal nutrition may be exacerbated by the injury and recovery potential limited by returning from hospital to a nutritionally-poor environment, or one lacking stimulation. Nelson and Naismith (1979) found 11 per cent of normal children under 12 years old, living in poor areas of London, were mildly to moderately malnourished. Large families on low income have an average nutritional intake below the recommended daily allowance (RDA) of calories and iron, with only marginal intakes of protein, thiamin and riboflavin (Bull, 1985), and calcium (Wenlock, Disselduff and Skinner, 1986). A review of the published work on nutrition in adolescence

(Greenwood and Richardson, 1979) concluded that specific nutritional deficiencies commonly occur, particularly with iron, zinc, and vitamins A and C. Iron deficiency disturbs 5-HT metabolism in rats and humans, and, may impair attention and learning ability (Mackler, Person, Miller *et al.*, 1978; Massaro and Widmayer, 1981). Mild undernutrition alone may be associated with adverse effects on physical, social and educational development. Whether these effects are the direct consequence of mal-nutrition or of other environmental factors such as sensory stimulation is unclear (Cravioto, Delicardie and Birch, 1966). Poor housing, overcrowding, lack of parental attention and stimulation may all influence growth at any stage of development, whilst stresses and changes in family circumstances after head-injury (Waaland and Kreutzer, 1988) may render borderline nutrition inadequate. Improved function might be expected only after the potential offered by a better nourished brain had been exploited by a stimulating environment. Both environmental and nutritional deprivation may produce similar effects, whilst environmental stimulation can offset many of the adverse effects of malnutrition (Tizard, 1976). The child at risk for head injury may, therefore, be at risk for poor optimal recovery because of a combination of inadequate nutrition and environmental stimulation.

The question of normal dietary adequacy generates much controversy (Barrett and Frank, 1987); whether diets high on refined food may have sufficiently low mineral and vitamin content as to impair biochemical function, or that in most cases the diet is adequate, often supplying minerals and vitamins in excess of our needs. There are no suitable biochemical indices of deficiency for some vitamins and minerals, and the RDA's are based on scant information. Dietary analysis in terms of RDA's may be misleading as they are primarily intended as statements about healthy populations rather than sick individuals. In addition the information can only be understood if the underlying philosophy is appreciated. Apart from those for energy, RDA's include safety margins to take account of individual variations such that they should cover 95 per cent of populations. Thus, individuals who consume less than the RDA are not necessarily deficient. Furthermore, variations in requirements mean that we should expect some individuals to be perfectly healthy on a low intake of some vitamin or mineral while others may be deficient on an intake above the RDA. Intakes of less than 50 per cent of the RDA have been considered clear evidence of inadequacy in surgical patients (Older, Edwards and Dickerson, 1980). It is nonetheless difficult to delineate clear relationships between nutrition and motor function or learning ability, or to separate the effects of an acute episode of traumatic malnutrition from the associated social and nutritional environment in which the child usually lives. Sub-clinical deficiencies which may arise from head injury, therefore, may persist indefinitely.

In the presence of suboptimal nutrition, persisting metabolic and neuro-transmitter inefficiency, and the range of cognitive and behavioural disorders following head injury, it seems reasonable to consider dietary or pharmacological manipulation as a means of effecting positive changes in brain function (Wurtman, 1983). Eames (this volume) has cautioned of the inherent dangers in this general line of reasoning but, it should at least generate research designed to counteract the biochemical abnormalities and identify the recovery processes.

Decreased levels of a specific neurotransmitter in the brains of patients with neurological or psychiatric diseases may be causally related to the clinical manifestations of that condition. The potential significance of positive dietary manipulations on motor function is exemplified by recent reports in Parkinson's Disease (Pincus and Barry, 1988). An increase in plasma LNAA levels and a reduction in the therapeutic response to L-dopa may follow a dietary protein bolus (Juncos, Fabrini, Mouradian *et al.*, 1987). In a small series of patients, Pincus and Barry (1987) have shown a good correlation between a reduction in Parkinsonion disability score (61 per cent change) and a reduction in the plasma concentration of LNAA (71 per cent change) on a low protein diet. From the time of awakening until four pm the protein intake was restricted to 7 g. A regular protein intake was provided for supper with no restriction in snacks until bedtime.

Manipulation of central cholinergic mechanisms has been reported in dementia, Huntington's chorea, tardive dyskinesia and Gilles de la Tourette syndrome (Drachman and Sahakian, 1979; Tanner, Goetz and Klawans, 1979). For example, prominent neuronal loss in dementia may lead to a reduction in choline acetyltransferase activity, deficiencies in 5-HT and other neurotransmitter systems (Chung-a-On, Thomas, Tidmarsh *et al.*, 1985). Malabsorption of tryptophan may result in lower plasma concentrations and in the ratio of tryptophan concentration to the sum of the concentrations of the other LNAA's, as well as low status with respect to vitamins C, B1, D and folate, and calcium. Nutrient deficiencies may modify the manifestations of other metabolic abnormalities (Dickerson, 1988b). A few reports have appeared of choline producing minor improvements in social behaviour, learning and memory of some patients with Alzheimer's disease, but administering lecithin with a normal diet (Etienne, Gaughier, Dastoor *et al.*, 1979) failed to yield significant results, although only seven patients were investigated, and with inadequate cognitive assessments. Choline or lecithin administration may also benefit any condition improved by the acetylcholinesterase inhibitor Physostigmine, such as post-concussional amnesic states and, possibly, learning disabilities. The potential importance of cholinergic mechanisms in learning and memory has been widely reported (Deutsch, 1971; Meck and Church, 1987) and, in general, cholinergic antagonists, such as atropine or scopolamine, impair memory and cognition in a consistent manner (Barbeau, Growdon and Wurtman, 1979); the inadequate neuropsychological measures employed, however, may restrict the significance of findings (e.g., Drachman and Sahakian, 1979). Single cases of adult post-traumatic memory disorder are reported (e.g., Walton, 1982), with variable improvements in orientation and memory. Goldberg, Gerstman, Mattis *et al.*, (1982) suggested that improvements in memory

following treatment with lecithin and physostigmine may be due to diminished interference. It appears that the learning of new verbal material exceeding memory span is most
sensitive to anticholinergic effects (Spring, 1986), which suggests the importance of
prefrontal involvement (Perecman, 1987) and highlights the potential significance of post-
traumatic change in this vulnerable region. Furthermore, the high capillary density of this
region may render it particularly vulnerable to metabolic and nutritional deficiencies.

One should not be mislead into simplistic thinking in this field, however, which
requires a broad flexible view of the relation between neural structures and cognition.
A cholinergic diet, for example, is likely to elicit biochemical effects in systems other
than ACh, as well as behavioural, sleep and cognitive actions, emphasizing that cholinergic influences affect practically unlimited numbers of functions both peripheraly
and centrally. As previously suggested, REM sleep disturbances may be present at
various stages of recovery from severe head injury, and there is potential benefit from
neurochemical manipulations by dietary or pharmacological means (Karczmar, 1979).

Meal frequency, quality and quantity may have important influences upon post-
traumatic cognitive performance (Spring, 1986). Children who ate a carbohydrate
breakfast, for example, performed worse on a test of vigilance than those who fasted,
but also worse than those who ate protein (Conners, Caldwell, Caldwell *et al.*, 1985).
Without breakfast, children performed variably, but with notable improvements in
arithmetical performance following breakfast consumption (Conners and Blouin,
1983). It is unclear, however, whether the results may be due to a change in meal
pattern, and it would be necessary to study children who habitually omitted this meal.

Experimental studies on the effects of sugar consumption on children's behaviour
suggest no change or a decrease in activity. Correlational findings still raise the
question of why restless, aggressive children with vigilance deficits apparently find it
reinforcing to eat large amounts of sugar. Consumption may meet a metabolic need for
calories or engender a desirable calming effect by enhancing brain uptake of tryptophan
(Spring, 1986). The possible role of food additives in behaviour remains controversial
(e.g., Rapoport, 1984), and methodological difficulties, including the basis for
diagnosis (Rippere, 1983), restrict the conclusions from such work. Aspartame (L-
aspartyl-L-phenylalanine) is a prevalent, non-nutritive sweetener composed of the
amino acids aspartic acid and phenylalanine, and the alcohol methanol (Pardridge,
1986). Among the adverse effects reported are mood changes, insomnia, and seizure
precipitation from high dose ingestion. Frey (1976) reported that children aged 7 to 12
years, with access to aspartame-containing products, consumed up to 77 mg/kg/day.
Children will consume relatively large doses of aspartame, owing to their lower body
weight. Ingestion of aspartame leads to linear increases in peak blood phenylalanine
levels, which may provide a mechanism for the sweetener to influence CNS neurotransmission. The form in which aspartame is ingested, for example as a slurry rather
than liquid form, may have a profound effect upon GI absorption of phenylalanine and
on its peak blood levels (Stegnik, 1979). The head-injured child may be more or less

sensitive to the effects of dietary additives, in the presence of post-traumatic neuro-chemical changes and behaviour disorders.

The much publicized Vitamin-IQ study (Benton and Roberts, 1988), has been criticized for the unreliability of its nutritional methodology and for its statistical flaws (Emery, Geissler, Judd *et al.*, 1988; Taitz, 1988), but it purported to show a significant increase in non-verbal intelligence of adolescents receiving a mineral-vitamin supplement. A recent replication and extension (Naismith, Nelson, Burley *et al.*, 1988) failed to find any significant difference between groups in IQ, memory, or psychomotor speed. The relative insensitivity of these measures, however, may be disproportionate to the nature or size of effect one might reasonably expect. It may be that speed of information processing, cognitive efficiency or propensity to learn are the areas which are facilitated by dietary supplementation.

Conclusions

Children with head injuries present a number of complex inter-related metabolic disturbances. The specific requirement for, and effects of nutritional support cannot be separated from the child's nutritional condition or the pre-injury environment and must be considered as only part of the total environment for recovery. Superimposed on the normal requirements for growth and development are the metabolic problems induced by trauma, the changes in nutrition that may directly result from focal brain injury, and the effects on neurotransmitter metabolism which are secondary to tissue damage and nutritional insufficiency.

The optimal milieu for recovery after head injury has been poorly investigated, and the conditions essential for maximizing further development in the head-injured child remain ill-defined. From a functional viewpoint, the effects on neurotransmitter metabolism may be considered crucial, but these are unlikely to persist solely because of dietary factors rather, they may be compounded by post-traumatic changes in sleep and behaviour, prophylactic drug use, disruption of social development or on-going social relationships, general levels of home stimulation and parental management (Kraemer, 1985). A continuum of insufficiency and impairment of brain growth, development and mental ability may exist for the head-injured child. For example, a 6 year old boy suffers a moderate head injury but appears to recover well apart from difficulties in speech and reading; father is away at sea; mother has a second job as a pub cook, so the child is left with grandparents early each evening, put to bed at a reasonable time, but is awoken at about eleven pm, driven four miles home, and expected to be bright and capable at school the next day. Not only is the sleep pattern disrupted irregularly but invariably, meals are often rushed, and there is less time to play with mother. All relatively minor and quite normal occurrences in themselves perhaps, but what of the possible additive effects upon a recovering and developing CNS?

The possibilities for nutritional intervention beyond that of routine support are, of course speculative at the moment, but may reasonably involve the additive or inter-changeable effects of nutrition and environmental stimulation in the support of recovery and further development. Consistent with a rational approach to rehabil-itation, adequate nutritional intake may be necessary, but not sufficient. Sensory activity may be essential but nutritional support a necessity in order to obtain it (Ricciuti, 1981). Whilst nutritional intervention may not provide a magic wand for the head-injured child, it might be possible to increase the probability of positive change by nutritional intervention. Studies of single amino acids such as tryptophan, tyrosine and choline or lecithin in relatively large doses may have little meaning in strictly nutritional terms for they are not representative of how people eat. The effects of ordinary meals on behaviour are usually smaller than those in studies of single nutrients, so that sizeable numbers of subjects, adequately sensitive measures and tight methodological controls are required (Spreen, Tupper, Risser *et al.*, 1984). Dose-response parameters are largely unknown in this sort of investigation, making it difficult to determine portion sizes for experimental studies. Whilst less dramatic responses to food than to the pharmacologically pure forms could be expected, food effects upon brain function may still be of more significance, at least in longer term maintenance of recovery achieved. It is important to note that if the specific neuro-transmitter receptors are damaged, or other neuronal populations are also destroyed which contain converting enzymes, for example, then increasing a particular class of neurochemical activity is unlikely to be uniformly successful, particularly in cases of severe diffuse head injury. Parents of head-injured children whose recovery is slow, and who appear not to achieve what might be expected of them or whose behaviour has become intolerable, are likely to grasp at the straws provided by any potential treatment (see Hall, this volume), and dietary change may offer them a relatively accessible and absorbing option to pursue (Taitz, 1988).

A great deal of research is necessary before nutritional and dietary factors are implicated in recovery from paediatric head injury. If post-traumatic deficits in nutritional status persist, compounded by social, cognitive and emotional difficulties, then dietary evaluation and management may be one avenue to explore, to help maximize progress and outcome. The effects of dietary stress on an individual child will not simply be matters of nutritional pathophysiology, but rather will be moulded and modified by his genetic endowment, stage of development, home stimulation, social and emotional climates. With increasing knowledge of neurotransmission and parallel concern about subclinical nutritional deficiencies, the development of coll-aborative research studies in this most complex field would soon help to delineate the validity of nutritional factors in determining the optimal milieu for recovery in paediatric head-injury. Head-injured children grow up to become relatively disabled adults, with the added possibility that, in the presence of structural damage, the normal ageing process may be exacerbated. Consequently, instilling good dietary habits in childhood may at the very least be beneficial to long-term mental function.

Chapter 6

Disorders of hearing and balance

Ewa Raglan

Introduction

It is apparent that accidental head injury is common in children, with road accidents and falls the most frequent causes (Rowbotham, Maciver, Dickson *et al.*, 1954; Freedman, Saunders and Briggs, 1986). As with other areas of post-traumatic disturbance, there is limited information pertaining specifically to otoneurologic function after head injury in children.

The incidence of otoneurological symptoms is high after head injury, although their type and time of onset varies. In some patients the symptoms and signs may occur immediately after trauma and may be permanent or transient; whilst in others they may occur later and be progressive, transitory or reversible. This suggests that there are various forms of trauma to the temporal bone and central neural pathways which could be responsible for a deterioration of otoneurologic function. Different patterns of pathologic change may be produced by variation in the force of impact to the head, and in the vectors of head movement resulting from the blow. Head injury from road traffic accidents may involve multiple impacts of varying direction and force, and result in both angular and linear acceleration-deceleration. A blow to a freely mobile head produces a great amount of swirling and rotary displacement of the brain, while a blow to an immobile head, as when it is supported by a hard surface, may produce little movement of the brain (Pudenz and Shelden, 1946). When the brain moves independently from the skull, the VIIIth. nerve sustains shearing injury, as it exits from the brainstem and enters the inner ear. Under these conditions the higher cerebral pathways are subject to contusion, laceration, haemorrhage and their sequelae (Makishima and Snow, 1975). Extensive lesions in human cerebral white matter and brainstem may result from the stretching and tearing of nerve fibres caused by the shearing forces of angular acceleration (Strich, 1961). Early experimental work reported degenerative changes in the cochlea and vestibular nuclei of guinea pigs following cerebral concussion produced with a pendulum apparatus (Windle, Groat and Fox, 1944). Similarly, Schuknecht, Neff and Perlmann (1951) reported hearing loss and degenerative changes in the organ of corti, following blows to the immobile head in behaviourally conditioned cats. Immediate, severe and permanent symptoms occur if the nerves of the cerebral auditory and vestibular pathways are damaged, or the VIIIth. nerve is torn. Progressive and permanent symptoms with delayed onset may occur if occlusion of the vertebral and basilar artery is incomplete, but sufficient to cause ischaemia of an end organ, and if there is degeneration of the central auditory and vestibular pathways. The symptoms may be largely reversible even if they are immediate and severe, providing the neurones of pathways remain vital and the continuity of the VIIIth. nerve is preserved. Transient otoneurological symptoms may be due to increased intracranial pressure from cerebral oedema, or intracranial haemorrhage. Progressive sensorineural deficits may be consequent upon changes in the composition of the inner ear fluid, due to accumulation of platelets, white and red blood cells (Makishima and Snow, 1976).

Auditory and vestibular disturbances following head injury have been extensively studied. Hearing disorders may include partial or complete loss of hearing, and tinnitus; whilst vestibular disorders may include dizziness, vertigo, or disequilibrium. Both types may be peripherally or centrally induced. Since the 1970s, accumulating clinical and experimental reports have suggested that auditory and vestibular tests are becoming more important in the assessment, management and rehabilitation of head-injured patients. Although auditory and vestibular damage commonly occur together, either may occur independently of the other. Auditory evaluations can be divided into three main areas, peripheral auditory system, central auditory processing, and brainstem function, each discussed briefly in turn.

Peripheral auditory system

Peripheral hearing loss is common (Papurov and Cholakov, 1970; Toglia and Katinsky, 1976) and may be due to perforation of the tympanic membrane, ossicular discontinuity, oval or round window fistulae, or temporal bone fracture. The nature and extent of hearing loss depends on the presence and type of temporal bone fracture. Longitudinal petrosal fractures (Figure 6.1) are usually associated with ipsilesional conductive hearing loss, in 30 per cent of patients with neurosensory loss, in the contralesional ear due to inner ear concussion (Toglia and Katinsky, 1976). Transverse fracture (Figure 6.2) is usually accompanied by sensorineural loss, associated with loss of labyrinth function, although there is frequently neurosensory loss in the opposite ear. Cases without temporal bone fractures usually present with bilateral sensorineural loss, the incidence of which varies between 20 to 56 per cent (Toglia, Rosenberg and Ronis, 1970; Berman and Frederickson, 1978; Tuohimaa, 1978; Griffiths, 1979); Pearson and Barber (1973) report 78 per cent of patients with hearing loss mainly at 4 and 8 kHz. In the post-concussion audiograms of cats subjected to head injury, hearing loss was more severe in the higher frequencies from 3 to 8 kHz. The poorest point for the mild loss centered around 4 kHz and the frequency spectrum widens as the severity of damage increases (Schuknect, Neff and Perlmann, 1951). The histopathology demonstrated injury similar to that caused by prolonged exposure to high intensity noise.

If the head-injured patient is conscious and responsive, then pure tone audiometry and speech discrimination tests will give an index of peripheral hearing sensitivity and speech recognition. In the unconscious patient, brainstem evoked responses (BSER) and impedance audiometry can be used. This procedure involves tympanometry and

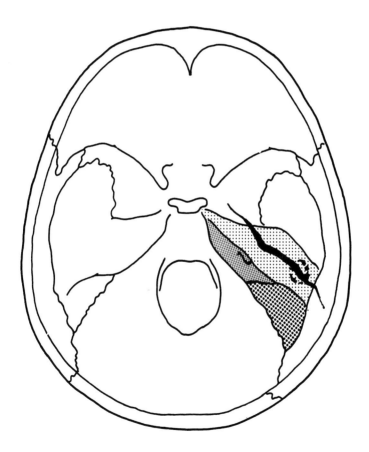

Figure 6.1: Longitudidnal fracture involves mainly the middle ear, causing conductive hearing loss

stapedial reflexes, and can be used to measure middle ear function, estimate hearing sensitivity, and assess the integrity of the VIIth. and VIIIth. nerves, and caudal brainstem. The detected pathology may require immediate medical attention, whilst the means of communication with the patient and need for amplification can be established. Knowledge of the peripheral hearing level may influence the interpretation of subsequent neuropsychological evaluations, especially in relation to the patient's further placement.

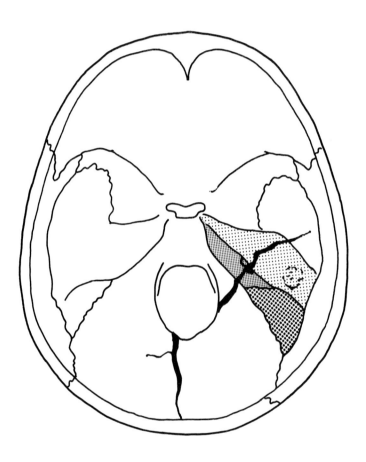

Figure 6.2: Transverse fracture involves mainly the inner ear and results in neurosensory hearing loss and loss of labyrinth function

Central auditory system

The central auditory nervous system battery (CANS) is useful in detecting injury to the auditory area of the brainstem or cerebral cortex, monitoring recovery of the auditory processing skills and providing a framework for counselling the patient about his communication capabilities. The majority of tests require the patient to identify a speech message that has been made difficult to understand through distortion, filtering, compression or adding a competing noise. Head-injured patients may complain of extreme difficulty with hearing in rooms having high levels of background noise, and may have difficulty in following complex auditory directions or commands, and localizing sound sources (Katz, 1985). Conventional audiometry will frequently reveal normal hearing sensitivity and speech recognition, whilst the CANS test battery may reveal more subtle auditory processing deficits. Such evaluations may be carried out in conjunction with the neuropsychologist's delineation of attentional disorder.

Tinnitus is a common complaint following head trauma, occurring in approximately one third of cases (e.g., Proctor, Gurdjian and Webster, 1956; Galliard, 1961), although unrelated to the severity of head injury. It may present as the noise heard in the ear or head, and may remain as the residual disturbance, causing considerable distress to the patient.

Brainstem function

The brainstem evoked response (BSER) is an accurate and objective measure of function in the auditory nuclei and brainstem auditory pathway, reflecting the conduction time of the signal between the brainstem generators (Figure 6.3).

Brainstem lesions affecting the auditory pathways may slow down the conduction times and prolong the interpeak latencies. Rowe and Carlson (1980) performed BSER on twenty-seven patients with mild head injury, who complained of post-concussional symptoms but no hearing loss; they found prolongation of interpeak latencies in 11 per cent of patients, from day one through to eight months after injury. This finding, combined with the results of vestibular assessment may assist us in delineating the central and peripheral components of post-traumatic disorders. Auditory brainstem response abnormalities are not uncommon after severe head injury and they can prove clinically useful in assessing the short-term neurological outcome (Hall, Musan and Gennarelli, 1982).

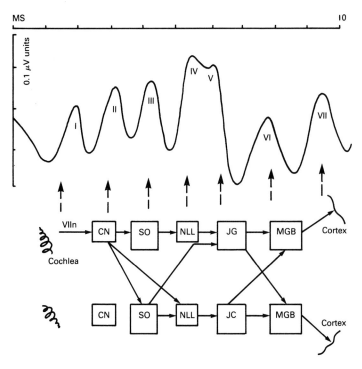

Figure 6.3: Schematic diagram to illustrate the neural generators of the BSER.VII n., acoustic n., CN, cochlear nucleus; SO, superior olivary complex; NLL, nucleus of lateral lemniscus; IC, inferior colliculus; MGB, medial geniculate body.

Vestibular symptoms

Vestibular symptoms include vertigo, dizziness and loss of balance. Vertigo, an hallucination of the spinning motion is caused by sudden loss of labyrinth function. The presence of concomitant auditory disorder suggests a peripheral origin for vertigo, whilst the absence of auditory symptoms combined with the presence of other neuro-logical symptoms suggests that it is of central origin. Dizziness, described as the sensation of swaying or floating, is the effect of the mismatch between the sensory input from the labyrinth, the eyes and proprioception. It gives the sensation of disorientation in space and could be due to peripheral or central dysfunction. There are two main post-traumatic vestibular syndromes; vestibular failure and benign paroxysmal positional vertigo. Sudden, unilateral vestibular failure occurs as the result of transverse fracture of the temporal bone and usually presents as sudden severe vertigo, loss of balance with tendency to fall to the affected side, and observation of spontaneous nystagmus to the normal side. Benign positional vertigo is a common clinical syndrome after mild head injury. Symptoms may develop up to a few weeks following injury, and occur in certain head positions. The episodes are typically short and characterized by the presence of positional nystagmus in the Hallpike manoeuvre — when a patient is rapidly changed from a sitting to a supine position with the head either to one side or hanging.

Two types of nystagmus may be differentiated; peripheral and central. Peripheral positional nystagmus is associated with marked vertigo, which begins after a latent period. With a new position, the nystagmus and vertigo eventually fatigue, usually within one minute. A rapid return to the sitting position causes another brief burst of nystagmus beating in the opposite direction, and vertigo. Repositioning in the pro-vocative supine posture again invokes nystagmus and vertigo, but to a lesser extent. Repetition of the movement ultimately results in disappearance or habituation of the nystagmus and vertigo. A possible mechanism has been postulated by Schuknecht (1969), who suggested that trauma may loosen the otoconia from degenerated utricular otolithic membrane, which then would fall on the cupula of the posterior semicircular canal making the organ sensitive to the effect of gravity. Central positional vertigo which is invariably reproducible, begins immediately on movement to the provoking position; the nystagmus neither fatigues nor habituates, and its direction varies. The central type is associated with brain stem or cerebellar disease (Luxon, 1988).

The neural trauma may affect cerebral connections of the vestibular system at its different levels, or the vestibular nuclei efferents to the external ocular muscle nuclei through the medial longitudinal fasciculus and the reticular formation, to the cerebellum, to the temporal lobe cortex and to the motor units of the spinal cord. It may affect the pathways of the slow and fast eye movements, the former arising from the vestibular (vestibulo-ocular reflex) or optic (pursuit) stimuli, the latter generated by the paramedian pontine reticular formation for horizontal saccades and by the pretectal region for vertical saccades. The abnormalities of these movements may be detected by performing the clinical tests of vestibular function, including tests of vestibulo-spinal function (romberg, unterberger gait), examination of vestibulo-occular function (bithermal caloric stimulation, rotational tests) and study of saccades, the smooth pursuit and optokinetic systems (visuo-ocular control). The abnormalities may be documented using electronystagmographic (ENG) recordings (Luxon, 1988).

As the immediate sequelae of the head injury, vertigo and dizziness are common, and their incidence varies from 20 to 90 per cent in different studies (see Table 6.1). Dizziness as late sequelae after head injury has been reported in 20 to 76 per cent of adults; conversely, dizziness after head injury in children has rarely been found. Mitchell and Stone (1973) reported seventy-one children with temporal bone fracture, of whom only 1.4 per cent complained of vertigo. Shapiro (1979) reported forty-eight children with temporal bone fractures, and only one child had vertigo for one week.

Table 6.1: The incidence of auditory and vestibular subjective and objective manifestation in the chosen studies in adults and children.

Study	No patients	Time after Head injury	Hearing loss	Symptoms of Dizziness/ vertigo	vestibular lesion peripheral	central
Griffiths 1979	84 majority 11–30 years	Immediately	56%	24%	–	–
		6 months later	22%	1%	–	–
Berman & Frederickson 1978	129 mean age 35	Immediately	20%	34%	43%	7%
		2 years later	–	59%	–	–
Makino & Matsushita 1981	75 age 10–70	Immediately	–	90%	–	–
		1–2 years later		32%	improvement in 22% patients 26%	
Gannon et al., 1978	50	Immediately	16%	60%	53%	46%
	50	Immediately	20%	78%	17%	60%
Tuoshimaa 1978	82 mean age 34	6 months later	20%	20%	53%	12% all patients returned to work
Vertiainen et al., 1985	61 children	Immediately	–	2%	21%	43%
	138 children	4 years later	–	1%	6%	12%

Dillon and Leopold (1961) reported fifty children with post-concussional symptoms, of whom nine suffered dizziness.

It is apparent that despite the subjective improvement in symptoms the objective vestibular tests may be still abnormal. This vestibular deficit remains and may be responsible for recurring symptoms under certain physiological or pathological stress (Toglia, 1972). Immediately after the trauma there is no difference in the occurrence of subjective dizziness or vertigo in documented peripheral or central vestibular lesions. Central ENG abnormalities as sequelae to the head injury, were found to be as frequent in children as in adults. Tuohimaa (1978), and Vertiainen, Karjalainen and Karja (1985), have reported that recovery occurs in most cases during the first six months after trauma, and definitely within two years, with no recovery occurring later. The frequency of the occurrence of objective vestibular symptoms in children and adults is similar, but children certainly have fewer vestibular symptoms. This may be due to two possible reasons; firstly the child may be better able to compensate for damage caused by the head injury, than is the adult after head injury; secondly, the psycho-social factors play no significant role in the occurrence of late symptoms, as opposed to in adult cases (Kay, Kerr and Lassman, 1971).

Concluding remarks

The post-traumatic symptoms of dizziness, unsteadiness, hearing loss and tinnitus certainly have an organic and proven vestibular and auditory base, with no psychogenic aetiology. Most cases of head injury in children and adults should have the audio-vestibular assessment because the incidence of hearing loss and vertigo following neural trauma is greater than has been appreciated to date. The practical impact of even mild audiological or vestibular disturbances to the child in school may be of very considerable importance to classroom performance, and social behaviour.

Chapter 7

Recovery of speech and language deficits after head injury in children

Janet A. Lees

Introduction

The recovery of language skills after head injury in children may considerably affect the personal adjustment, educational placement, social integration, family and peer relationships and all aspects of further development. There have been few studies in this complex field and, as with other areas of investigation into children's head injury, we must draw upon other brain-injured populations to seek objective and experimental verification of our clinical observations. The conclusions of previous studies of language disorder following head injury in children are limited because they are usually based in rather heterogeneous populations, poor diagnostic classifications, and inadequate assessments, whilst the time-course of recovery is seldom considered and outcome is not differentiated by aetiology. The latter point alone makes it very difficult to draw any valid conclusions from those studies (e.g., Guttman, 1942). This chapter reviews the available evidence and presents preliminary data from an on-going study.

Problems of classification

There is often confusion over the terminology used for language problems in childhood, both in the literature and clinically (Urwin, Cook and Kelly, 1988). The following classification categories are suggested.

Developmental language problems

Those which are manifest from the beginning of the child's language development and may be part of, or associated with, other developmental problems such as learning difficulties, cleft palate or conductive hearing loss. Bishop and Rosenbloom (1988) suggest that a wide spectrum of disorders is seen in clinical practice. Many terms are used and some of these are confusing; one term previously favoured, but not used by speech therapists, is developmental dysphasia. This 'is particularly unhelpful, since it implies that we are dealing with a condition analoagous to that found in adults . . . whereas in fact the only similarity between these disorders is that language is impaired in both' (Bishop and Rosenbloom 1988, p. 17.)

Acquired Childhood Aphasia (ACA)

The loss or impairment of language consequent upon a brain injury, following an initial period of normal language development. This category may be divided into two main aetiological groups:

(a) Traumatic (ACA-T): children with either unilateral localized cerebral lesions, such as cerebrovascular and neoplastic disorders, or bilateral diffuse insult, such as infection or head-injury, are assigned to this group. It may be advisable to further delineate ACA-T into these specific sub-categories.

(b) Convulsive aphasia (ACA-C): children in this group are also referred to as Landau-Kleffner Syndrome (Landau and Kleffner, 1957), the exact pathology of which remains unknown. It is thought not to be related to head injury and is referred to here for the sake of completeness.

Acquired childhood aphasia

Previous studies of Acquired Childhood Aphasia-traumatic origin (ACA-T), typically included heterogeneous populations, with both unilateral — localized, and bilateral — diffuse lesions. Similarly, language investigations and follow-up were poorly documented. Neuroradiological techniques have generally not been helpful in localizing the lesions responsible for such language impairment, although the increasing availability of more advanced techniques, such as MRI and PET, offers some hope for the near future (Levin Williams, Crofford *et al.*, 1988). The continuing controversies concerning the development of cerebral dominance and its effect on ACA have also been sadly neglected.

Early studies of ACA-T emphasized the rapid and complete recovery of speech and language skills of children after cerebral injury and this has been a major factor in its differentiation from adult aphasia. Guttman (1942) marked the beginning of modern discussions of this subject; he reported a mixed group of thirty children with ACA-T, including six head injuries, six tumours, twelve cerebral infections and one cerebrovascular condition, concluding that children with benign lesions recovered their language functions within four weeks. If aphasic signs remained after that time, however, a more guarded prognosis for final outcome was indicated. Alajouanine and Lhermitte (1956) referred to the common belief that ACA-T is a rare and transitory disorder with consequently few or absent sequelae. Their typically heterogeneous group of thirty-two children included thirteen head-injured, twelve cerebrovascular abnormalities, two tumours, and five cases of unknown aetiology; of these children six were reported to have normal speech within six months of onset, and twenty-four had regained normal, or nearly normal language one year after onset. Recovery of written language was considered to lag behind that of spoken language. The authors concluded that recovery for two-thirds of the children was an indisputable fact, and that the speed of recovery of the aphasia depended on the site, extent and 'reversibility' of the cerebral lesions. Nonetheless, continuing and severe motor sequelae and EEG disturbances in the majority of these children were also reported. The speed of recovery from aphasia in relation to the child's age at onset was further discussed by Collignon, Hecaen and Angelergues (1968), who examined twelve children, including nine head-injured. Comprehension problems recovered more completely than difficulties in expressive language. Of the four cases who showed the least recovery, three were over 10 years old at onset. Cases with no apparent recovery were taken to reflect the presence of substantial bilateral lesions, although this was not confirmed radiologically. Extending this work, although again with poor pathological classification and delineation, Hecaen (1976) reported twenty-six cases, of whom sixteen were head-injured, finding no clear relationship between occurrence and duration of coma, and the persistence and severity of language deficit. Complete recovery was reported in five of the head-injured children within two years of injury. Hecaen suggested that his findings supported Lenneberg's (1967) view that there was a critical period for the acquisition of language. Despite the conflicting evidence of studies reported between 1976-83, a subsequent review (Hecaen, 1983) did not represent substantially altered views, i.e., lesion localization and aetiology were considered the most important factors in recovery, despite the absence of anatomical delineation.

Of the recent studies which include the results of X-ray computerized tomography (CT) to confirm the site and size of lesions, Van Dongen, Loonen and Van Dongen (1985) reported three patients with fluent aphasia, two of whom were head-injured, the third with a space occupying lesion. Although the lesions appeared to be localized to Wernicke's area, the authors agreed that the lesions from head injury could have been more diffuse. The language data included an analysis of the phrase length, prosody and rate of spontaneous speech, all of which are important in an analysis of fluent aphasia. Unfortunately, no comparable data on these aspects of speech in non-fluent aphasia in children exists to allow comparisons between subtypes of aphasia.

There is long-standing controversy regarding a higher incidence of ACA following right hemisphere lesions in children than in adults. In reviewing the evidence Carter, Hohenegger and Satz (1982) concluded that, when early studies in which the incidence is conflictingly reported are excluded, the ACA data are consistent with electrophysiological, neuroanatomical and behavioural data in supporting the developmental invariance position; that is, for the majority of humans the left cerebral hemisphere is predisposed before birth for dominance in language function. They criticize many of the early studies for not separating cases by aetiology in order to differentiate possible bilateral lesions in the absence of suitable radiological techniques.

The question of recovery of language in children and adolescents with acquired language problems after head injury has been poorly reported. Van Dongen, Loonen and Van Dongen (1985) discussed the recovery of three right-handed girls, aged 9 to 11 years who presented with fluent aphasia over a two-year period. Two were said to have recovered within one year, whilst in the other case, virtually no improvement was observed. Ewing-Cobbs, Levin, Eisenberg *et al.* (1987) found no sparing of function in terms of the recovery seen in head-injured children aged 5 to 10 years, relative to adolescents aged 11 to 15 years. Conversely, they suggested that written language performance was more depressed in children than adolescents, although this may have resulted from many factors, including attention and speed. These results confirmed those of Woods and Carey (1979), for children who were said to have clinically recovered from ACA-T but in whom significant residual impairments were found on most language tests at the four year's follow-up. More recent confirmation comes from a group of children and adolescents with a history of ACA-T between one to ten years post onset (Cooper and Flowers, 1987). As with other studies, the problem of heterogeneity is evident, with only four children reported as head-injured. Particular deficits did not characterize this latter group as a whole and, for individuals, deficits ranged from no impairment, through mild to significant deficits; notably, two-thirds of the group were receiving additional but unspecified help in school. This has continued to be the general finding of recent studies of head-injured children and adolescents. Jordan, Ozanne and Murdoch (1988) examined children at least twelve months after head injury and confirmed that overall language performance scores were significantly lower than those of a non-neurologically impaired control group. The major criticism of these more recent studies is the short follow-up time for evaluation of residual deficits. One year after injury is not necessarily the end of any recovery phase and good progress may still continue at that time. Similarly, residual problems may become more noticeable many years later as educational placements and expectations change, and intellectual demands become greater.

The condition of ACA-T may also be differentiated from both the adult disorder and developmental language disorders by its reported symptoms. Ford (1937), considered it impossible to reconcile speech disturbances resulting from cerebral lesions in infants with any type of aphasia seen in adults. He described the main features as indicative of a motor aphasia, noting the absence of a sensory aphasia even after temporal lesions. The main principal types of linguistic impairment described in the literature are as follows:

1   Auditory-verbal comprehension deficit: difficulty understanding spoken language.
2   Word-finding problems: difficulty recalling specific words.
3   Jargon aphasia: incomprehensible expressive language.
4   Semantic and phonemic paraphasias: word errors. Semantic (memory) or phonemic (sound) relationship to target word.
5   Perseveration: persistent, undifferentiated repetition of a previous error response.

The most striking feature of ACA-T reported by Alajounanine and Lhermitte (1965) was the general reduction of expressive activities in all communicative modalities. Dysarthria was observed in 69 per cent of cases, closely correlated with the severity of the hemiplegia and probably to bilateral lesions, although it is not possible to define the aetiological groups more precisely. Simplified syntax and the degree of aggrammatism found in children did not represent that observed in adults. Disorders of receptive language, jargon aphasia, perseveration, paraphasic errors, neologisms and verbal stereotypes commonly observed in adult aphasia were reported as only rarely occurring in ACA. Written language was disturbed in all cases and more severely than verbal language. Agreement that both verbal and written language difficulties are predominantly expressive came from Collignon, Hecaen and Angelergues (1968); their description of dysarthria as a rare symptom, however, may reflect a clinical difficulty in differential diagnosis of speech and language problems. More formal evaluation revealed, however, verbal comprehension problems which ranged from complete receptive aphasia in three cases, to well preserved comprehension in six cases and moderate problems in three others. The predominant expressive difficulty was mutism, a poverty of vocabulary and difficulties with naming. Mutism has been reported as the usual initial feature of paediatric ACA-T, but less commonly in adults. Levin, Eisenberg and Miner (1983), describe a fairly typical post-traumatic history of a 12 year old girl who remained mute for more than three weeks after injury. Whilst loss of communicative initiative may be the most marked initial feature after head injury, verbal naming difficulties may occur frequently and tend to persist. A poverty of readily available vocabulary may therefore be evident in later stages of recovery (Hecaen, 1976). A wide range of paraphasias may arise, including semantic or phonemic paraphasias, perseverations and verbal stereotypies, which may occur as temporary initial features, or as more persistent long term aphasic disorders (van Hout, Evrard and Lyon, 1985).

Assessment

It is strongly recommended that language investigations should be undertaken as soon as possible, for example within the first week or two of verbal communication after injury. Failure to do so may result in neglecting temporary paraphasias, which may partly account for the lack of previous reports of paraphasias. When seeing children in the early stages after head injury, other factors may limit the amount of language assessment that can be undertaken, including medical stability, mobility and physical difficulties, concentration and memory problems, and emotional lability. The experience of seeing children from acute onset through long term follow up has led the author to the view that in-depth linguistic investigation at all stages of recovery is important if we are fully to document the natural history of ACA-T, particularly in head injury. The complex combination of both aphasic, motor, sensory, cognitive, behavioural, social and educational difficulties which may occur following head injury presents a considerable problem to the rehabilitation team. A greater understanding of the nature, course and outcome as well as the assessment and possible treatment of these children is required by both speech therapists and other professionals seeing them. From assessing children several years after reported recovery of ACA-T, the author supports the view that language tests can and do reveal residual impairments in higher level language functions at this late stage, which are not usually apparent on informal observation. The presence of such difficulties has implications for the child's family, provision of speech therapy services, and future school placement. Language disorders will interact with cognitive difficulties, for example, and further aggravate the problem of placing the head-injured child appropriately.

The size of the problem

The number of children presenting with ACA is not as great as those presenting with developmental language problems. In a retrospective study Robinson (1987) found that only 3 per cent could be described as having an acquired basis (early cerebral infection) for their disorder, none of whom were head-injured. The remaining cases were described as developmental disorders. In recent years, however, the number of children referred with acquired language problems has increased and the largest group are now those with head injury. This appears to be due to two factors; firstly better intensive care facilities leading to more survivors after severe head injury in children and, secondly, the introduction of the 1981 Education Act which makes provision for the assessment of children with special needs.

A recent postal survey of speech therapists yielded greater information about children with acquired language problems (McMillen, Mule and Lees, 1987). Acute care and rehabilitation hospital services were compared in the New England and New York states (USA) and the United Kingdom. In both countries, patients reportedly received more intensive treatment in hospitals with designated rehabilitation units. The USA focus of intervention differed consistently with head-injury as opposed to cerebro-vascular accident (CVA) cases, whilst in the UK similar techniques were used with both populations. Although discharge placements were similar, a higher percentage of UK patients went home and returned to school with special educational support, as opposed to attending a rehabilitation centre. This largely reflects the scarcity of rehabilitation centres for head-injured children in the UK. A higher percentage of USA patients were referred for continuing therapy in speech, language and cognition. Both UK and USA speech therapists played major roles in cognitive, language and speech management, as well as discharge planning, indicating their important contribution to rehabilitation. Speech and language therapists in the North-Eastern United States used different treatment techniques with young head injury and CVA patients, focusing on cognition with the head-injured. In the UK both populations received similar treatment techniques, and the relative lack of cognitive therapy was due to a greater input from teachers and psychologists. The high number of respondents reporting varying session lengths may be representative of this population's diverse needs. Although adult tests and informal measures were frequently used, they were outnumbered by child language tests, at least in the UK. Many of the tests cited were designed for children with developmental language problems, reflecting the general paucity of tests geared towards children and adolescents with acquired insults. Most UK facilities reported discharging children from rehabilitation programmes to former schools as common practice. Experiences suggests that two factors tend to affect this decision; firstly, community health and local education services are unfamiliar with the needs of these children; secondly, the UK state education policy seeks to educate children with special needs in mainstream schools where possible. Alternative programmes following discharge from acute rehabilitation seemed to be more common in the USA, suggesting that they have started to recognize the specific needs of this population.

Current research

A longitudinal study of ACA (Lees, 1989) was established in 1985 to focus on the evolution of language difficulties. At the time of writing, thirty-four children aged 5 to 16 years presenting with ACA of either traumatic or convulsive aetiologies had been followed for up to two years. Comprehensive neurological investigations, audiological, psychological and language assessments were undertaken. The following questions were specifically addressed:

What are the characteristics of ACA-T?

Informal descriptions of the aphasia indicated that the main types of linguistic impairment occurred at some stage during the course of their aphasia as follows:

Table 7.1: Features of ACA, by aetiology

	ACA-T (other)	ACA-T CHI	ACA-C	Others	% of total
Numbers of children	5	17	4	8	
AV Comp	4	10	4	4	65
WFD	4	12	1	3	59
Jargon	1	0	1	1	9
Paraphasic semantic	3	4	1	1	26
Phonemic	3	3	1	0	20
Perseveration					
— receptive	0	4	1	0	15
— expressive	2	3	1	1	20

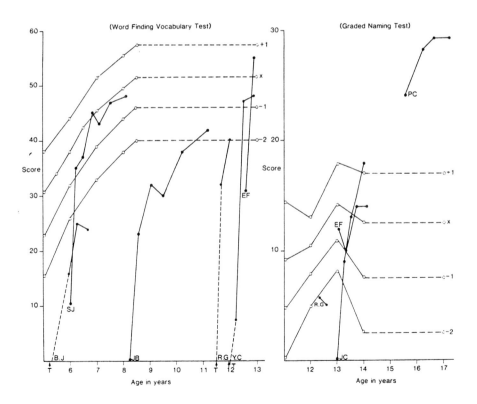

Figure 7.1: Recovery of Confrontational naming as measured by WFVT and GNT for 8 children with ACA, from onset

This limited data supports the view that auditory-comprehension problems and word-finding deficits are the most common features of ACA. Auditory-comprehension deficits were described in 65 per cent of the children, which is substantially higher than most other reported series. Acute expressive aphasia was uncommon, occurring in only 15 per cent of cases seen at onset. When informal observation alone is used to reveal a child's difficulties, high level auditory-comprehension problems can easily be missed. Expressive language difficulties are obviously easier to detect from informal observation. The most commonly cited reason for referral is word-finding difficulty. For children referred with residual difficulties only in written language, however, adequate examination often reveals high level difficulties with spoken language. The symptoms of jargon, paraphasia and perseveration were previously thought to be uncommon in ACA having been reported only in small numbers in studies since 1978. The current data suggests, however, that such symptoms occur in a sizeable minority of cases. Jargon aphasia seems to be a short-term problem and generally resolves into the more usual receptive difficulty with paraphasias in expressive language well before three months after onset. Perseveration is more common after head injury and is usually a feature of the first six months of recovery. Its persistence after one year is usually a poor prognostic sign, indicating the child's difficulty in self-monitoring of errors. Unfortunately, the small numbers in the different groups studied so far, have prevented the demonstration of significant between-groups differences. This evaluation is continuing, however, and full data analysis will be reported in due course.

How does the linguistic deficit change during the course of recovery after head injury?

Figures 7.1 and 7.2 show the recovery of auditory comprehension (Bishop, 1983) and confrontational naming (Renfrew, 1972; McKenna and Warrington, 1983), plotted over two years from onset. For the head-injured children, the dotted lines indicate time from trauma to first testing. All head-injured children were tested when neurologically stable, and the other children within five days of aphasic onset. The figures indicate that, apart from case number 8, all children initially presented with severe aphasia, with expressive and receptive language test scores more than two standard deviations below the mean. All children showed the greatest recovery within the first three months, whilst most continued to make good progress for at least one year, after which the rate gradually declined. Cases 1 and 3 continue to have severe language difficulties more than two years after onset; cases 2 and 4 continue to have significant difficulties which affect progress at school. All children are in mainstream education and receive varying educational support, depending on local authority provision.

Table 7.2: Summary profiles of eight cases with ACA-T

Child	Sex	Age at onset	Aetiology	Hearing	WISC-R[1] PIQ	VIQ[2]
1 BJ	M	5:3 years	CHI	normal	75	–
2 SJ	M	6:0 years	left cerebral haemangioma	normal	100	78
3 JB	F	8:3 years	left middle cerebral artery infarct	conductive loss 30dB	86	52
4 RG	F	11:5 years	CHI	normal	95	73
5 YC	F	12:0 years	CHI	normal	untested	
6 EF	M	12:8 years	Landau-Kleffner	normal	*below 69	
7 JC	F	13:0 years	left temporal AVM	normal	77	79
8 PC	M	15:0 years	left frontal cerebral abscess	normal	124	110

*(tested within one week of onset, however, returned to school and reported to have made average academic progress).

[1]Wechsler Intelligence Scale for Children-Revision
[2]Verbal & Performance Scale I.Q.

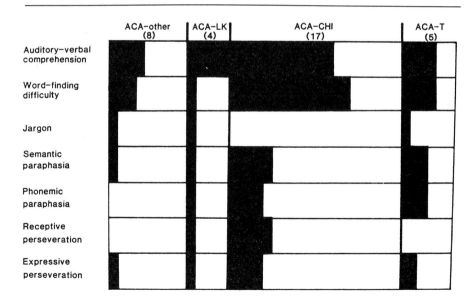

Figure 7.2:   Reported features of ACA, by aetiology

What is the prognosis for recovery, what are the residual problems?

Few children continue to make dramatic progress in the second year, when the recovery curve appears to slacken. Specific deficits become defined as general communication difficulties or problems with written language, and the child may learn to make personal adjustments and compensations. The overall prospect for complete recovery after significant head injury is bleak, if it is ever possible, although some children may regain average levels of performances on some tests. Of fifteen head-injured children seen more than two years after injury, one third continued to have severe problems with auditory-verbal comprehension, 20 per cent with word-finding, and 40 per cent continued to have moderate problems with auditory processing and word finding. Over half of the fifteen children were also having specific spelling difficulties. It is important to note, however, that five children were specifically referred more than two years post onset because of residual language difficulties. Only two children were reported as not having any difficulties two years post onset, neither of whom were head-injured. This suggests that long term auditory processing and lexical recall difficulties are the main residual language problems of head-injured children. This preliminary data does not support the view that language development is relatively resistant to the effects of closed head injury (Levin, Benton and Grossman, 1982). The outstanding question is whether any remaining deficits are amenable to treatment.

Speech therapy: what, when and how?

Appropriate and adequate assessment and diagnosis is the necessary prerequisite to any speech therapy intervention. This is often not so straightforward with a head-injured child, however, because of the complex association of motor, cognitive, perceptual, emotional and communication problems, the fact that very little formal assessment material is available specifically for these children and the changing nature of their deficits. Further restrictions are encountered because of the uncommon nature of the problems and the relative inexperience of staff in this specialized area.

The test materials used with head-injured children by twenty-six British speech therapists (Table 7.3) include those designed for developmental disorders (Reynell Developmental Language Scales, Reynell, 1977) and those for use with adults (Frenchay Dysarthria Test, Enderby, 1983). The minimum requirement for evaluation is a test of auditory-verbal comprehension and one of confrontational naming. In the former, the Test for Reception of Grammar (Bishop, 1983) is recommended, because of its simple administration, attractiveness to the child, its applicability with motor handicaps, and ease of analysis. Several confrontation naming tests may be recommended, depending on the age of the child, including the Word-Finding

Table 7.3: Language assessment materials used in rank order of popularity

	No.	%
Test for Reception of Grammar	13	50
Frenchay Dysarthria Test	12	46
Reynell Developmental Language Scales (rev)	10	38
British Picture Vocabulary Test	8	30.7
Symbolic Play Test	5	19.2
Aphasia Screening Test (child)	4	15.4
Alphasia Screening Test (adult)	3	11.5
Sentence Comprehension Test	3	11.5
Porch Index of Communicative Ability (child)	3	11.5
Illinois Test of Psycholinguistic Ability	3	11.5
Derbyshire Language Scheme	3	11.5
Graded Naming Test	2	7.6
Renfrew Tests	2	7.6
Goldman-Fristoe Articulation Test	2	7.6
LARSP	2	7.6
Boston Aphasia Test	2	7.6
Token Test	2	7.6
Robertson Dysarthria Test	2	7.6

Vocabulary Test (Renfrew, 1972) and the Graded Naming Test (McKenna and Warrington, 1983). The child version of the Aphasia Screening Test (Whurr and Evans, 1986) is a popular screening measure which may be useful with younger children and those in the very early stages of recovery.

Reassessment is clearly important in measuring recovery and fundamental to evaluating the clinical efficacy of therapy, so it is crucial to use an appropriate protocol. Where the situation is changing rapidly, particularly in the initial recovery period, it is important that therapeutic intervention keeps up with this. Where the situation is rather static, such as in the later stages of recovery, reassessment can identify those persistent and specific deficits. The implications of a carefully reviewed deficit-specific approach for therapy, are numerous. For example it can be graded in a stepwise manner, based on the child's strengths and needs. When working through the range of auditory processing difficulties it is important to begin therapy in a distraction-free environment to minimize auditory interference, working progressively through more complex situations which a child may encounter with less ease, including the various sound environments found at home and school. A structured approach to auditory comprehension and syntax are preferred when teaching the rule-based systems of language. Both the Colour Pattern Scheme (Leao 1970) and the Derbyshire Language

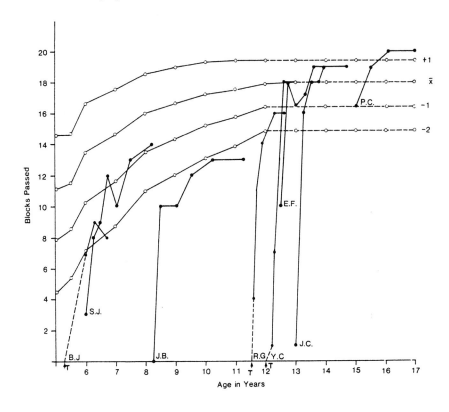

Figure 7.3: Recovery of verbal comprehension as measured on TROG of 8 children with Acquired Childhood Aphasia, from onset

Scheme (Knowles, Masidlover and Smith, 1982) are useful for this. A consistent approach in the use of cueing by therapists and carers to aid confrontational naming and word-finding allows the child to generalize these skills more readily. Work in adult aphasia (Howard, Patterson, Franklin *et al.*, 1985) suggests that different types of cues may be effective over different time periods. Similarly, experience suggests that children may pass through different stages at which different types of cues aid recall. The child is encouraged to develop a capacity for self-monitoring of errors related to specific deficits, which can be more readily generalized and of greater long-term benefit. Long periods of individual therapy in traditional treatment centres may not always be the most appropriate management for teenagers with chronic problems. The therapist needs to be as flexible as possible when considering the place, timing and style of therapy offered, including imaginative use of holiday groups.

It is not appropriate to leave a child who has severe communication difficulties without speech therapy support in the initial period of rapid recovery. Both the child and family will need informed and sensitive help in order to cope with the communication difficulties which arise. Alternative or augmentative communication may sometimes be appropriate to ease problems in the acute period. It is not, however, a straightforward matter of supplying a communication aid and leaving the child, family and other staff to get on with it. It is important to consider that the child's reaction to a sudden loss of communication and other skills may be catastrophic. Underlying language and cognitive problems may mean the child cannot understand how to use the device where complex instructions may be required, or he or she may lack the desire or motivation to communicate. The family may insist on normality of approach and equate alternative communication with the acceptance of handicap, but the associated motor, visual and perceptual problems may limit choice of system or device. The speed at which the problem changes may mean that any device is only appropriate for a short time and needs frequent changing or adjustment, hence the importance of regular reviews. Consequently, two methods are recommended; firstly, gestural support for communication, either informally or in the framework of the Makaton vocabulary (Walker, 1980); secondly, child-specific communication boards, which should be as appropriate to the child as possible. Personal photographs are often a good idea to stimulate interest, aid recall and involve the family in the project.

Speech and swallowing

Associated oral motor problems, such as feeding and dysarthria are commonly seen in ACA associated with head injury. At the severe end of the spectrum most children will spend part of the initial recovery period receiving naso-gastric feeding. In some exceptional cases long-term naso-gastric feeding or gastostomy may be required. Detailed investigation of swallowing problems is important during rehabilitation, and radiological investigations which include videofluroscopy are recommended. This allows the therapist to see where oral problems are occurring, either during the oral preparatory stage (in the mouth), the oro-pharyngeal or pharyngeal stage (the swallowing mechanism) or the oesophageal stage of swallowing. Problems in the latter stage are not usually considered the domain of the speech therapist and, where videofluroscopy reveals a need for intervention at this level, it is usually surgical. Problems at other stages may also be contributing to dysarthria and require speech therapy. There are, however, several problems of dysarthria management in head-injured children. Firstly, the problem of assessment is similar to that encountered with the head-injured child's language, in that very little specific assessment material is available. Two types of assessment predominate, (a) use of adult material: in this respect the Frenchay Dysarthria Test (Enderby, 1983) is most commonly used, but has limited success with children under 8 years of age; (b) use of informal material: most therapists use their own informal assessments, which should include assessment of head position and general posture, in conjunction with a physiotherapist, the presence or absence of oral reflexes, control of respiration and phonation, movement of the facial musculature, dentition, swallowing and control of saliva. The major problem in the use of informal assessments is in developing an objective evaluation scheme which allows adequate documentation of the situation, with sufficient accuracy and reliability for repeat assessments. A second problem of treatment is complicated by the fact that most head-injured children do not present with any one 'pure' type of dysarthria. Usually the motor pattern is mixed and is quite different from the oral motor problems of cerebral palsied children, from whom most speech therapists initially derive experience of assessment and treatment in this area. Treatment of dysarthria at any stage of recovery requires a consistent and intensive programme, carried out several times each day by staff or family, under the direct supervision of a speech therapist.

Problems with written language

Persisting problems with written language may appear to be the major residual deficit after head injury in children. Ewing-Cobbs, Levin, Eisenberg *et al.*, (1987) reported that head-injured children demonstrated greater difficulty with written language tests than head-injured adolescents, regardless of injury severity. None of the studies of written language problems in this population, however, have investigated the level of impairment, or the strategies used by the children to overcome reading problems, both of which are important considerations when planning remedial programmes. Thorough language investigation is required to confirm that other difficulties really do not exist. Children referred with persisting spelling problems frequently also have high level auditory comprehension problems, auditory discrimination problems and other difficulties with the discrimination and manipulation of phonemes, and word-finding problems. A thorough investigation of reading and spelling strategies used by the child will reveal which routes for the transposition of phonemes to graphemes (speech to spelling) is functional, what knowledge of errors the child has and what self-correction strategies are employed. With school-aged children, access to their pre-accident class work will be of invaluable assistance. Although it may be difficult to establish pre-traumatic levels in younger children it is important to look for evidence of any family spelling difficulties. Some of these can be dealt with quite simply by learning of irregular spelling rules, keeping a spelling book and disciplined use of a dictionary. Management of written language difficulties is a joint concern for the speech therapist and tutor or class teacher, if an appropriate remedial programme is to be implemented.

Conclusion

Of the different types of acquired childhood aphasia which a speech therapist may see, the most common and complex are presented by head-injured children. Whilst the majority of these make good initial progress, very few can be said to recover completely. Specific types of language disturbance can occur after head injury in childhood, which frequently resolve into difficulties of auditory processing and lexical recall. These, in turn, may significantly affect educational needs. Other specific long term problems include dysarthria (including swallowing and phonation) and spelling. The view that younger children with head injury recover better cannot be upheld. The speech therapy required by head-injured children will change during the course of recovery and it is important to review continually these changing needs. Investigations into the evaluation, treatment and recovery of head-injured children of speech and language disorders are absent (Jordan, Ozanne and Murdoch, 1988). Although evaluations of post-traumatic cognition are just beginning, we are far behind in the area of language. Yet this is an equally important area of development and normal function for the child. Consequently, we should adopt a far more scientific and methodologically rigorous approach to our research in this area.

Chapter 8

Life in the slow lane: attentional factors after head injury

David A. Johnson and Karen Roethig-Johnston

Introduction

There is confusion surrounding use of the term attention and the various aspects of related behaviour. It is not surprising to find considerable differences in meaning between the reports of parents, teachers and psychologists, all confounded by a child's individual variability; for example, the child cannot attend to classroom instructions, but can watch television over an extended period of time and frequently provide some detailed information. Attention is one of those ubiquitous psychological concepts which we bandy around freely as if referring to an easily identifiable, well defined and unitary function or ability. The variety of attentional problems with which one is presented clinically, however, suggests that attention cannot be considered as a single neurological entity or process. Careful examination of attentional performance suggests distinct components, which may reasonably reflect different aspects of neurological function (Nissen, 1986). Accurate and meaningful delineation of those component processes is essential if we are to understand the nature of cognitive disorder in the head-injured child, and to implement effective rehabilitation. Whilst it is difficult to define adequately what we mean by attention, it is nonetheless necessary to attempt a working definition. Attention is certainly a universal function (Ferrier, 1880), highly dependent upon the integrity of the nervous system (Posner and Presti, 1987) and fundamental to its smooth, efficient and integrated function. Recent models of attention (McGuinness and Pribram, 1980; Mesulam, 1981; Stuss and Benson, 1986) generally postulate different but related networks for a sensory modality, with a central role for arousal, and a higher level control system responsible for the allocation of resources and regulation of performance; sensory input is thereby transformed, reduced, elaborated, coded, stored, retrieved and used. The central nervous system (CNS) has a naturally finite capacity to deal with the continuous stream of information normally received (Luria, 1973; Moskovitch, 1979). To deal accurately and efficiently with information at any stage of processing, from orienting (Lynn, 1966) through to long-term memory storage (Squire and Zola-Morgan 1988), the individual must select and apply the appropriate strategies with which to focus and divide attentional resources. The broad dichotomy of involuntary (automatic) and voluntary (controlled) attention (James, 1899; Schneider and Shiffrin, 1977) may help to elucidate these processes further. Automatic attention operates involuntarily without conscious control, and relies on stored experience and skills in long-term memory. Attentional resources are required for fast and efficient processing, with conservation and extension increasing with automaticity. The higher level function of controlled attention operates when the amount, complexity or novelty of input exceeds available resources; it is more voluntary, usually serial, slower and demands more attentional resources, especially consciously controlled mental effort and strategy use.

Models of attention involve complex systems of inter-related pathways between the brainstem, limbic and cortical regions, which may be asymmetrically represented within the right cerebral hemisphere (Heilman and van den Abel, 1980; Reivich, Gur and Alavi, 1983, Tucker and Williamson, 1984; Weintraub and Mesulam, 1987), before the cognitive functions are measurable (Hiscock and Kinsbourne, 1987). Outwith the capacity limitations of the CNS, there are complex interactions between the structural and metabolic aspects of the brain which may alter attention and experience qualitatively (Rapin, 1982). Essentially all information processing is mediated by neurotransmitters acting at specific receptor sites (e.g., Clark, Geffen and Geffen, 1986). The vast majority of central monoaminergic systems, for example, originate in the brainstem, so it is not surprising to find substantial changes in their activity after head injury, due to either structural or functional alteration. These same neurochemical systems have been implicated in a wide range of attention-related measures, so it is reasonable to suggest that such neurochemical abnormalities may form part of the substrate for persisting cognitive deficits. Abnormalities within the catecholaminergic and cholinergic systems, for example, may be particularly important to early recovery, and may persist for varying periods after head injury. The cholinergic system may have an important role in the stimulus-evaluation stage of information processing and a general priming function in behaviour (Panksepp, 1986). For example, the anticholinergic scopolamine slows reaction time and latency of the P300 waveform (a positive evoked response potential) in a dose-response fashion, suggesting inhibition of a cholinergic based stimulus-evaluation (Callaway, 1984).

Arousal

The concept of arousal-activation is crucial not only to the notion of attention, but also to behaviour and rehabilitation (Klove, 1987). The brain normally regulates its level of arousal as a function of the demands for attention (Kahnemann, 1973). With increasing task complexity, so the demands for greater control, effort and self-regulation increase. The brainstem reticular activating system forms the basis of this self-regulatory complex (Lindsley, 1960), with its dense reciprocal connections to the subcortical (thalamic and hippocampal) and highly developed cortical (fronto-parietal) systems. Impaired control of arousal will preclude normal information processing and registration. The under-aroused CNS is unable to process information adequately before this is partially lost or decays. Conversely, over-arousal lessens performance beyond an optimal point, when CNS capacity becomes overloaded. The respective consequences would be storage of partially coded information or automatism. Tonic arousal is reflected by the diurnal cycle, typically disrupted by severe head injury; phasic arousal occurs more rapidly, affecting the speed with which we are aware of and respond to stimuli. To sustain attention requires phasic arousal and expenditure of mental energy, which cannot be sustained indefinitely, either because of limited capacity or lack of control over other stages. Attention essentially represents control over different levels of brain activity, therefore, which combine to form a system of knowledge, or long-term memory. Knowledge allows a greater efficiency in the acquisition of information; with practise, cognitive and behavioural skills become easier to acquire and increasingly more automatic, thus allowing time to acquire new and potentially useful information. We suggest that, from a broad perspective, attention appears to represent the ability of the alert CNS to orient, process information, direct and sustain selective mental effort, over specific time periods and for particular tasks.

Development

The development of attention is of primary importance to understanding its disruption after head injury in children. Evidently complex behaviour such as attention is initially moulded by interaction with the adult, who provides a clear external structure to facilitate the infant's responses. Anderson (1988) suggests that a basic information processing mechanism is essentially unchanging over the ages 7 to 12 years. Aspects of speed of information processing may change through development and processing speed or capacity may be a causal factor in developmental change. Throughout development there are increasing demands upon the child for greater concentration, strategy development, selective control, physical and mental effort. Consequently, children come to use increasingly sufficient and efficient procedures (Kail and Bisanz, 1982). The same procedures may be used by individuals at different ages, but the components are performed more quickly with age. Repeated use or practice as the child develops may lead to greater proficiency in devising efficient strategies for task performance, which then becomes increasingly automatic. Successful performance on any task demands the use of effective strategies, especially under time constraints. For example, the head-injured child may be unable to regulate cognitive processes and sustain performance on a specific task, such as reading.

Head injury and attention

The complex area of development and information processing, its relation to strategy use, general cognitive ability and educational progress clearly has widespread implications for the head-injured child (Hunt, 1980). As such performance factors change, so the underlying neurological organization must also alter. It may be seen that the child's development of self-regulation and self-awareness (Bromley, 1977; Gibson and Rader, 1979) generally reflect the development of attentional control and subordinate neurological systems.

Post-traumatic disruption of the postulated processes underlying attention may seriously interfere with memory and other cognitive functions, as well as social behaviour and school performance. The extent of such impact remains speculative, but the available outcome studies suggest that few head-injured children are able to fully resume normal school activities. Attention seems to be particularly vulnerable to the effects of head injury; Ommaya (1979) suggested that the resultant slowing of electrophysiological responses after trauma, for example, may underlay the hypothesized slowing of information processing (van Zomeren, 1981) and some aspects of memory deficit (Geschwind, 1982). In her recent review, Gronwall (1987) suggests that the pattern of attentional behaviour shown after head injury will vary according to the severity and time since insult. The acute pervasive confusion and disorientation, covering retrograde and post-traumatic amnesia (Russell, 1959), is difficult to measure reliably in children, but is likely to be qualitatively different than in adults. During the subsequent period of early recovery, a general slowing of information processing and behaviour may persist, which probably reflects deep and widespread neurological disruption. There may also be specific disruption of higher level regulatory functions causing, for example, poor inhibitory control. Van Zomeren and colleagues have postulated two major types of attentional pathology after head injury.

Focused attention deficit:

Focused attention is essentially an active process of selection (James, 1899; Schneider and Shiffrin, 1977; van Zomeren and Brouwer, 1987). A deficit arises when automatic response tendencies conflict with the responses demanded in the task. Diminished control from frontal lobe dysfunction may particularly produce such difficulty

(Buchtel, 1987). Consequently, it is important to determine how and when the patient can withstand distraction from interference, a point most pertinent to the environmental design of treatment and school rooms.

Divided attention deficit

Divided attention refers to the process of having to allocate our attention between two or more tasks, such as driving and listening to the radio, writing notes from a lecture, and so on. Divided attention is particularly restricted by information processing capacity, the amount of information with which the CNS can cope at any one time. A deficit occurs where poorer performance is due to speed limitations on the consciously controlled processing.

The notion that attentional deficits increase relative to trauma severity would be consistent with the centripetal hypothesis of head injury, predicting relative degrees of cortical and brainstem involvement (Ommaya and Gennarelli, 1974; Ommaya, 1979; Thibault and Gennarelli, 1985; Levin, Williams, Crofford *et al.*, 1988). It would also support the increasing evidence for pathological changes in brainstem and basal forebrain regions following relatively mild head injury. The implication of disruption to a high level control system (Buchtel, 1987; Posner, 1987) is inherently attractive and clearly supported by the considerable attentional pathology yielded by such an anatomically prone region as the basal forebrain, for example. Thus, the structural damage and functional disruption typically caused by head injury may reduce both the attentional capacity and processing efficiency of the CNS.

Assessment

In order to help the head-injured child, we must understand how alterations in information processing arise from the specific brain systems affected by trauma. Children who demonstrate common behavioural deficits may well be shown to possess common aberrations in brain function but, of course, they need not share common aetiologies (Dickstein and Tallal, 1987; Johnson, 1989, Taylor, this volume). There are three main areas of investigation, each with their inherent methodological difficulties: cognitive testing, neurophysiological recording, and self-report. The reader is referred to recent reviews for a comprehensive criticism of published studies (Papakostopoulos, 1985; Gronwall, 1987; Papanicolaou, 1987).

Cognitive assessment

Relatively few studies have adequately evaluated attentional disorder in the head-injured child, despite its omnipresence and seemingly critical nature; their selection of measures is generally inadequate or inappropriate (e.g., Leahy, Holland and Frattalli, 1987). Attentional disorder after head injury has been poorly demonstrated using achievement tasks that primarily tap structured cognitive resources (Stuss and Benson, 1986). For example, many clinicians and educators attempt to measure attention using formal measures of intellectual ability (e.g., Fay and Janesheski, 1986), administered in highly controlled settings, which may overestimate the head-injured child's actual level of functioning in more natural settings (Telzrow, 1987). These approaches are insensitive and inaccurate for individual diagnoses and prescription (Yule, 1978; Chadwick and Rutter, 1984). They clearly do not provide reliable or meaningful estimates of neuropsychological function, nor sufficient guides to rehabilitation. The persistent reliance on global IQ figures, especially when pro-rated, is a meaningless practice which is to be deplored and discarded (Rapin, 1986; Lezak, 1988a). It should be self-evident that no single subtest, test or averaged score is a reliable guage of either attentional processes or neuropsychological function. Authors have tried to relate spurious IQ estimates with the practical significance of the head-injured child's specific difficulties on speeded tasks (e.g., Filley, Cranberg, Alexander *et al.*, 1987). Whilst deficits in speeded motor performance are consistently reported (Bawden, Knights and Winogren, 1985) we still have little idea of the precise nature of the neurological or cognitive substrates involved; neither shall we reach that understanding by the uncritical, seemingly perpetual use of intelligence tests. We should heed Teuber's insistence on the insensitivity of many traditional psychological tests in evaluating aspects of cognition which may show little disruption after mild or moderate head injury, or predominantly focal injury to the prefrontal region (Perecman, 1987; Welsh and Pennington, 1988). The range of available tests is limited, however, and there is concern about the downward extension of adult tests for children (Fletcher and Taylor, 1984).

Post-traumatic and retrograde amnesia are difficult to assess at the best of times, and usually evaluated retrospectively (Russell, 1971). Unfortunately, prospective measures such as the Children's Orientation and Amnesia Test (COAT; Ewing-Cobbs, Fletcher and Levin, 1985) appear not to have been widely developed, despite the clinical need. More recently, Crovitz and colleagues have attempted to develop empirical formulae relating to length of retrograde amnesia, post-traumatic amnesia and time since injury (Crovitz and Daniel, 1987). Attempts to increase the confidence in prospective estimations of traumatic amnesia urgently require extension to the paediatric population.

Attentional efficiency is usually measured in terms of response speed on relatively simple tasks, such as digit cancellation (Coughlan and Hollows, 1985), reaction time (van Zomeren, 1981), or inspection time (Barrett, 1988). At least one clinical measure, the Stroop Test (Stroop, 1935) appears to be tapping inhibitory control and focused attention. In a recent review, however, van Zomeren and Brouwer (1987) concluded that head-injured adults do not have a specific difficulty in focusing on the colour dimension of this test's ambiguous stimuli. Similarly, Chadwick (1976, unpublished data) suggests that head-injured children are slower on all trials of the Stroop, but not disproportionately so on the last response-conflict interference trial. Tests such as the Stroop or reaction time are invariably constructed locally in slightly different formats. Although there are some limited developmental norms available (e.g., Comali, Wapner and Werner, 1962), evaluation of psychometric properties is lacking.

A slowing of reaction time is a general finding in many different neurological populations (Benton, 1986). It appears to be a non-specific effect which, at least after head injury, may persist in the absence of sensori-motor impairments. Van Zomeren (1981) discusses his work on choice reaction time (CRT) in considerable detail, noting that the primary difficulty of head-injured young adults occurs when presented with the choice of making one of a number of possible responses. Factors such as task complexity and memory set size may interact with the severity of injury and stage of recovery to significantly increase the patient's reaction time, hence the importance of serial assessments and accurate delineation. Clear re-test effects are evident on adult CRT performance after head injury. Conversely, no differences in RT three days after injury were found between mild head-injured children (6.5 to 9 years, and 9.5 to 12 years old); both age groups were slower than controls at one month after injury, however, suggesting that they did not benefit from practice effects (unpublished data from Ramsden, 1980, cited by Gronwall, 1987). CRT performance may yield important qualitative information beyond that of overall response speed. For example, a four-choice RT task will yield response differences for left-right and decision-movement dimensions, as well as variability in scatter of responses.

In vigilance tasks, the subject is required to respond rapidly to infrequent signals presented over an extended period of time. The capacity to maintain attentiveness to stimuli in vigilance situations is a primary reflection of an integrated and highly regulated neurological system (see Reivich, Gur, and Alavi, 1983). Even for normal subjects the loss of control over one's thought processes during a vigilance task must eventually lead to a slowing of response and missing some of the stimuli, although they should be able to respond reasonably quickly if a rapid shift is made between one component and another (Buchtel 1987). Results of investigations in this field are summarized by van Zomeren and Brouwer (1987), who conclude that whilst head injury patients show poorer signal detection and longer reaction times to signals, their performance over time was as stable as the control group. There are relatively few studies which have adequately addressed the problem of individual variability, however, which may be a major source of information for individual treatment.

In the series of studies on outcome from head injury in children, Rutter's group

(Chadwick, Rutter, Shaffer *et al.*, 1981) used a paced auditory serial addition task (PASAT), based on the equivalent test for adults (Sampson, 1956). Unfortunately, Chadwick used this potentially valuable measure only once, at twenty-seven months follow-up, and obtained no significant results. It is reasonable to suggest that greater effects might have been observed with serial examinations. Performance on this type of task appears to require selective and sustained attention, stored memory components, and mental transformation. It clearly has inherently strong control requirements for inhibition of automatic response tendencies, such as adding the answer to the next stimulus number, and sustained performance under time pressure (the fastest trial presents 61 digits at a rate of one every 1.2 seconds). A revised version of Chadwick's task, the Childrens Paced Auditory Serial Addition Task (CHIPASAT), is currently being developed (Johnson, Roethig-Johnston and Middleton, 1988). The initial normative data for CHIPASAT suggested that speed of response increases exponentially with age, older children achieving more correct responses in every trial, concurring with the nature of developmental change for information processing reported by Kail (1986). One explanation for the younger child's slower speed of response and greater sensitivity to presentation rate may be their less available automatic processing, demanding more attentional resources to perform the task. Such resources may increase gradually and continually with age, reflecting a general maturational change which, in turn, would alter the physiological limits on attention. Our current evaluations of attentional pathology suggest that, after head injury, children have generally less efficient attention, performing at lower age levels on CHIPASAT in early stages of recovery for example, but subsequently following a limited developmental curve. Less effective, immature strategies may also be used by the head-injured child, such as using fingers to add the numbers.

Other potentially useful tasks may be derived from experimental procedures (see Sheer and Schrock, 1986), although practical considerations of portability and ease of administration may initially limit their clinical application. For example, computerized tasks of mental rotation (Kail, 1986), inspection time (Anderson, 1988) or tachistoscopic reaction time (Bakker and Vinke, 1985) may prove useful clinically, given adequate standardization and availability. Swanson (1987a) cautions on the ecological validity of research in this area, suggesting that insufficient concern has been given to the context in which attentional performance is demanded.

Neurophysiological assessment

The central role of arousal in attention provides an important framework for investigating neurophysiological changes after head injury. As the physiological state of the brain presumably determines which stimuli will influence behaviour, post-traumatic disturbances may exert considerable effect upon processing. Neurophysiological measures of attention primarily involve evoked response potentials (ERP), that is changes in the EEG caused by sensory stimuli, and support for a slowing of processing speed is indicated (Curry, 1981, Oken and Chiappa, 1985; Squires and Ollo, 1986). There has been particular interest in the P300 waveform, which is generated in response to infrequent, attended, task-relevant stimuli and appears between 300 and 700 milliseconds after stimulus presentation; the latency regarded as an index of stimulus processing time. There are conflicting reports, however, on the relationship between ERP's, severity of injury, cognitive function and recovery. Papanicolaou, Levin, Eisenberg *et al.,* (1984) claimed that prolongation of P300 latency represented physiological correlations of a neurobehavioural state associated with post-traumatic amnesia, subsequently resolving with that amnesic state. Conversely, Olbrich, Nau, Lodermann *et al.,* (1986) reported that P300 latency was the most sensitive indicator of persisting post-traumatic brain dysfunction in a small heterogenous population of head-injured adults. A significant association between P300 latency, orientation and memory were reported, with prolonged P300 latencies persisting, despite psychological test performances returning to normal levels. Such disparate findings are hardly surprising, given the population heterogeneity and appalling contrasts of measures utilized in many studies. Neurophysiological measurements may provide a useful means for delineating attentional deficits, but only when applied in conjunction with adequate neuropsychological assessments, in a neuroscientific context.

Self report measures

These are relatively unexplored and may be extremely difficult to validate with the younger or more severely head-injured child. Given the considerable importance of attention to classroom performance (Wittrock, 1986), however, this is a potentially important area for investigation (see McMillan, 1984; Sunderland, Harris and Gleave, 1984), which may yield valuable information on the head-injured child's general and specific difficulties.

It appears that any one assessment approach has failed to yield adequate knowledge on attentional substrates and the various aberrations following head injury. A combined investigative framework offers great potential by merging areas of neurological and neuropsychological expertise (Friedman, Klivington and Peterson, 1986). It is necessary to refine our evaluation and analyses of the component processes of attention, without necessarily reaching a stage of extreme reductionism. Different components of attention may develop and mature at different rates (Chi and Gallagher, 1982) and so be more, or less, vulnerable to the deleterious effects of head injury. One result of which may be that age and severity of injury will dictate the type and level of treatment approach. Careful delineation remains the fundamental rule for effective rehabilitation; it is of no use to rely on reports, irrespective of source, that the head-injured child doesn't, won't, or can't pay attention. Their performance on any assessment task will be a complex matter, involving interaction between speed of information processing, control processes and knowledge. The mechanisms implicated in such interactions might include differential hemispheric activation, conscious effort, capacity restrictions and strategy use (Swanson, 1987a,b).

Attention and memory

The capacity and speed of attentional processes may form an integral relationship with memory performance after head injury. Both learning and memory should be regarded as complex neural functions, depending upon many different-stage and widely distributed operations (Hebb, 1949; Luria, 1973; Gaddes, 1986), which are highly vulnerable to the effects of head injury. These cognitive functions are clearly dissociable phenomena and have crucial roles in development, cognition, and daily life.

The potential for learning, whereby we acquire new knowledge about events in the world, parallels the complexity and integrity of the CNS, with its inherent capacity for plasticity, which allows changes in brain function in response to experience, i.e., the ability to learn and remember (Black and Greenough, 1986). Memory refers to processes through which we retain that knowledge (Morris, Kandel and Squire, 1988). Development of learning and memory implies composite changes in each of several components (Kail, 1979), reflecting the child's increasing understanding of memory tasks, the acquisition of appropriate strategies to cope with such demands and, of course, their own memory systems. More recently, Baddeley (1988) questioned the separability of different types of memory, and whether subsystems are represented by different neural substrates, or reflect different processes within a single neural system (Squire and Zola-Morgan, 1988), although their differentiation should not necessarily be rigid. For example, procedural learning occurs in incremental and automatic fashion with no conscious awareness of what exactly has been learned. This leads to a disposition to behave in a particular way, as with perceptuo-motor skills. Information becomes available by feedback through performance, allowing the child to access information by engaging in the procedures in which the particular knowledge is embedded. Alternatively, declarative learning encodes information about specific events, which allows conscious recollection of past episodes and inferential thinking. It is particularly dependent upon limbic and diencephalic structures, such as the hippocampus (Squire and Zola-Morgan, 1988). A higher level control system has also been postulated (Stuss and Benson, 1986), integrating information from more than one source, co-ordinating, planning and controlling behaviour. Such a system would be consistent with anatomical and neuropharmacological evidence implicating a prefrontal focus (e.g., Irle and Markowitsch, 1987; see recent review by Mishkin and Appenzeller, 1987).

The capacity and speed of access for information already in short-term memory, which co-ordinates and temporarily stores information in use, are important practical considerations for the head-injured child. Speed of access is usually measured by scanning experiments such as the Sternberg paradigm (Sternberg, 1966), in which reaction time is found to be a linear function of the number of items in the memory set, and the slope of this function is considered a measure of the speed of access to information in short-term memory. A consistent relationship between speed of information processing and capacity of working memory in children has been reported (Chi and Gallagher, 1982), with the suggestion that the speed at which letters and words are processed, for example, may determine the remaining capacity in working memory for comprehension (Das and Varnhagen, 1986). This is clearly crucial to the process of learning and memory, and the child's normal development. Slow information processing might lead to problems with memory in a number of ways. Firstly, a slower rate of processing may lead to inefficient encoding of information (Cermak, 1982). The way in which information is encoded in memory is often a key predictor of the ease and accuracy with which the child will recall information on demand, solve problems, and so on. Secondly, processing of semantic or multiple aspects of information may be disproportionately slow (Meudell, Mayes and Neary, 1980). The child must be capable of estimating his own limitations and of realising the need for some deliberate plan in situations where memory capacity will be exceeded. An important interaction may arise between previously stored information or knowledge, and strategy utilization, the former restricting strategy use within a given domain. Such a relationship between speed of processing, complexity of information and memory seems intuitively plausible but, differential impairments after head injury remain to be shown.

Memory and head injury

Memory may become disproportionately impaired after head injury (Levin, Goldstein, High *et al.,* 1988) and, considering general cognitive development, the head-injured child's poor memory performance may easily result in declining attainments (Chadwick, 1985). Despite their apparent vulnerability to insult (Levin, 1985) and presence as major long-term sequelae (Fletcher, Miner and Ewing-Cobbs, 1987) there have been few objective studies. Learning and memory in head-injured children are reported sporadically, generally without regard to developmental status, and typically refer to a single process. An early study (Richardson, 1963) found memory impairment at eighteen months after head injury, despite the inadequate measures, small population, and wide age range investigated. Similarly, despite poor methodology, Gaidolfi and Vignolo, (1980) found persisting memory deficits ten years after injury. Levin's group in Galveston continue to make substantial contributions to the evaluation of learning and memory in head-injured children. Levin and Eisenberg (1979), have confirmed Fuld and Fisher's (1977) demonstation of impairments in consistent long term retrieval (CLTR) on the Selective Reminding Task (Buschke and Fuld, 1974). Such impairments were found even in mildly head-injured children, increasing with severity of injury, and together with reduced capacity for increasing the amount of information recalled on successive trials in the more severely injured subjects. Signal detection analysis of visual recognition memory performances (Hannay, Levin and Grossman, 1979) revealed increased false positives in severely head-injured children at six and twelve months follow up, with younger children demonstrating more errors than did adolescents. Levin, Eisenberg, Wigg *et al.*, (1982) hypothesized that young age would confer no advantage with respect to memory after head injury. They compared four groups (n = 15), aged 2 to 12 years and 13 to 19 years, with Glasgow Coma Scores below or above 8. In the Selective Reminding Task, animal names were used in the younger group, and unrelated words in the older group, which would predictably yield different results (see Lezak, 1983). Levin found that severely head-injured children had residual disability in recognition memory, as compared with age-matched children with milder injuries. The more frequent impairment of recognition memory may reflect its greater vulnerability at young age, and demands for sustained attention, or undeveloped verbal-semantic memory. Reductions in long-term memory were also found in both children and adolescents with severe head injury. Retrieval on the Selective Reminding Task involves a strategic search through the contents of memory, which may be confounded by strategy use or speed differences. The characteristics of subgroups of head-injured children remain unknown, however, including whether the head-injured child displays the same recall and learning curve typical of amnesic adults. Further difficulties stemming from prefrontal involvement may include metamemory or its development, or strategic control over the learning process. Deficits may become disproportionately evident when the child tries to acquire amounts of information exceeding that which can be kept in mind through active rehearsal, or when trying to retain information across delay. Increasing difficulties may also arise as the time since injury increases, due to either primary or secondary structural changes (Cullum and Bigler, 1985; Levin, Williams, Crofford *et al.*, 1988). Serial evaluations are necessary, however, before reaching conclusions on recovery curves and developmental progress.

Sleep and memory

Post-traumatic cognitive difficulties, particularly the integral processes of learning and memory, may interact with disturbance of sleep pattern. One phase of the sleep cycle, rapid eye movement sleep (REMS), deserves particular attention in research because of the possible interactions between vestibular and reticular systems. The normal sleep-wake cycle requires intact and functioning brainstem, subcortical and cortical structures. It is not surprising, therefore, that trauma sufficient to disturb consciousness will also disrupt general cerebral function to produce persisting changes in sleep (Parkes, 1985). The potential interactions between arousal, REMS, learning and memory, (Marti-Nicolovius, Portell-Cortes and Morgado-Bernal, 1984) and their common neurochemical pathways, may provide important guidelines for clinical remediation in the head-injured child (Quera-Selva and Guilleminault, 1987; Shiromani, Gillin and Henriksen 1987).

Implications for school performance

Irrespective of ability, attention is an essential component of learning, the fundamental activity required of all children in building a pool of experience, skills and knowledge sufficient to enable them to cope with increasingly complex and new situations. Similarly, the capacity to consolidate and retrieve information has obvious implications for school performance and academic attainments. Post-traumatic difficulties can easily lead to substantial educational problems, the results of which may arise only years after the original head injury, when it is effectively too late to help. These matters are now beginning to be adequately examined, but it seems that whilst the nature of problems faced by the head-injured child may indeed parallel those of his adult counterpart, extra difficulties are imposed by developmental limitations and restricted capacity. Consider-able controversy remains as to if and how attentional pathology relates to a general decline in intellectual abilities (see Hunt, 1980; Gronwall, 1987), or similarly, which specific difficulties in cognition and behaviour result from impaired regulatory control (Buchtel, 1987; Swanson, 1987a). The head-injured child, for example, may show difficulties in focusing and sustaining attention, in controlling distractability, and generally thinking at a normal pace within the classroom. Indeed, distractability alone may be due to any number of things, including inability to inhibit strong response tendencies, or ignore competing and irrelevant stimuli (see Kewman, Yanus and Kirsch, 1988), which may particularly slow some components of attention (Ewing-Cobbs, Fletcher and Levin, 1985; Clark, Geffen and Geffen, 1986).

Encouraged by the often dramatic early improvements of the head-injured child, parents are optimistic for a total recovery, and they institute the quickest possible return to his pre-accident lifestyle. Yet, the capability of a child merely to attend school does not necessarily imply a good recovery. An initial period of special consideration and extra tuition by the school is frequently more geared towards filling in the gaps caused by his absence, rather than addressing his actual post-traumatic difficulties. Regrettably, the educational system does not teach attending or remembering skills and often assumes that these are automatic and remain intact after head injury (Cohen, 1986). Many educational placements are based on the ubiquitous and meaningless IQ or similar achievement average. There can be little doubt for anyone who has worked with head-injured children that many can achieve IQ's within the normal range in the presence of unremitting deficits in attention, learning and memory. Those children cannot, in any reasonable mind, be expected to perform adequately in the classroom. The perpetual classroom command to pay attention and answer questions will, at best, serve to arouse the head-injured child momentarily, but he may lack the internal control or self-regulation to respond appropriately, to switch attention back to the task in hand, focus and sustain performance, all in time to process what the teacher has said subsequently. The speed of information processing and limited capacity will partly determine what is noticed or attended to, and what goes unnoticed or lost. This suggests, for example, that the head-injured child may be only able to process a fraction of what is said by the teacher, before the remainder is lost, subject to interference, or decays. The ability to attend discriminately may be particularly disrupted by prefrontal impairment. In social or group situations, the cues and clues to appropriate interpersonal interaction may be missed if appropriate attention is not paid to the environment. An interesting suggestion (Buchtel, 1987) is that head injury patients may have particular difficulty in the inhibitory control of separating 'attending to' from 'looking at'. As is typical of disruption to prefrontal function, automaticity overrides weak inhibitory control, so that the head-injured patient is frequently observed to look at whatever is going on around him, irrespective of task engagement. Clearly this would restrict classroom learning and social performance in the head-injured child. A further difficulty may arise in retrieving specific information from memory on demand. Even with an intact memory system, retrieval based on partial information is often difficult at the best of times, requiring more effort and controlled searching; the nature of which the head-injured child finds difficult. In the attempt to keep up and perform according to expectations, the head-injured child must try to concentrate harder and longer but, with limited resources, the likely outcome is fatigue, attentional failure, and increasing task failure. Cognitive and physical fatigue may arise under conditions of normal time pressure, such as producing work on time, when the head-injured child must expend greater effort to perform tasks that used to be automatic. Fatigue, in turn, produces greater distractability and yet further decline in performance. Post-traumatic difficulties in attention, learning and memory affect not only classroom performance but, at the end of the school day the head-injured child is more tired and exhausted, less able to play or willing to socialize. He is more likely to choose less demanding, solitary and passive activities, such as watching television, flipping through magazines or simply resting. The head-injured child is forced into life's slow lane; he quickly falls behind in performance, learning and development, losing contact with his peers. Without systematic evaluation, post-traumatic difficulties may prove fundamental obstacles to the child's progress (Levin and Eisenberg, 1979).

Conclusions

Consideration of the literature on attention and memory deficits after head injury and, particularly, observation of performances by head-injured children, suggests that a non-specific slowing in the speed of information processing may occur, with associated difficulties in higher level control processes. In very broad terms, the spectrum of disorders appears to parallel that of trauma severity, and supports the hypothesized regions of pathology in most cases of diffuse accidental head injury. To understand more precisely the nature of these disorders in head-injured children, a crucial step is the application of a combined framework of investigation, relating cognitive processes to neural systems, ranging from cellular activity through to the level of task performance (see Levine, 1984; and Levine, Guermay and Friedrich, 1987). Education is primarily concerned with plasticity, yet it is precisely this attribute of head-injured child which may be limited. Despite the omnipresence of post-traumatic difficulties in attention, learning and memory we seem quite unaware of, and unconcerned by, their potential impact upon the child's educational progress and achievement. Educational authorities at all levels seem predisposed not to take those difficulties with any serious-ness nor consider their long term implications. In order to prevent the seemingly unstopable slide into a dim future we must press for the recognition of the difficulties and regular evaluation of the head-injured child (Friedman, Klivington and Peterson, 1986).

Chapter 9

Disorders of self-regulation in head-injured children

Eric Taylor

Introduction

The starting point of this chapter is the clinical observation that children referred with psychiatric symptoms after a head injury, often find it difficult to concentrate, show disturbances of memory, and are disorganized in their personal life and their attempts to solve problems. This pattern of disability is similar, at least superficially, to some of the symptoms presented by children with the hyperkinetic disorder of childhood (Taylor, 1986). If the similarity is real, then it would suggest ways of helping the re-habilitation of children with brain injury. There is considerable knowledge about the effects of treatments for hyperkinetic disorder, and a very extensive body of research about therapy for the more broadly defined condition known as Attention Deficit-Hyperactivity Disorder (Taylor, 1985). The treatments range from cognitive approaches, to training children in attention, to the use of amphetamines and related drugs. If they are relevant to the needs of children with head injury, then such treatment approaches may improve outcome.

This chapter therefore considers impairments of attention and self-control after brain injury in children. From reviewing the literature, one may ask, firstly, whether the clinical observation of population similarity is valid. Referral practices to specialized clinics can produce misleading associations in their clientele. Is there any specific tendency for physical injury to cause changes in attention and self-organization? If so, are they similar to the changes seen in hyperkinetic children? The next questions will be whether these symptoms have a clear pathogenesis, and if there is evidence of specific correlates, such as frontal lobe dysfunction or neurophysiological unresponsiveness. Since direct information on this point is lacking, it will be necessary to draw on circumstantial evidence from investigations of children with hyperkinesis that is not caused by trauma, and from children with localized frontal cerebral injuries. Finally, I shall try to make recommendations for clinical practice and for future research.

Psychiatric symptoms after head injury

The strongest conclusion that can be drawn from the clinical literature is that there is too little evidence to be confident about the overall profile of symptoms, or about any subgrouping. The minimum requirements for a study of this topic are a reliable and comprehensive means of assessing behaviour and mental state, a series free of selection bias, and an appropriate control group. No study completely achieves this, and most of the clinical literature fails to meet any of the three requirements. One needs to rely heavily upon the studies reported by Rutter, Chadwick and Shaffer (1984), in which serious head injuries were identified from the surgical units to which they were admitted, so that no selection on psychiatric grounds was involved. They were compared with children who had also suffered trauma, but had received injuries elsewhere than to the head. The results of behavioural ratings and systematic accounts by parents indicated that there was no pathognomonic brain damage syndrome. Rather, there was an increased risk for a wide range of psychiatric problems, as is the case for other types of neurological disability.

Conversely, studies of attention and activity impairment make it clear that they are common and non-specific symptoms of many types of psychiatric disorder (Taylor, 1986), whether or not they result from structural damage to the brain. The ideas that brain injury only causes attention and activity disturbance, and that attention and activity are only disturbed by brain injury, are clearly wrong. Those ideas were not, however, very plausible to begin with. Different types of brain injury are likely to have varied effects, some of the effects will be remote from the original cause, and psycho-social effects are likely to be strong. The wide variety of problems with which children may present emphasizes the need for subtyping the disorders. Other contributors to this volume will address the role of family relationships, the reactions of teachers and peers, and the child's own attitudes in the genesis of disorder. It is clear, however, that some psychiatric morbidity in children after head injury is a direct consequence of the injury. One of the next stages in research will be an attempt to find subgroups of disorder in which a more specific pathogenesis can be traced.

Hyperactivity and disinhibition as subtypes of disorder

Restless, inattentive behaviour (hyperactivity) and related problems, have been linked to head injury for at least fifty years. Blau (1936) described children seen in psychiatric practice where symptoms followed rapidly upon trauma to the head. One of the patterns of disturbance was an enduring picture of disinhibited and hyperactive behaviour with impairment of social relationships. There could have been several reasons for such a symptom pattern developing; there was not enough detail in the study to be clear that the changes were indeed the result of damage to the brain or that they were accompanied by characteristic alterations of attention. Black, Jeffries, Blumer *et al.*, (1969), found that hyperactivity was a frequent characteristic of children who had been injured: it increased in severity over the weeks and months after the injury and then declined, suggesting that it was a consequence rather than a cause of the injury. Overactivity and inattention were common behaviour problems, but they were not specific and the same would have been found in any group of children with behaviour disorders. Conduct disorder and emotional disorder symptoms were also common, and a number of children became less active after their injury. Rutter, Chadwick and Shaffer (1984) described a study of head-injured children that was noteworthy for the detail of psychiatric and psychological assessments, the adequacy of the control groups, and the availability of information on the pre-injury status of the children. Nearly all the symptoms of psychiatric disorder were more common than in matched controls. The most characteristic symptom, one disproportionately common in the head-injured group and virtually absent in controls, was a disinhibition of behaviour and social interpersonal relationships. This led to behaviour quite inappropriate to the situation, and perhaps even a failure to appreciate what constituted appropriate behaviour. Disinhibition often went together with forgetfulness, impulsiveness and carelessness.

Parallels between head-injured and hyperkinetic children

The children who show the symptom cluster of disinhibition and disorganization following injury could represent cases of a distinct subtype of disorder. Their symptomatology is in some ways reminiscent of hyperactivity in children who have not sustained severe head injury. In one study of neurologically normal children who had presented to psychiatric clinics because of disruptive conduct, a standardized psychiatric interview was used to obtain ratings of mental state (Taylor, Schachar, Thorley *et al.*, 1986). Social disinhibition was associated with hyperactivity and inattentiveness, and indeed these items emerged as a single factor in a factor analysis. A further study made it clear that this was not a matter only of rater artefacts, such as a halo effect. When videotapes were taken of a separate series of children who were undergoing the same standardized interview, detailed time-sampling observations could be applied to the presence or absence of specified behaviours (Luk, Thorley and Taylor, 1987). Severely hyperactive children were more likely than their matched controls to show behaviours such as personal questioning of the examiner, inappropriate personal remarks, touching the interviewer or moving very close, loud talking and expansive gestures. All these observed behaviours correlated positively with the interviewer's global rating of social disinhibition, and were presumably among the reasons for that rating being made. It is not clear whether this disinhibition is in fact identical in form to that described in the Institute of Psychiatry series of severely head-injured children (Brown, Chadwick, Shaffer *et al.*, 1981). Disinhibition in the latter series was indeed similar in that it involved outspokenness, over-personal remarks and embarrassing behaviour in public; but it also included getting undressed in social situations where it would usually be considered inappropriate so to do, which is not at all a usual complaint about the ordinary group of hyperactive children. This may be a matter of severity rather than of qualitative difference, but it does suggest some caution in assuming identity.

Other differences between the head-injured with inattentive behaviour, and children with a diagnosis of hyperkinetic disorder should be noted. One of the defining characteristics of hyperactivity is restlessness and this was an uncommon symptom in the series of Brown, Chadwick, Shaffer *et al.* (1981); it was even less common in the severely head-injured than in control groups. Similarly, fatigue is often described in head-injured children, seldom in those with hyperkinesis. More research is needed to determine whether the pattern of impairment in attention after head injury is the same as that seen in hyperkinetic disorder, or in attention deficit-hyperactivity disorder.

Neuropsychological deviations in hyperactive subgroups

It would be helpful to know whether the subgroup of head-injured children who have disorders of attention and self-regulation have a similar pattern of neuropsychological or neurophysiological deviation to that of children with hyperkinetic disorder. It is difficult to study this question directly, however, for a number of reasons; firstly there is no certainty about what constitutes a specific group of head-injured children. There are also controversies over the definition of hyperkinetic disorder and attention deficit-hyperactivity disorder, and there is consequently a lack of consensus on whether there is in fact any characteristic impairment of cognition in hyperactive children (Prior and Sanson, 1986). Accordingly, the question needs to be addressed indirectly; and one way is to describe the available knowledge about the functional impairments of those with head injury and those with a behaviourally defined syndrome of hyperkinesis or attention deficit.

The cognitive changes after severe head injury have often been described, but they have not yet been given sufficiently experimental analysis that could help to illuminate their nature (Johnson, 1989). Van Zomeren, Brouwer and Deelman (1984), describe some of the attentional changes seen in adult subjects. The speed of information processing may be reduced, and memory is often impaired. However, there is very little evidence to suggest that there is a deficiency of selective attention, and studies of alertness, during vigilance and reaction times do not sustain the view that there is a reduced level of arousal. On the contrary, Brouwer (1985) suggests that head-injured adults show increased tonic alertness, at least in the experimental situation. The possibility of impaired phasic alertness is suggested by this work, in terms of lowered preparation for action. The possible relevance of this notion to impairments of higher level cognition, resulting from frontal lobe pathology, is intriguing but, as yet, speculative.

As in adults, so in head-injured children, the cognitive deficits have not yet been given any specific basis. Severe head injury appears to produce a general effect upon a range of different tests, including most of the subtests of the Wechsler Intelligence Scales for Children (Chadwick, Rutter, Brown *et al.*, 1981). Relatively little can be said beyond this. The speed of visuomotor and visuospatial function can be impaired more specifically, and is reduced in some children who show no other difficulty (Chadwick, Rutter, Brown *et al.*, 1981); and in other investigations slower motor speed of performance, language deficits and memory impairment have been particularly common (Levin and Eisenberg, 1979). The common behavioural description of poor concentration does not seem to be supported by clear evidence of a selective attention deficit; but of course there is a great gulf between behavioural concepts of poor concentration and any process of attention yet suggested by theory (Taylor, 1986). In view of the slowness of children in several tasks, it would be helpful to mount research into the psychophysiological responsiveness of injured children to stimuli.

One possibility, which deserves to be tested, is that children with disturbed attention following head injury show the pattern of diminished responsiveness to novel or signal stimuli, that seems to characterize children with Attention Deficit-Hyperactivity Disorder (ADHD) (Taylor, 1986). Several studies comparing ADHD cases with age-matched controls from the general population have found a reduction in autonomic indices of phasic response to simple auditory and visual stimuli (Hastings and Barkley, 1978). This is in contrast to the lack of clear evidence for an alteration of tonic arousal; and the pattern is rather similar to that noted above for head-injured adults. It would be premature to conclude that similar neurophysiological mechanisms are at work after head injury to those in ADHD, but the speculation can be made. The research, however, has left unclear the exact associations of decreased unresponsiveness in those with ADHD. Possibly, autonomic and EEG changes are characteristic of an impaired ability to concentrate, but they could also be associated with different aspects of the syndrome, such as motor clumsiness or defiant or aggressive behaviour.

It is also possible that amphetamine-type drugs will have a similar benefit in learning problems after head injury to the effects which have been demonstrated in children with ADHD (Taylor, 1986). Anecdotes of injured children suggest that their test performance may be enhanced by methylphenidate treatment; but I know of no controlled trial in such a group of subjects. The value of medication deserves more assessment (see Eames, this volume).

Is the pattern of neuropsychological test deficits in ADHD similar to that of children with impaired attention or disinhibition following head injury? The question is difficult to answer, in spite of the abundance of experimental work into the psychological abilities of children diagnosed as showing attention deficit disorder. The findings are contradictory to a degree: reviewers have been able to conclude both that ADHD is associated with specific disabilities in the maintenance and focusing of attention over time (Aman, 1984) and that there is no problem in anything that a psychologist could regard as attention (Prior and Sanson, 1986)! The field has been bedevilled by inconsistent and invalid definitions of cases and by artefacts resulting from the comparison of psychiatrically referred cases with controls drawn from the general population. It is worth mentioning results from a recent study in which standardized measures were applied to a population sample (Taylor, 1988). The investigation used a multiple-stage design, in which a community sample of 3,215 boys aged 6 to 7 years were screened with rating scales by teachers and parents; comparison groups were selected on the basis of their rating scale scores for intensive study; and diagnostic groups were defined on the basis of the intensive measures and compared on a range of cognitive, neurological and psychosocial measures. Disruptive behaviour was common, and subgroups of boys with different types of disruptive behaviour could be selected for detailed study. It was possible to set up contrasting groups with pure hyperactivity, pure attention deficit, pure conduct disorder ('pure' in the sense that they were free of other types of disorder, including head injury), mixed hyperactivity and conduct disorder, and a control group that did not meet criteria for any of these types of disorder. The groups were valid in that the detailed measures taken at the second stage confirmed that they differed from one another in the expected ways. Hyperactive boys performed slightly less well than the non-hyperactive conduct-disordered on tests of attention such as a continuous performance test of vigilance, a digit span test, and the MFF-20 test of impulsiveness versus reflectiveness (Cairns and Cannock, 1978). They were more active and inattentive in their behaviour during testing, but there were few other differences from normal controls. A mixed group of hyperactive-conduct disorder boys showed a more severe impairment of concentration and were delayed in learning to read. The biggest cognitive impairment was found in a group of non-hyperactive boys with attention deficit: they also showed lower Verbal and Performance IQs (Wechsler, 1974) and poorer language development than controls. The cause did not seem to be connected with early injury to the brain or delays in motor development: if it was an immaturity of development, it was a rather isolated one. The detailed behavioural measures of the second stage were then used to define a group of boys each of whom was individually characterized as showing hyperkinetic disorder. They were separable from those with non-hyperactive conduct disorder by an early onset of problems and a strong association with cognitive impairment, motor clumsiness, language delay and perinatal risk. In short, both hyperkinetic disorder and non-hyperactive attention deficit were associated with poor performance on many psychological tests. The nature of their neuropsychological deficit was not a simple failure of the mechanism of sustaining focused attention. The length of the test was not a determinant of whether impairment would be shown, and errors were as likely at the beginning of tests as at the end. Indeed, it may be doubted whether the deficit can usefully be described as one of a central process of attention at all. There was certainly a tendency to make more errors in several tests. While central learning was particularly poor, however, incidental learning was not any better. This seems to refute the notion that the deficit comes from an excessive breadth of attention. If that were the case, then less good performance on the intended task should be associated with better processing of peripheral and task-irrelevant information: this was not found. Whatever the difficulty is in test performance, it does not result directly from a shift of processing resources towards irrelevant stimuli at the expense of important ones. Indeed, the striking aspect of inattentive behaviour was the range and severity of cognitive impairment with which it was associated. We suggested that an unfocused and disorganized style of behaviour could have caused children to live in a less stimulating environment, and therefore to have reached a lower level of cognitive development. This explanation would obviously not apply to the situation in which a sudden event such as head injury causes an acute reduction of performance. We also suggested that disorganization was often interpreted by parents and teachers as evidence of antisocial behaviour, even when there was no other kind of defiant or rule-breaking behaviour. For head-injured children too, their problems in self-control can sometimes be misinterpreted as a motivated disobedience or as a moral failure.

It seems, therefore, that several patterns of inattentive and disorganized behaviour can be recognized clinically. One of them is the restless, distractible, impulsive pattern of hyperactivity. Another is the dreamy, unresponsive style of child with a 'pure attention deficit'. Both these are likely to be seen in some head-injured children but the most characteristic style after brain injury is one of disinhibited and forgetful behaviour. In the state of present knowledge, all appear to be associated with a general rather than a specific cognitive impairment. Further study will be needed, both to analyze the behaviours involved and to test hypotheses about the nature of the cognitive impairment. It will then be clearer whether these patterns need to be treated differently, or all have the same pathological basis.

Case study

One case history illustrates the differences between the types of dysregulation. Ian was born with congenital agenesis of the lower cranial nerve nuclei, and in consequence had much trouble in learning to eat and swallow: from the first year of life he was noted by physicians and nurses to be exceptionally active, exploratory and boisterous to the point of uncontrollability. By the age of 7 he was identified as a very difficult classroom problem and a 'whirlwind of activity'. At that time he was given standardized cognitive and behavioural research measures of activity and attention (Taylor, Schachar, Thorley *et al.*, 1986), which documented a very limited concentration span. In interview he changed activities about every fifteen seconds, and persisted in tasks introduced by the examiner for about ten seconds only; he was over-friendly, and physically affectionate to strangers; his Verbal and Performance IQ's were both in the 'bright average' range. This, of course, was a typical presentation of hyper-kinetic disorder and there was a good response to treatment with methylphenidate. He began to learn to read, but remained rather impulsive and isolated among his peers. A year later, he fell out of a tree where, characteristically, he was playing on his own and probably without much thought of danger. He sustained a severe closed head injury and was in a coma for twelve days, during which time there was extensor rigidity in all limbs. He eventually made a good neurological recovery, but was left six months later with a 20-point drop in Performance IQ and an increased difficulty in coping with classroom demands. Repeat testing (off medication) demonstrated that his new pattern of problems was not simply an intensification of his former disorder. Attention span was at a similarly low level; reaction time was longer; and both forward and backward digit span were particularly impaired, suggesting limited capacity. His activity level in structured situations was actually much lower than previously. He was less impulsive, and it was more difficult to arouse his interest in new things or toys. Qualitatively his impulsiveness and distractibility had changed to one of forgetfulness and lack of interest. Methylphenidate no longer seemed to be of much help, and was discontinued without adverse results.

Mechanisms of association between head injury and impaired self-regulation

There are several possible reasons why children whose brains have been injured might be at risk for changes in attentive and controlled behaviour. The behaviour problem could have contributed to an accidental injury; the accident could make other people behave differently to the affected child; treatment could be harmful; or the injury could be the direct cause of the problem.

As the above case history has emphasized, some children are hyperactive before the injury. This may be the result of psychosocial or constitutional factors. There are many causes of head injury, including the actions of parents and other adults. Craft, Shaw and Cartlidge (1972), found that 4 per cent of their cases of head injury in children were caused by parental assault. There are many psychosocial associations even of accidental injury to children. Multivariate studies that allow for several social variables have shown that stresses in the family (including household moves and other family life events) and a lower educational level in mothers are linked to accidents (Langley, 1984). Accidents do not happen to a random cross-section of children, but qualities of the victims predispose them to injury. Being a male is the clearest factor, and indeed deaths from accidents in this age group are three times as common in boys as in girls. This large risk is presumably mediated through the different behaviour of boys and the different degrees of control that are applied to boys and girls. Boys tend to take more risks and to be more venturesome and impulsive. Even within groups of boys with antisocial behaviour, those with a hyperkinetic pattern of symptoms are distinguished from other clinic referrals by a higher frequency of accidents (Taylor, Schachar, Thorley *et al.*, 1986).

The recent epidemiological study of hyperactivity, already cited, included a systematic study of accident frequency in longitudinally followed cohorts of hyperactive and non-hyperactive children (Davidson and Taylor, 1987). This replicated the finding that accidents are more common in the severely hyperkinetic; but it did not find milder degrees of hyperactivity to be a risk factor at all. Most hyperactive children are allowed out of the house at a younger age than their fellows, but this does not translate into an increased prevalence of accidental injury. Accordingly, one should not assume from the presence of hyperactivity in an injured child than it must have been the cause of the injury. Neither should one over-estimate the contribution of the caretakers' actions. Overprotection and restrictiveness are likely to be a common pattern of family relationships after head injury, but they are likely to be risk factors for social adjustment generally rather than for the self-control deficits considered in this chapter (Taylor, Schachar, Thorley *et al.*, 1986).

The actions of doctors may well play a part. Anticonvulsant medication is often given prophylactically, and is well known to cause disorders of attention and activity. Phenobarbitone has a particularly poor reputation, and several controlled trials have shown that it does indeed cause aggression and other behaviour disorders (Wolf and Forsythe, 1978) and impairs memory (Camfield, Chaplin, Doyle *et al.*, 1979). Carbamazepine has a better clinical reputation than phenobarbitone, and does indeed have positive psychotropic properties in some circumstances. It should not be forgotten, however, that in other circumstances even this anticonvulsant can be harmful. When given to non-epileptic hyperactive children it tends to impair concentration and behaviour control (Esser, Schmidt and Witkop, 1984). Furthermore, many of the drugs given to control aggressive or agitated behaviour disturbances, such as the phenothiazines and butyrophenones, have sedative properties (Taylor, 1985). They tend to impair concentration, especially when given at higher doses. It is important that attention and self-control should be accurately monitored during any such therapy.

Finally, brain injury may cause direct damage to brain systems involved in the processes of self-regulation and maintenance of attention. Frontal lobe pathology is evidently one possible explanation: the secure tethering of this part of the brain may well make it more vulnerable to direct neuronal damage in closed head injury, involving the mechanism of rapid acceleration-rotation-deceleration forces. In contrast, a study of localized, compound head injuries with skull depression and dural tears did not suggest that there was any simple relationship between the part of the brain injured and the emergence of behavioural or cognitive symptoms (Chadwick, Rutter, Thompson, *et al.*, 1981). One of the few associations between locus of damage and a high prevalence of disorder was found for right frontal (and left parietotemporal) injuries; but the symptoms were affective rather than those of hyperactivity. Nevertheless, the lack of specific anatomical or known neurochemical correlates of disorder is not an argument against the physical causation of disorder. On the contrary, the associations of disorder with severity of injury and with the development of epilepsy suggest that an organic pathogenesis is important.

Concluding remarks

The methods of operant conditioning and cognitive therapy have both proved effective in studies of hyperactive children with normal brains (Yule, 1986). The increase of attention span is particularly helpful by enabling children to practise educational tasks more effectively. Their effect might well seem feeble if they were assessed in unselected groups of children recovering from trauma, for only a majority will have the attentional and behavioural dyscontrol considered in this chapter. Single case studies, and trials directed to this subgroup, would have the power to assess the effect of this component of rehabilitation and treatment.

Chapter 10

Learning and behaviour change

Judith Middleton

Introduction

When a child returns home and resumes education following a head injury, clinical experience suggests that subtle as well as gross behaviour changes begin to emerge which were perhaps not so evident in the unfamiliar but relatively structured hospital ward. For the child's future development it is crucial to examine the nature of such changes. Before looking at the ways in which learning and behaviour change following head injury however, it is necessary to examine critically the basic assumption that there is a direct link between brain injury and changed behaviour. It is reasonable to assume that some behaviour and learning difficulties may be partly related to brain injury, but equally it would be wrong to suppose that there is direct evidence that specific deficits relate to particular damage to the central nervous system (CNS). Fletcher and Taylor (1984) list four fallacies relating to the type and strength of the brain-behaviour inferences that are commonly made in child neuropsychology. Firstly, there is the assumption that those procedures appropriate and valid for adults are equally so for children; however, children are not small adults, especially in terms of CNS organization. A second assumption is that tests which have been developed for adults measure the same abilities in children; this appears to ignore the fact that as children get older the organization of their abilities changes. Thirdly, there is the assumption that brain injury in children can have specific and distinct behavioural consequences. Although the discovery of relationships between brain and behaviour is useful, it does not constitute direct proof of isomorphism. Closed head injury seems more likely to result in generalized disruption of brain function in children, than in adults (Rutter, 1981). Furthermore, injury to the same part of the brain in children and adults may give rise to different behavioural changes. Finally, there is the error of over-interpreting behavioural tests or observations. The core of the problem here is mistaking dysfunction as a description of brain, rather than of behaviour. For instance, acting out in the classroom is not a description of frontal lobe injury, although this may be a contributory factor, but a description of a child not being able to cope in a classroom environment for any number of reasons.

Unfortunately, the use of more sophisticated diagnostic tools such as computerized tomography (CT) and Magnetic Resonance Imaging (MRI) do not necessarily help in identifying much of the pathology of the brain or in correlating it with dysfunctional behaviour. For instance, a survey of ninety-eight children who received a CT scan following head injury (Rivera, Tanaguchi, Parish *et al.*, 1987) found that no combination of clinical findings in the emergency room was able to predict all abnormal CT scan results. Increasing developments in MRI may prove more sensitive. Levin, Amparo, Eisenberg *et al.*, (1987) compared CT and MRI results in relation to neurobehavioural deficits of both mild and moderate head injuries in adults. MRI was more sensitive in disclosing lesions (i.e., showed more and larger lesions) than CT scan. Further, MRI and neuropsychological testing undertaken one and three months later showed considerable reductions in lesion size which paralleled improvements in cognition and memory. The implications of these findings will hopefully provoke further research into the issue of brain-behaviour inferences following head injury in children.

Learning and behaviour

With these cautions in mind, it is now useful to look at the close relation between learning and behaviour. The great majority of our behaviour is learnt. Children learn and develop by observing and imitating; by actively experimenting and receiving feedback from their behaviour and the environment; by curiosity; and through being specifically taught by adults and their peers. Throughout these stages, it is possible only to infer that learning has occurred from observing behaviour. The process of learning itself cannot be observed directly.

As behaviour is planned, initiated, effected, stored and retrieved in the CNS, when the brain is injured by head trauma it is likely that behaviour will also be affected, especially during early recovery. What inferences can we make about changes in the learning process? This question is important, as changes in the ability to learn are likely to change behaviour. Yet teachers and parents often comment that a child's behaviour has changed since the accident, and that there have also been learning difficulties, as if the two were completely independent. Consequently when a child's behaviour is different following a head injury we must consider if the ability to learn has also changed, carefully delineating the respective contributions of each.

The dichotomy between behaviour and learning is not necessarily useful, however, and may indeed be counter-productive, in as much as a child may exhibit maladaptive behaviour following head injury which reflects both cognitive and emotional changes. Changes in the process of learning can lead to a reduced self-image and frustration giving rise to difficult behaviour which, in turn, may interfere with learning capacity.

Learning — content and process

An important issue to consider is what is meant by learning. The same description covers both the content or product of what is learnt, as well as the process of learning. It may be that a child can superficially reproduce the content of previous learning which, therefore, appears relatively unchanged. Conversely, a child may return to the same classroom after an absence of a few months, and changes in the observed content of performance may be seen as due to the gains the class as a whole have made in his absence. In other words, poor comparative functioning may be seen as lost classroom experience which can be made up with hard work and extra tuition. The major problem, however, is that the process of learning new material may become dysfunctional. Figure 10.1 illustrates a simplified model of the processes between the initial stimulus or intention to act and the response or act itself. Motivation, levels of arousal, perception, attention, speed of information processing, memory and organization may be variably dysfunctional after head injury and need to be carefully assessed. Post-traumatic disruption of any one of these cognitive processes will detrimentally affect learning and so cause changes in observed behaviour.

Models of learning

To illustrate this, it is worthwhile looking at the effects of disruption in the learning process by considering three theoretical models in which learning is inferred from changed behaviour:

Classical and operant conditioning

In the classical model (Pavlov, 1960) neutral antecedants become associated with, and then elicit patterns of behaviour, when children learn to behave (Y) in the presence of a stimulus (X). In the operant model (Skinner, 1953) children learn that doing Y causes something (Z), pleasurable or not, to follow. As Figure 10.1 illustrates, these extremely simple sequences imply a number of necessary steps. Firstly, children must be able to focus, attend to and experience X and Y, or Y and Z. Secondly, they must be able to link Y and Z etc., and then encode, store and recall those steps having a link. Thirdly, they must have the ability to plan, initiate and execute the action which will bring about a desired action or goal. Motivation to act is important and the speed with

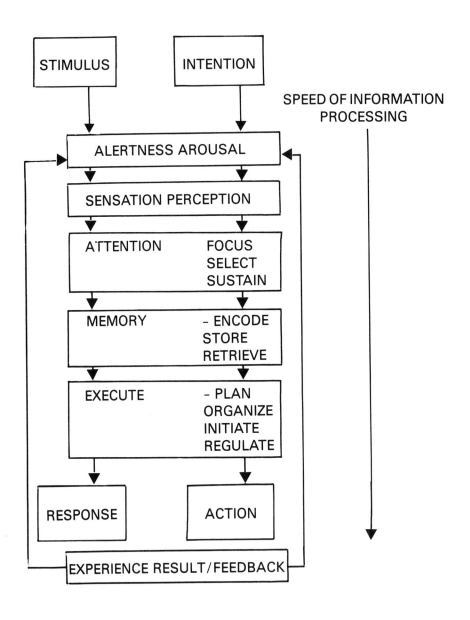

Figure 10.1: Steps in Processing Between Stimulus/Intention to Act and Response/Action

which this information can be processed may also be crucial. This entire process, once learnt, may be at an automatic level. For example young children do not usually make a conscious effort to learn how to walk and talk, and once these skills are learnt they walk and talk with little thought or conscious effort. As children develop they increasingly use greater conscious control to facilitate the learning process. Thus, when they begin to read and write, greater application and effort is needed in order to learn these skills, which gradually become automatic with practise. Analyzed in this way, the simple Stimulus-Response or Response-Response sequence is seen to be more complex than would first appear.

Goldstein and Oakley (1985) reviewed reports of association learning (classical and operant conditioning) and memory in humans and animals, and argued that this type of learning can remain unchanged even in the presence of diffuse cortical brain damage, as it may be mediated by subcortical brain structures which may be largely spared. Clinical evidence (Wilson, 1981; Woods and Eames, 1981) is cited to support the conclusions that, despite gross CNS damage, behaviour can be modified and learnt. That is not to say that tasks or the content of learning do not need to be adapted to the child's level of understanding and information processing, nor that the learning environment has to be substantially different from any normal reinforcing situation. Rather, the emphasis should be on individually tailored interventions at all times, with high levels of stimulation and training. A good example is the case of a 13 year old boy who sustained diffuse cortical damage from a severe head injury sustained in a road traffic accident. He was in coma for over two months and still had no bladder control eight months after injury. The parents had been told that only surgery would help his incontinence problems and, even so, the probability of a complete cure was not very high. Although his comprehension was very limited, a structured, twenty-four hour behaviour modification programme was devised in which continence was consistently rewarded. As successes increased and his ability to communicate slowly returned, the programme was adapted to teach him to control when he need to empty his bladder. Thirty-five weeks later he was completely continent and able to indicate when he needed to go to the toilet. This case history clearly illustrates that, despite severe impairments, some learning is possible even at a very basic but socially essential level. A reduced speed at which learning or relearning can take place means that structure and persistence are essential but can be effective.

Although association learning may remain intact following head injury, any one of the steps between attending to a stimulus or planning an action and its execution may become disrupted. When a child cannot recall that Y follows X he is unlikely to do X to obtain Y unless at random. To the observer this could appear as simply a lack of motivation to learn. Similarly, a child may be able to recall what to do in order to obtain Y, but is unable to initiate or organize that action. The observer might assume he has not learnt that Y follows X, while in fact that is not so. Thus, our interpretation of his failure may be wrong. If we openly express this to the child, suggesting that he is not trying when this is not true, for example, then his motivation may be reduced. He may become frustrated, his performance may decline and he may fail to try in future — a self-fulfilling prophecy of failure.

Observation and imitation

A child also learns through observing and listening to the world about him. Watching others act, he learns through imitation and experiment (Bandura, 1969). He will assimilate and modify what he observes, increasing his repertoire of behaviour and his ability to control and adapt to his environment. Consequently any perceptual deficit is likely to affect his ability to learn. Attempting to learn an action through observation and finding it either totally or even partially impossible to replicate because it has been misperceived may prevent any further attempts. Equally, the pace at which the observed action is performed may be too fast for the child's reduced speed of information processing. The need to sustain attention for any reasonable length of time may be outwith his capabilities. He thereby fails to observe the crucial, small steps comprising the action and, thus, is unable to perform the task.

Cognitive models

Another way of looking at the same phenomena is from a cognitive model (Piaget, 1954). A child may predict that if he behaves in a certain way, he will achieve certain desired consequences. In early childhood this process may be non-verbal; in time the child will be able to think about the steps and, later still, reflect on his own process of learning. At any age, if his experience proves him right then he will have learnt that his behaviour can be effective in gaining desired goals.

Prior to a head injury a child will have learnt a repertoire of behaviours, stored in long term memory, which will have enabled him to control his environment to a greater or lesser extent. Following injury, the processes which he used to predict, effect and experience control over his environment and behaviour may be dysfunctional. Attentional, memory and perceptual difficulties may distort his ability to predict his own and others' behaviour. Problems with initiating, planning and organization may make him unable to effect or control an intended action. For instance he may be hungry and have a meal in front of him, but be unable to organize and control the necessary sequence of arm, lip and tongue movements in order to take a mouthful of food. Even if he is able to predict and effect an action, sensory and perceptual deficits may prevent him from experiencing the consequences of his behaviour without distortion. Food may appear tasteless, thus lessening the desire to eat, whilst feelings of hunger or satiation may be disturbed leading to hypo- or hyper- phagia. In such circumstances the child's understanding and motivation to predict and to learn from experience may be changed. His previously successful cognitive model has essentially become ineffective.

In summary, subsumed in each of the above models of learning is a complex process, where the importance of appreciating the multiple influences and steps in even the most simple action a child effects needs to be emphasized in order to understand how just one dysfunctional facet of the learning process may give rise to pervasive difficulties.

Contributory factors

Changes in behaviour and learning ability displayed by children with head injury need to be seen within a wider context than that described above. Goldstein and Levin (1985) argue that research into children's head injury has often failed to look at potentially important factors such as premorbid functioning, personality and age. Figure 10.2 illustrates the context in which we need to see problems in order to understand these changes. Developmental age at injury and time since injury; premorbid functioning and personality; present environmental expectations and changes in the process of learning will all influence changes in behaviour (Rutter, Chadwick and Shaffer, 1984; Levin, Ewing-Cobbs and Benton, 1984; Shapiro, 1985; Haas, Cope and Hall, 1987), as will the child's self-awareness and self-image.

Environmental demands and expectations

When a child who has suffered a head injury leaves hospital, he generally returns to an environment which is essentially unchanged. The hospital ward will generally have been unfamiliar to the child's earlier experience, but is also likely to have been adapted to meet his present needs. Consequently, some of his behaviour may not have appeared particularly dysfunctional, because of environmental adaptations, and any apparent changes could be attributable to a normal reaction to the strangeness of the hospital environment. The demands of both home and school, however, may be unchanged unless they are particularly adapted to individual needs. Where adaptations have been made, it is most likely that these are focused around any physical disability resulting from the head injury. Changes in behaviour may become more apparent at home, although parents may deny difficulties or accommodate to them unconsciously. For instance, parents described a 9 year old boy with a severe head injury as having no behaviour problems, but failed to indicate that on trips to the supermarket he climbed into the deep freeze. Thus, children's behaviour becomes part of a changed system influenced by, and inflencing, parental expectations and attitudes.

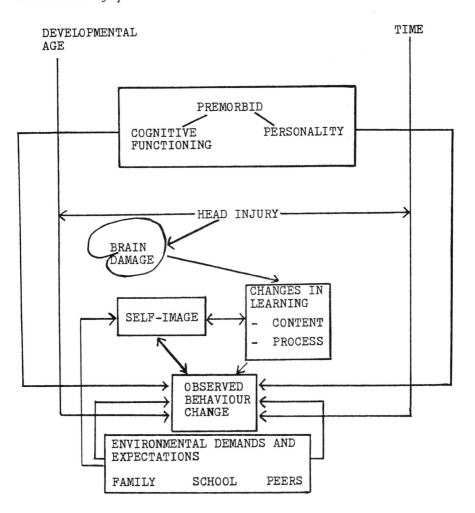

Figure 10.2: The Context of Head Injury

Once a child appears to have made a good physical recovery and, to all intents and purposes looks better, parents are often keen for early return to school with expectations that he will function normally to the challenges of the classroom, challenges which he had previously met. At this point any changes in behaviour may become more apparent, because of the discrepancy between normal demands made in the classroom and the now limited capacity of the child's brain. Conversely, where there is prolonged coma with very severe damage, then expectations of some parents and professionals may be greatly reduced, which can lead to self-fulfilling prophecies. A child who is consequently left to recover spontaneously with no effective intervention or rehabilitation may make limited progress. The case of an 11 year old girl illustrates this point. She was reportedly in persistent vegetative state for seven months after head injury, being cared for on a paediatric ward where she was apparently left to recover spontaneously. The expectations for her recovery, by some hospital professionals, were low and so she was given minimal therapy and made little improvement. Transferred for rehabilitation where she was expected to make some improvement, she underwent intensive therapy from an interdisciplinary team. Rehabilitation helped her to partially regain some skills and, although she required surgery for her contractures, two years after her accident she walked out of the unit with help, and whispered a faint good-bye. A single case study design showed that very carefully structured step-by-step teaching improved performance which did not change prior to training. Positive expectations and the necessary and consequent changed environmental demands modified her behaviour and learning.

Parents of children with severe head injuries may also become over-protective and less strict in their discipline following the injury (Brown, Chadwick, Shaffer *et al.*, 1981). If, for example, a child is seen as sick, limits may not be set on inappropriate behaviour as they had been in the past. This can mean that the very structure and boundaries which are necessary in order to help the child learn, predict and make sense of his world are removed or inconsistent. For example, inappropriate sexual behaviour may be tolerated or excused in the home or on the ward, but failure to set very clear limits on this behaviour does not help the child to learn to discriminate between situations. Rather, he learns that this behaviour is tolerated and, once outside the protected environment of ward or home, it can lead to serious consequences. At the same time he may be protected from taking even the smallest risks, such as going outside to play alone, which will be necessary at some point in order to learn independence because of fears (sometimes justifiable) that he has no sense of danger.

Family expectations and demands will change with time. It is possible that the family will need to go through some form of bereavement process for their previously normal child in order to accept him with long-term impairments (Hall, this volume). Their expectations will change as they go through this natural process, hence the need to re-assess the family situation continually.

Age

The time from injury to his return to home or school may be a matter of only a few days but, in cases of severe injury, it can be months or even years. Analysis of changes in behaviour, therefore, needs to take into account a child's age at injury and whether his behaviour is now seen as delayed and/or deviant from what might be expected, had the injury not occurred.

Although children were initially thought to have a better predicted recovery than adults after brain injury (Lenneberg, 1967; Smith and Sugar, 1975), the evidence now suggests the contrary, with children under the age of eight years having poorer expected recovery than adolescents and adults (Levin, Ewing-Cobbs and Benton, 1984). To understand changes in learning with regard to age at injury, questions must focus on whether a child has lost a skill he possessed at an earlier age; whether he has retained it but its development is delayed; or whether he has acquired behaviour which may be deviant because of the development of his injured and, therefore, abnormal brain. Fletcher, Miner and Ewing-Cobbs (1987) argue that age *per se* is not a mechanism of recovery. Using Zigler's model (1969) of cognitive development, they propose that as children learn different levels of skills, at varying rates, at different stages in their development, disruption of learning at one of the sensitive periods of acquisition may interrupt and distort the consolidation of learning a particular skill and the acquisition of later skills. The crucial question, they propose, is not one of whether the effect of age exists, but why it should occur.

Premorbid functioning and personality

When we consider children with head injuries, it is not just the uniqueness of the injury, the extent and site of damage to the brain, the length and depth of coma or PTA that is important, but also the uniqueness of the individual to which the damage is inflicted. A child's age is one factor in this but, premorbid cognitive functioning and personality can also influence recovery and the propensity to learn.

Rutter, Chadwick and Shaffer (1984) reported that children with mild head injuries, when compared to orthopaedic controls, had a history of learning difficulties prior to injury, while those with severe head injuries did not. It was concluded that although severe head injury caused impairment, there were no demonstrable cognitive sequelae following mild injury where PTA was less than twenty-four hours (Chadwick, Rutter, Brown *et al.*, 1981). One of the major problems in this study is the insensitivity of the clinical measures (Johnson, 1989) and over-reliance on intelligence quotients (IQ). The absoluteness of such findings is also challenged by Boll (1983), who argues that impairments in attention, memory and information processing can follow even relatively mild head injury. Similarly, Gulbrandsen (1984) found significant neuropsychological differences between children with mild head injuries and a matched control group.

Whatever the degree of impairment, it is clear that a child's premorbid level of functioning is an important factor when considering learning and behaviour during recovery. Premorbid difficulties may be exacerbated when the injuries are more severe, and at least temporarily if the injury is mild. Knowledge of premorbid behaviour and personality as well as of previous cognitive functioning is also crucial. Rutter, Chadwick and Shaffer (1984) have reported that following PTA of up to seven days no personality changes were found suggesting a rise in the incidence of new psychiatric disorder but, following severe head injury, the incidence was greatly increased. Clinical experience also confirms that a child's pre-injury personality may influence behaviour and recovery and is, therefore, a crucial factor in understanding post-traumatic changes. Boll (1983), however, suggests that emotional irritability and lethargy can follow relatively mild injury, both of which can produce long-term effects on behaviour and learning. A tired child is likely to be irritable, less likely to learn, and generally more vulnerable to classroom stresses. This will compound attentional deficits and increase the probability of distractability which, in turn, will affect his learning and performance. Poor understanding of what is happening can increase frustration and lead to angry outbursts. Judgments and expectations may then follow, with the result that relatively mild problems can have serious consequences.

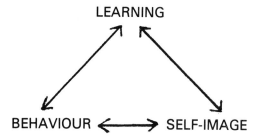

Figure 10.3: Learning, Behaviour and Self-Image

Self-image

A crucial factor which is often omitted from the assessment of factors contributing to recovery is the child's self-awareness and ability to reflect on the catastrophic changes that have occurred. As discussed above, difficulties in learning will alter observed behaviour. With a certain level of awareness the inability to learn and behave appropriately may also alter self-image (Figure 10.3). It may not be surprising to find a greatly increased incidence of psychiatric disorder in children following severe, rather than mild, head injury (Rutter, 1981). Children's self-image and the processes whereby they can understand themselves and their world (i.e., their cognitive skills) may be severely dysfunctional. If they have some insight into their problems, then the greater their difficulties are likely to be and, consequently, the greater may be their grief. This is in addition to any change in mood or social inhibition caused by focal injury to the brain, particularly the frontal lobes. Green (1985) humanely discusses three single cases from the basis of Personal Construct theory (Kelly, 1955), highlighting the need to understand the changed cognitive constructs of the child or adolescent in order to understand changed behaviour. Luria's (1972) account of the struggle to understand the shattered world and consequent self-image of a young soldier who received a penetrating head injury illustrates the close interaction of cognitive and emotional changes following head injury. The difficulties with which this man had to contend, with his adult's understanding of the world, will likely be far greater for the young adolescent and, particularly, the child who is trying to make sense of what has occurred to him. If this crucial aspect is ignored, then learning and behaviour changes in children with head injuries cannot be fully understood.

Conclusions

Other contributors to this volume have discussed the evidence of the effects of brain injury on learning and behaviour, findings which are commensurate with clinical experience in this field. Children with severe head injuries have poor attention and memory, perform more slowly and need time to take in and process instructions. Their ability to organize and plan is reduced. Even if these problems are only relatively slight they may nonetheless have quite profound and devastating effects on their learning capacity in the classroom where the pace of teaching can rarely be adjusted to that of a single child. Trying to keep up, let alone catch up, easily causes fatigue which affects performance. Frustration can arise when learning tasks become just that little bit too much to take in. A consequence of which may be a fall in motivation, or perhaps anger, changes in behaviour which can all too easily be simply attributed to not trying, laziness or acting out.

The problem for parents and professionals then is to determine the reasons for the changes in behaviour. Why can a child now not cope with previously met challenges? A central issue is the extent to which changes in behaviour are related to changes in learning ability, or to other factors. We need to consider the relative importance of many inter-relating factors:

1   the child at the time of the injury (age and premorbid functioning)
2   changes in the external world (expectations and attitudes)
3   changes within the child (cognitive and learning difficulties)
4   the child's understanding of the changes that have occurred, his ability to cope with them and the consequent effects on his behaviour.

Only when the relative importance of all these factors have been carefully assessed, can appropriate rehabilitation begin. What is important is the realization that the maximum potential recovery can be facilitated in the appropriately structured environment, that learning can take place and some behaviours can be changed following even severe head injuries (see Wood, 1987). This does not only mean that lost skills, such as speech, may be regained but, also that new ones can be learnt, such as an alternative means of communication. As the above cases illustrate, some basic personal and daily living skills, as well as complex skills, may also be relearnt if tackled with persistence and in a step-by-step approach.

Chapter 11

Psychiatric aspects of children's head injury

Peter Hill

Introduction

This chapter deals with the disorders of emotion, behaviour and personal relationships that may follow head injury in children. For convenience of presentation, they are grouped under three headings: predisposing factors, adjustment to acute trauma, and the long-term sequelae of head injury.

Predisposing factors

It is customary to think of the relationship between head injury and psychiatric problems as one of straightforward cause and effect. Usually this is appropriate; most children and adolescents who suffer traumatic head injuries and subsequent psychiatric disorder would have been psychologically normal before their injury. There is an appreciable minority, however, who were already affected by behavioural abnormalities before their injury, or who lived in unusual family situations which may have increased their likelihood of being injured.

The most powerful instance of this is head injury caused by non-accidental injury at the hands of parents or other carers. In such circumstances, the likely co-existing abnormal parental attitudes and practices will be a fertile breeding ground for psychiatric disorder in the child and, indeed, most children who are physically abused are subsequently found to show psychiatric symptoms, independently of whether the physical abuse caused a head injury (see Martin, 1980). Skulls may be fractured by direct blows, and Oliver (1975) has described how shaking, swinging or throwing babies can result in secondary microcephaly and severe mental handicap. Buchanan and Oliver (1977) estimated that 2.5 per cent of hospitalized severely mentally handicapped children were there as a result of shaking or battering. In such circumstances, both the head injury and emotional or behavioural disorder would be consequences of abnormal parenting.

It is interesting to note that of children who sustain head injuries in road traffic accidents, rather more have pre-existing behaviour disorders than would ordinarily be expected. Klonoff and Low (1974) estimated that roughly one-third of their series of school-age children admitted to hospital with a head injury had previously shown evidence of difficult or abnormal behaviour. In Craft, Shaw and Cartlidge's (1972) survey of children admitted to hospital with a head injury, fifteen out of 110 head-injured schoolchildren had pre-traumatic scores on the Rutter B (abnormal classroom behaviour) (Rutter, 1968) scale of over 12, compared with only three of 110 control subjects selected from the same school class as the head-injured children. Similarly, Brown, Chadwick, Shaffer *et al.* (1981) found that approximately one-third of children with mild head injury (post-traumatic amnesia between one hour and one week) had pre-traumatic psychiatric disorder, compared to children with severe head injury, whose rate of pre-traumatic psychiatric disorder was only slightly above that among controls. Apparently common factors amongst the families of children suffering accidents, include poor supervision of children secondary to parental preoccupation, illness, pregnancy or depression (Brown and Davidson, 1978) and extroverted, impulsive behaviour by the child (Manheimer and Mellinger, 1967) along with poor provision of opportunities to play within the home (Backett and Johnston, 1959). None of these factors alone appears sufficient to explain the excess of pre-traumatic psychological disturbance among children with mild head injuries. There are indicators which suggest, however, that they stand as proxies for an assortment of vulnerability factors for childhood psychological disturbance, including parental psychiatric disorder, adverse childhood temperamental features, and social disadvantage. What is not clear is why pre-traumatic emotional and behaviour problems should be over-represented among children with mild head injury but not appear to be excessive among those with severe head injury. Presumably there is some as yet unclarified distinction between the circumstances or mechanism of mild and severe injuries. For instance Klonoff (1971) suggests that the characteristics of children suffering mild head injuries are more similar to children experiencing injuries caused by falls than to those involved in road traffic accidents.

Reaction to acute injury

Following an accident in which a child sustains a severe head injury, a sequence of neurological and psychological reactions is likely to occur. The quality of these will vary according to the age of the child, the severity of the injury, the consequent neurological complications, and the responses of parents and hospital staff. As far as psychological reactions are concerned, there is value in adopting a framework, such as that suggested by Prugh (Prugh and Eckhardt, 1980), which proposes three stages of a generic, phasic response to acute, serious injury: impact, recoil and restitution. In severely head-injured children it is necessary to preface the stage of impact by a stage of coma and emergence from coma, and allow for the effects of confusion, memory loss and disinhibition on the child's attempts to adapt. In milder cases, particularly those wherein there are other tissue injuries or loss of function, the reaction is closer in style to the cases of respiratory paralysis secondary to poliomyelitis to which Prugh and Tagiuri (1954) originally applied their model.

Impact

This stage is dominated by a fear of annihilation. Concomitant confusion or delirium intensifies such fear and reassurance will only have a short-lived effect. As a result there is likely to be a defensive regression in order to elicit nurturance. This compounds the clinical picture of functional deficit secondary to neurological damage or dysfunction. There may be a massive withdrawal into mutism and helplessness, a state of psychic shock with a good prognosis which mimics the effects of gross neurological damage around the third ventricle and can lead to a diagnosis of akinetic mutism or 'locked-in' syndrome. Emerging from this state, after a period which can vary from a few days to several weeks rather than months, the child remains exceptionally self-centred and more helpless than either his years or injuries can account for. Associated with this, in Prugh's system, is a propensity for psychological denial. Personal experience suggests that this is more likely to follow, than accompany, gross regression and indicates that the child is becoming aware of his own helplessness. Unrealistic ambitions are voiced, such as becoming an air hostess, a champion cyclist or a pop star. Positive affirmations that paralysed limbs 'don't matter'and 'will be all right' may be stated with euphoric emphasis. Disentangling this from the specific effects of frontal lobe injury may be difficult, indeed often unnecessary since denial at this stage is likely to be helpful for the child in coming to terms with his injuries. Only when it prevents a child from making an active effort in activities or exercises will it impede rehabilitation.

Recoil

This phase follows impact, and represents the beginning of positive adaptation and coping, with an abandonment of regression and denial. Typically, the child becomes less preoccupied with himself and attempts to exert control over his environment. He asserts himself by demanding and arrogant behaviour. This may essentially be a defence against depressive feelings and pessimism as to the eventual outcome, as the bossiness interspersed with brief solitary weeping is commonly observed. Some teenagers and a few children will be overwhelmed by their misery and appear listless and depressed, eating erratically and sleeping poorly. This may be especially likely when the head injury was the result of carelessness, such as no rear light on the bicycle, so the guilt is rational to a certain extent. Irrational guilt arising from an assumption that the accident was a punishment is more likely to be an issue in primary or pre-school children, since they are more prone to egocentric and magical thinking.

Not all apparent misery results from guilt, or is a product of the child's sense of loss of previous integrity. Some children will have lost parents, siblings or friends in the accident which produced their head injury. Their unhappiness needs to be recognised as grief at the loss of others and dealt with supportively. This is the most difficult time for parents and nurses. It may last weeks or months, sometimes recurring as the child who has made unsteady progress relapses back into it, in the face of disappointments and setbacks.

Restitution

This third phase in Prugh's model is characterized by gradual accommodation to the disabilities resulting from injury. It is understood to be the development of a conscious, realistic adjustment to the situation but will inevitably be coloured by the child's personality and the support he receives. This means that it may not be entirely healthy and there is a risk of erratic and inadequate coping, such as unhelpful stubbornness, ingratiation or unrealistic independence.

Prugh's model is untested scientifically and, therefore, like all stage models it should not be taken too literally or rigidly. Clinical experience suggests that elements of different stages may exist simultaneously in one child. Furthermore, it is not established that, as a rule, a child must progress through one stage before the next. So long as it is recognized as a conceptual tool which can generate hypotheses, rather than a rigid blueprint, there seem good grounds for using the model to understand some of the post-traumatic behavioural disturbances in children. Prugh and Eckhardt (1980) suggest that it can be helpful in generating management implications. For instance, the withdrawal and mutism which may be encountered in the impact stage should be seen as adaptive and not a challenge to be countered by attempts to 'break through', since these may serve only to intensify it. The recommended response to demanding and apparently hostile behaviour during the recoil period is to set limits to it, whilst understanding that such difficult behaviour need not be taken personally. Encouragement to express feelings of loss or misery through speech or drawings may allow the recognition and working through of depressive feelings so that these need not be defended against by excessive omnipotence. It may be helpful to enable the child to participate actively in his own management and care, allowing him to make choices for example, in order to lessen his sense of helplessness. Within the restitution stage, an attitude of firm encouragement is argued to be preferable to a laissez-faire approach which might reinforce the child's feelings of worthlessness and poor self-esteem which can follow his realization of his loss of skills or altered social presentation of self. Similarly, it is suggested that forcing a child prematurely into rehabilitation may carry the risk of provoking depression or anxiety at anticipated failure. Whilst there is clearly some sense in such proposals, the separation of rehabilitation from early clinical care is questionable; there should be a seamless progression from one to the other.

Long-term psychiatric sequelae of closed head injury

Adjustment to the acute crises of hospitalization following injury may be associated with emotional and behavioural disturbances, as described above. Some older children and adolescents may show a short-lived episode of agitated, excitable or disinhibited behaviour as they emerge from post-traumatic amnesia, but this is not particularly common. Most research interest in psychiatric pathology has centred around the longer term consequences of head injury. To avoid selection bias, studies have usually been structured as a follow-up of a group of head-injured children. Any such series will contain a preponderance of mild head injury cases, reflecting their greater clinical incidence. For example, Rune (1970) mailed questionnaires about possible head injury to all families with 7 to 16 year old children in a small Swedish town. Non-responders were telephoned so that ultimately a 100 per cent response rate was achieved. Fifteen per cent of the children were reported to have suffered a severe blow to the head (and there were grounds for thinking this an underestimate) of which only about a quarter were admitted to hospital; 9 per cent of the children had been concussed and 5 per cent had lost consciousness, although only just over one-third of the latter were admitted to hospital. Information on the children and their families was obtained from a variety of sources, but the psychiatric signs and symptoms asked about were very few, assessment at interview was extremely limited, and the diagnoses given (e.g., 'psychic insufficiency') have no parallels with contemporary psychiatric practice. Nevertheless, from examining this report's tables one may infer a general rate of about 12 per cent for psychiatric disturbance among children hospitalized with head injury, compared with a rate of 4 per cent among controls. This appears to be a significant comparative difference but a small overall prevalence. Children who were not admitted to hospital with their head injury and did not suffer significant loss of consciousness, occupied an intermediate position for psychiatric disturbance.

It makes sense, therefore, to concentrate on children who have been admitted to hospital as the most vulnerable group for the development of psychiatric disorder. Black, Jeffries, Blumer *et al.* (1969), conducted a follow-up of 105 consecutive cases of head injury among children up to the age of 14 seen at the Johns Hopkins Hospital. All had skull fractures, documented loss of consciousness or neurological dysfunction.

One year after injury, eighty-seven cases were studied from the point of view of behaviour. The most common and troublesome problems were with irritability and tantrums, hyperkinesis, poor attention and headache. All showed a statistically significant increase over pre-traumatic levels, with prevalence rates typically doubling, but only a minority of children were troubled in each case. Even in the case of headache, the most common symptom, post-traumatic prevalence was only 27 per cent compared to a pre-traumatic rate of 10 per cent. The authors suggested that 36 per cent of children acquired new symptoms or exhibited severe aggravation of pre-morbid traits. Half of these were headache, suggesting a rate of 18 per cent for behavioural problems attributable to the injury. This figure is derived from the total sample; within the group studied, behavioural sequelae were less likely with age, but headache was more so. There was no difference in the rate of problems according to whether abnormal behaviour existed before the injury or not. The value of this study is the description of a cluster of post-traumatic symptoms and behaviours which clearly differ from those commonly seen following head injury in adults. Among children, for instance, vertigo, dizziness and anxiety were very rare. The study does not yield adequate information on psychiatric disorder since the children were not apparently interviewed, and there is no account of systematic interviewing of parents which would have yielded psychiatric diagnoses. Furthermore, the study was uncontrolled so that the possibility of behaviours emerging as a function of age cannot be excluded.

To meet such objections it is necessary to turn to the studies by Rutter and colleagues (see Brown, Chadwick, Shaffer *et al.*, 1981). These authors investigated thirty-one children with severe closed head injuries resulting in post-traumatic amnesia of seven days or more. They were compared with a matched control group of twenty-eight children with accidental orthopaedic injuries and a group of twenty-nine head-injured children with post-traumatic amnesia of less than seven days. This was a prospective study wherein the parents of children were given a semi-structured interview as soon as possible after the injury in order to obtain a picture of pre-injury psychiatric status. Structured assessments of the children and their families were then repeated at four, twelve and twenty-seven month intervals. The findings were fairly clear-cut; the mild head-injured group (PTA < 7days) were found to have a rate of pre-traumatic psychiatric disorder which was three times that found in the orthopaedic group (34 per cent compared to 11 per cent). It is important to note, however, that the orthopaedic group was matched only to the severe head injury group. Furthermore, the mild head injury group had higher rates of boys, social disadvantage and school achievement or adjustment problems than the other two groups. Nevertheless they showed no increase in the rate of psychiatric disorder over a one-year period following the injury. Those children with severe head injury (PTA < 7 days) showed a higher rate of new psychiatric disorder following injury, compared with the matched orthopaedic controls. The prevalence rate at the three assessment points was about 50 per cent, depending upon the precise method used to identify cases. Generally speaking, most of the psychiatric disorders arising after severe head injury showed no specific features and were generally comparable to psychiatric disorder as manifest in the general child and adolescent population. There were two diagnoses, however, which deserve special mention. At the twenty-seven month follow-up, three severely head-injured children were diagnosed as hyperkinetic. Two of these had previously been seriously disinhibited. This is somewhat awkward finding since, among hyperkinetic children generally, head injury is not a common cause of hyperkinetic disorder nor, evidently, do most head-injured children develop it. Indeed, restlessness and the total activity score (a composite) were significantly less common among the psychiatric disorders attributable to head injury than among disorders which predated injury. It is possible, however, that the diagnostic criteria for the recognition of hyperkinetic disorder overlap uneasily with social disinhibition. Certainly nothing emerged from this study which would even suggest that the hyperkinetic syndrome or hyperactivity as a sign complex were indicators of previous head injury.

The second diagnosis of note was that of disinhibited state, evident in five of the twelve cases of psychiatric disorder attributed to head injury. As the authors state, this is not a formal or conventional diagnosis, but it is familiar to all psychiatrists who deal with the consequences of head injury. The core feature was of marked socially disinhibited behaviour, including undue outspokenness without regard to social convention, frequently making very personal remarks, asking embarrassing questions, or getting undressed in social situations in which this would usually be regarded as unacceptable behaviour. In association with this core symptom were forgetfulness, overtalkativeness, carelessness in personal hygiene and dress, and impulsiveness. All children with this diagnosis had a PTA of more than three weeks. Apart from the general diagnoses, the incidence of specific symptoms arising post-traumatically was examined; only social disinhibition emerged as significantly more common among post-traumatic cases, although overeating, enuresis, overtalkativeness, general slowness, and stuttering were also commoner, but did not reach statistical significance. There was no evidence for any other pattern of symptoms indicating a more subtle disorder among head injury cases with no formal psychiatric diagnosis.

A salient feature of this study was the attempt to elucidate mechanisms of causation. Without presenting the arguments in detail, the elegance of the method must be taken for granted. The rate of post-injury disorder was over twice as high in severe cases compared with controls and these new disorders showed a proportional relationship with the duration of PTA, the degree of intellectual impairment and the presence of neurological signs. A causal association between severe head injury and psychiatric disorder was very strongly suggested, but there was no evidence that head injury with a PTA of one week or less was associated with new psychiatric disorder.

The work of Rutter and colleagues is undoubtedly a most thorough study of the effects of head injury on children's psychological health, yet some doubts remain. For instance, none of the children themselves were interviewed, which may have led to an under-reporting of emotional disorder, especially among adolescents in whom this is a well-recognised problem of method (Hill, 1985). Nor were any subjective assessments, such as self-esteem, carried out. The follow-up time seems short in view of a clinical suspicion that the lesser degrees of cognitive impairment may take several years to express themselves in academic or social failure. The small size of the sample probably led to the most severely injured children, those whose behvioural abnormalities can cause so much trouble for their families and rehabilitators (McCabe and Green, 1987), being under-represented or absent. At the other end of the severity scale there is some uneasiness over the finding of no new psychiatric disorder in the group with PTA lasting less than one week. One is reminded of Teuber's dictum that absence of evidence is not evidence of absence. There were no controls for this group which were, before injury, very different from the controls matched with severely head-injured children (more boys, more psychosocial adversity, more inner city addresses, more school achievement and adjustment problems, more antisocial, and so on). In fact, they were less thoroughly studied than the severely injured group. Although these limitations are discussed by the authors and judged unimportant, some clinicians (e.g., Middleton, 1989) remain sympathetic to the views expressed by Boll (1983). Whilst reiterating the familiar tenet that acceleration-deceleration of the head causes more damage to white matter by way of shearing injuries, fat embolism and local ischaemia, than penetrating injuries do; Boll points out that such injury may follow shocks and jars to the head even without a blow being struck. At the same time, animal studies show axonal degeneration follows only minor head injuries with only momentary loss of consciousness (Adams, Graham and Gennarelli, 1981). Consequently, it is argued that information processing difficulties and problems with learning in complex situations are likely to be common among children with minor head injuries who, therefore, have to spend more effort coping. Outward and objectively assessed normality is only achieved, therefore, at substantial effort and cost to the individual, rendering them more vulnerable to stress under which they may develop psychiatric pathology. Such views are, of course, speculative, but resonate with clinical experience. They might offer an explanation for the findings remarked upon by Black, Blumer, Wellner *et al.* (1971): hyperkinesis, affective symptoms and antisocial behaviour all increased during the first few months after injury in their study but then subsided to levels close to pre-injury status. Antisocial behaviour subsequently increased again, however, at four to five years after injury. Since antisocial behaviour in boys peaks in the early teens this may, of course, be merely an effect of age and have little to do with head injury, but it is in accord with the notion expressed by Bowman, Blou and Reich (1974), that psychological problems may not emerge overtly until a particular developmental stage places new adaptive demands upon the child and his nervous system.

Mechanisms

Rutter's group argue that causation of the emerging psychiatric disorders following severe head injury is likely to include indirect mechanisms (Brown, Chadwick, Shaffer *et al.*, 1981). In this respect the mechanism of causation differs from that involved in post-traumatic intellectual deficit which primarily results directly from injury and tissue loss. In the first place, some cases of psychiatric disorder which seemed causally associated with brain injury displayed no neurological signs and had no cognitive decrement. Also, post-injury psychiatric status was positively correlated with psychosocial adversity and pre-injury behavioural abnormalities to a certain extent, although not with post-traumatic physical disability.

Locus of injury, as an instance of a putative direct effect would seem to have little influence upon the rate or type of psychiatric pathology in children (Naughton, 1971; Shaffer, Chadwick, and Rutter, 1975). It seems at least possible from knowledge of individual cases, although not actually substantiated systematically, that the disinhibiton syndrome is preferentially associated with frontal lobe injury.

Cognitive deficit appears to be proportionally associated with psychiatric disorder. In Brown, Chadwick Shaffer *et al.*'s (1981) study, children with psychiatric disorder functionally related to head injury had a lower WISC Performance IQ (Wechsler, 1974). This may, of course, just be a reflection of severity of brain injury but there is the possibility that low intelligence reduces the ability to learn appropriate coping strategies and adapt to stressors, as seems to be the case with children in the general population. The consequences of a loss of cognitive skills will also result in school failure or transfer, changes of friends and leisure pursuits, with a sense of loss and loneliness being common complaints among these children.

Abnormalities of brain function resulting in epilepsy, hypertonus or extensor spasms, for example, can disrupt subjective experience and give rise to stigmatizing changes in the child's appearance. Mood changes such as apathy, irritability and impatience have an obvious effect on interpersonal interactions as well as having symptomatic importance in their own right. It is often asserted (Boll, 1983), and clinical experience confirms, that head-injured children may show an asthenic fatiguability, a reduction of mental resilience or stamina which impairs their tolerance for stress, whether physical (illness, medication) or emotional.

Iatrogenic influences include the effects of hospital admission which may involve enforced separation which might distort attachment formation in the young child, will clearly distress parents (particularly when intensive care is required) to an extent which may produce long-lasting alterations of their perception of the child, for example as even more precious and vulnerable. Anticonvulsant medication can have adverse effects on cognition and behaviour (Corbett and Trimble, 1984).

Alterations of parental behaviour and attitude would follow from the above and from the parent's perception of their child as vulnerable because of his history of injury or his overt handicaps. Chadwick (personal communication) indicates that unpublished data from the Institute of Psychiatry study suggests that parental handling of children changes after head injury with insufficient use of discipline, excessive appeasement, over-restrictiveness and unnecessary helping (i.e., overprotection in the traditional sense) being particularly common. Handling abnormalities were associated with the presence of psychiatric disorder in the child but, surprisingly, were said not to vary with the type of disorder.

Events associated with the accident causing the head injury

Given that the most common cause of severe head injury to children is road traffic accidents, in a proportion of instances the child will have parents, siblings or friends who are killed or injured at the same time. Bereavement responses or changes in caretaking arrangements will follow.

Personality alteration

Remarkably little has been written on the personality changes which can follow very severe head injury in children (arguably a PTA of more than one month) although these are familiar to interested clinicians. There is a risk of creating a stereotype by listing common problems but, in so far as these commonly appear to be overlooked by schools in particular, a stereotype may have its uses.

Memory deficits are common and devastating. At a minimal level, conversation becomes difficult because the thread is easily lost. There may be problems with time keeping, school work or shopping; with moderate deficits, self-care is limited on account of omissions and derailment whilst in mid-task. The consequences for educational and work careers are obvious and these adverse effects of poor memory will be intensified by slow mental information processing. At its worst, there is a delay of several seconds between question and answer, a further impediment to social conversation and a likely element in the progressive drift into social isolation which seems such a frequent problem for head-injured adolescents.

Social disinhibition, a lack of reserve and diminished modulation of familiarity, is notable among very severely head-injured adolescents and some older children; tact and social judgment are typically lacking. At an anecdotal level it appears to be less common among younger children. Many cases will show an associated mild euphoria and facile manner. Apathy and a striking loss of initiative as far as planning ahead is concerned may be primary difficulties, or the result of poor attention. On the other hand, a dominant mood may be irritability, with aggressive outbursts triggered by trivial incidents. The latter may interact with an obvious self-centredness and a lack of concern for others. Although egocentricity is quite often a recognizable trait, this is by no means compatible with frequent interfering with other childrens' classroom activities or siblings' possessions. A blunting of emotional responsiveness makes continuing social education extremely difficult to carry out, whilst impulsive acts may bring a teenager into contact with school authorities or the law. Sexual disinhibition in concert with novitiate status in the affairs of social sexuality breeds crude sexual overtures such as exhibitionism or forceful groping.

In teenagers, the parallels with adults who have frontal lobe pathology are clear. In the absence of systematic studies, it is much less certain how variations in the clinical picture correlate with localized injury in children. Clinical experience derived from individual cases is unreliable because of the extensive cerebral damage most of the author's cases have sustained.

No discussion of personality changes can omit the pathoplastic effect of social development, particularly as it progresses in adolescence. Loss of skills and abilities following serious head injury, or even the knowledge that one's brain has been harmed, forces the teenager into a self-appraisal of his identity (McCabe and Green, 1987). As a result of this he may attempt to preserve status and self-esteem by trying to retain his previous reputation and power within his family and group of friends. This may involve bluster or impulsive acts intended to attract attention. Alternatively, he may decide to change his sense of self identity, perhaps by adopting an invalid role or becoming the local clown.

Treatment considerations

The first consideration must be prevention; it is not the burden of this chapter to promote the value of rear cycle lights, cyclist helmets, rear seat restraint in cars, safe playgrounds and traffic sense, but all of these measures deserve repetition.

Counselling of parents and teachers with respect to handling the severely head-injured child has not been evaluated, but this is a most important and urgent matter for investigation.

There is no reason to think that even severely head-injured children and adolescents with psychiatric disorders will not respond to the ordinary range of psychological and psychiatric interventions. It is sometimes casually assumed that brain injury requires preference to be given to a pharmacological approach, but there is neither logic nor data behind such an assumption. Indeed, McCabe and Green (1987) in their discussion of rehabilitation, make the point more positively: 'we consider severely head-injured adolescents with emotional and behavioural problems to be viable patients for psychological therapies'.

The principles of a behavioural approach, already widely adopted in rehabilitation, force an evaluation of deficits and thus provide a particularly apposite model for the treatment of behaviour disorders, as so many are likely to result ultimately from skill deficiencies. This may be especially relevant to the management of difficult behaviour during the early phase of rehabilitation, when an evaluation of antecedant events leading up to an outburst can reveal, for example, that the child is easily overwhelmed by auditory stimuli or, in the instance of hemianopia, surprised by people approaching from their blind side. Similarly, the application of a functional analysis based on learning theory may enable seemingly inexplicable abnormal behaviours such as head banging or shouting to be understood as learned responses to frustration or an otherwise intolerable situation. Agitation or emotional lability as a symptom following severe head injury has been seen to be an indication for tricyclic antidepressants (Barin, Leger and Backman, 1985) but such claims are based on anedcotal evidence only. In general, there would seem to be good grounds for withholding medication in such instances until ordinary counselling has been attempted. Some children and adolescents with inexplicable mood swings will, at interview with a trusted counsellor, reveal survivor guilt or profound feelings of shame that they have caused their families such distress, particularly when the accident occurred as a consequence of a prohibited activity.

The management of the disinhibition syndrome presents specific difficulties. Forceful prohibition by parents at the time of transgression coupled with rote tuition of social rules ('never talk about other people when they can hear you') is the minimum, but it is surprisingly often omitted. Sexual disinhibition may occasionally warrant anti-libidinal medication, but this should never be prescribed unless an attempt at social training has already been made. This promiscuity with which some severely head-injured girls exhibit may not result so much from disinhibition, rather an attempt to prove to themselves that they are sexually attractive. Whatever the mechanism, contraceptive advice is mandatory.

Future research

With the honourable exception of Rutter and colleagues, and earlier work from Baltimore and Vancouver, the territory of psychiatric disorder in the head-injured child and adolescent population has barely been mapped. Readers of this chapter will doubtless develop their own questions but, from examination of the issues covered, there would seem to be a particular need to address the following problems.

1   Precise characterization of the disinhibition, amnesia, dysfunctional attention syndrome which is widely recognized among very severely head-injured older children but not yet delineated. Neuropathological correlates need exploration by means of modern imaging techniques, especially NMR.
2   Development of effective treatment techniques for children and adolescents with such a constellation of difficulties.

3   Long-term prospective controlled follow-up of mildly head-injured young children in conjunction with documentation of life events, using interviews with children, parents and teachers, as well as neuropsychological assessment with contemporary instruments such as the CHIPASAT (Johnson, Roethig-Johnston and Middleton, 1988). This would enable an examination of Boll's (1983) hypothesis that overtly normal behaviour may be maintained only by extreme effort and will decompensate under stress.

4   Further exploration of changes in family relationships and interactions following head injury, so that these can be predicted from the point of view of preventative counselling.

Chapter 12

Return to school

Ruth Furlonger and David A. Johnson

Introduction

The general morbidity of head-injured children is high; they are widely dispersed geographically and probably do not constitute a significant group within any one local education authority (LEA). Yet it is likely that many such children are unknown to the LEA or actual school. Head injury is not an all-or-none phenomenon, but occurs along a continuum of severity, causing commensurate changes in cognition and behaviour, with parallel needs for help. In this chapter, we propose that head-injured children are an identifiable group with special educational needs, but for whom educational provision is very limited.

Parents may have specific concerns about their child's education from the earliest stages of recovery after head injury. They may assume, or at least hope, that the child will return to school and progress normally through the educational system. It is often difficult for parents to realize and accept that the child's neurological functioning will have changed and, consequently, that educational help may now be necessary.

The head-injured child may no longer progress at a normal rate for many reasons (Savage, 1987). Moreover, any lack of progress or decline in achievements may not become obvious for some time after injury, partly as scholastic measures are relatively insensitive and may not show immediate effects, and partly because of secondary neurological factors (see Goodman, this volume). An early study in this area (Klonoff, Low and Clark, 1977) found that delayed school progress was not present prior to injury in those closed head-injury children who subsequently required special assistance. That severity of head injury may relate to severity of cognitive deficit is not surprising, especially for children younger than 10 years at the time of injury. Heiskanen and Kaste (1974) reported that if a child had been unconscious for more than two weeks he was rarely able to make normal progress at school; of thirty-four children, unconscious for twenty-four hours or more, eight were unable to remain in a normal school, and the school performance of nine others was poor. The remaining seventeen were described as 'coping fairly normally', a statement which should ring alarm bells in any concerned parent or practitioner. Similarly, Flach and Malmros (1972) found that two-thirds of their children with simple fractures or concussion were able to perform normally in school during the eight to ten years after injury. They do not, however, adequately address assessment, recovery or developmental profiles in their examinations. Brink, Garrett, Hale *et al.* (1970) studied children aged two to eighteen years at injury, who had been unconscious for one week; in contrast to the eventual resumption of activities of daily living and ambulation in nearly all patients, neuropsychological testing disclosed persisting cognitive impairments. One quarter of the survivors were unable to resume any form of schooling, whilst over half were in special schools; only seventeen per cent were in normal schools, but were described as coping poorly within that setting. Such reports illustrate the paradox of the head-injured child, his outwardly good recovery in the presence of persisting disabilities hidden from sight (Johnson and Roethig-Johnston, 1988). This is particularly so for the child who suffers relatively mild head injury, which may also cause cognitive difficulties which disrupt learning and education (Boll, 1983). In their seminal work Chadwick, Rutter, Shaffer *et al.* (1981) found, at two-and-a-quarter years follow up, that children with post-traumatic amnesia (PTA) exceeding three weeks were rated by teachers as experiencing difficulties in their school work or had been placed in special schools. Many of the early studies have methodological drawbacks, particularly heterogeneous groups and inadequate assessments, which limit the practical validity of their findings. There should be no surprise that severely head-injured children with verified brain injury, particularly in the prefrontal cortex, are found by some authors to be achieving normally at school, given the insensitive assessments and methodological inadequacy which characterize so many of these studies.

Education for children in hospital

It has not always been readily apparent to outsiders why education in hospitals is important. School may be seen as a negative experience and parents may feel that sick children should be excused from the pressures of education. Considering the fundamental importance of education to the developing child, the particular vulnerability of learning and memory to the effects of head injury (Levin and Eisenberg, 1979) and their relative immaturity, it would seem that early teaching may offer an integral contribution to rehabilitation. Absence from school disadvantages any child, irrespective of age or reason; planned and progressive stages of education are missed, gaps arise in knowledge and understanding, and the logical process of skill acquisition is disrupted. Children normally returning from a period of absence are able to exert greater effort and catch up with work missed but, for the head-injured child, the fundamental nature of their neurological injury typically precludes such redoubled efforts and resumption of work, effectively slowing any further progress. They may return to school with disruption of both the capacity and the motivation to learn new things. Interest and motivation are important to learning for the normal child (James, 1899) and subjects will differ in their inherent interest but, after head injury, these factors are of greater practical importance in the classroom (Friedman, Klivington and Peterson, 1986). It is the ability for new learning which is universally disrupted following cerebral insult (Hebb, 1949). With the child's unique but limited store of previously acquired knowledge, disruptions of learning are, therefore, likely to be a limiting factor in further development. All learning occurs by the gradual and sequential acquisition of new skills consolidated with existing knowledge. For example, walking cannot be mastered before postural control and balance; arithmetical fractions cannot be understood before the rule of division. School curricula are based on the assumption that as children develop they acquire greater maturity in cognition, social and emotional behaviour, with increasingly complex and diverse skill acquisition. The demands made by normal learning upon the traumatized CNS are, therefore, quite substantial. In order to make an optimal return to school, the head-injured child must receive specialist educational help during his enforced absence and, concurrently, the teachers must be fully aware of the potential difficulties caused by the child's return. None of the teachers in Gulbrandsen's (1984) study, for example, had noted a change in the head-injured child's academic achievements, and quite a few did not even know of the accident. Regrettably, clinical practice repeatedly produces similar examples, irrespective of injury severity. It is important to remember that the child's absence consists not only of time spent in hospital, but also the interim time spent at home. For the more severely head-injured child this can easily result in a very protracted period of absence over months, or even years. Official provision for this period is a grey area, in which there appear to be no guidelines or rules. Some children may not receive any education during this enforced absence, simply because of inadequate resources and bureaucratic inefficiency.

Educational provision is organized by local authorities and includes hospital schools, home tutors and specialist teachers. The child's education in hospital may depend upon the size of the paediatric unit, length of stay and LEA provisions. The hospital tutor represents the minimal level of LEA provision but, in trying to implement this, one may find that the LEA is unable to contact or allocate a suitable tutor immediately. Tutors are often employed on a part-time basis, they frequently work in isolation, have insufficient time to liaise with other staff involved in the child's care, and teach age groups and subjects outwith their training. Many of the larger hospitals have tuition units or schools, with resident full-time teachers who are readily available and can share their expertise. Practically, there appears to be diffuse, ill-defined responsibility to inform the LEA of the child's status, in order to secure adequate resources for the child. Hospitals with no resident school unit or full-time teacher may not refer the head-injured child to any educational speciality. If the child's school, in turn, is not informed of the injury and absence then they will clearly not be in a position to make an early LEA referral. It is unrealistic to expect parents to know about or ask for a home tutor, particularly when they are already highly stressed by the child's accident.

Early approaches

The teacher's role with the head-injured child need not be that of formal pedagogue, rather a part of a multi-disciplinary team, liaising with medical staff, nurses, occupational therapists, physiotherapists, speech therapists, psychologists and parents, directly contributing to the overall rehabilitation process. Interdisciplinary contact concerning the child is of the utmost importance for the proper identification and delineation of learning difficulties arising from neurological injury. Whilst most teachers and educational psychologists use standardized tests in making assessments of their pupils, these may not be appropriately administered, and are typically inadequate for neuropsychological evaluation. Similarly, recent clinical assessments may seldom be forwarded to educational personnel unless specifically requested. This may lead to unnecessary duplication of assessments, with obvious restrictions on validity. Test performances of head-injured children must be interpreted differently from those of other children and, consequently, school placements should not be made on the basis of test scores alone. Whilst general ability scales such as the WISC-R (Wechsler, 1974) have obvious utility, the over-reliance on ubiquitous IQ estimates in neuropsychology is a practice to be deplored (Lezak, 1988a). There are many aspects of cognition detrimentally affected by head injury, which are not addressed by such general scales and yet are of fundamental importance to the child's classroom performance. As Rutter, Graham and Yule (1970) suggested, handicap must be judged in terms of what the child can and cannot do, rather than in terms of his relative position in class or on a test. This is most pertinent to the head-injured child who may have intact skills which are beset by difficulties in speed of information processing, distractibility, or sustained effort.

Most teachers are conversant with the concepts of intellectual function, classroom behaviour and academic competence, but may ignore the contributions of brain-behavioural relationships. Changes in brain function result in overt behaviour which, in turn, has an impact on the physical and social environment (Engel, 1980). Changes in the environment may act reciprocally to produce structural or functional changes in the brain, the latter being the focal point for all rehabilitation. It is suggested that, by having a basic understanding of such relationships, teachers can make important contributions to the child's progress after head injury (Friedman, Klivington and Peterson, 1986; Gaddes, 1986). It is vital that they are not misled by the child's outwardly good physical appearance into thinking that the soft and vulnerable tissue of the brain looks as good after injury. It may be difficult for teachers and other educational workers to identify cognitive problems of young head-injured children but, with the help of the neuropsychologist, it should be possible to distinguish between emerging, delayed or impaired skills and identify aberrant learning styles. Teachers should also be aware of the general difficulties facing head-injured children, as in fatigue, slowness, hand-eye co-ordination, impulsivity, distractibility and immaturity, as they affect classroom performance. The presence of focal brain injury may give rise to further specific problem areas, such as visuoperceptual or endocrinological disorder, and specialist advice on their assessment and management should be obtained as early as possible. Within the educational category of learning difficulties, for example, teachers identify reading as the most frequent problem (Croll and Moses, 1985), yet reading difficulties may be relatively common after head injury and involve at least two major pathological mechanisms, attention or visuospatial orientation. Consequently, early and accurate delineation is the *sine qua non* for intervention.

In order to achieve maximum learning from intact skills and abilities, early teaching must be individually tailored. This will help to focus and sustain attention, cope with the frustration caused by disabilities, and help establish a sound framework for future progress. Teachers play a vital role in re-accustoming the child to following instructions, improving listening skills, checking factual recall, developing and consolidating reasoning skills and conceptual thinking, and practising social skills, so consistently reinforcing appropriate behaviour. Molnar and Perrin, (1983) discuss a number of teaching methods, citing one school of thought which advocates remediation of defective perceptuo-motor skills as a prerequisite of higher level, more academic learning, which parallels the neurological approach advocated by J. Moore (1980). Learning may be facilitated by associating the most effective sense modalities with the desired mode of response. Hence, it is important to exclude input from any impaired sense modality which distorts normal perception and so interferes with learning. Working with the head-injured child one should ideally adopt an eclectic approach drawing upon the models of cognitive development (Russell, 1978), Luria's neuropsychological delineation (Luria, 1973), and current neuropsychological research (Finger, LeVere, Almli *et al.*, 1988). For the younger child, approaches to prosocial development could also be usefully incorporated (Mussen and Eisenberg-Berg, 1977). Professional considerations and common sense will dictate that when any one approach is ineffective, other methods must be tried.

A major problem for teachers and psychologists is the estimation of premorbid intellectual potential, as achievements may not have been formally documented, learning styles, skills and characteristic behaviours may not have been established. Contact with the child's school will give an accurate view of premorbid abilities, as any pre-existing learning or reading difficulties will be of greater significance after head injury. This information helps to assess the more practical effects of injury upon learning and behaviour, and to establish realistic goals, particularly in relation to later vocational choice. Statistical formulae have been calculated for an American population (Reynolds and Gutkin, 1979), but appear not to have been evaluated with English children.

Return to school

An integral part of the preparations for the child's return to school is a visit to advise on learning, emotional or social difficulties arising from the head injury. As suggested by the Gulbrandsen (1984) study, for example, the normal school teacher's awareness of health-related difficulties may affect the child's response to schooling. Croll and Moses (1985) found that a number of teachers complained of not being told of health difficulties by either parents or hospitals, and were unsure whether such difficulties were associated with learning and behaviour problems. There is no guarantee, of course, that merely providing the information guarantees its acceptance. Whilst sensory and physical disabilities may be acceptable to ordinary school integration, learning and behavioural difficulties are generally not. This seems automatically to preclude head-injured children. It is also possible that special education provisions exist to remove from the mainstream educational system pupils whom schools find unacceptable (Croll and Moses, 1985). Similarly, removal to a special school may be more in the interests of the school than the pupil. The fundamental importance of normal teachers' attitudes to children with special educational needs was recently highlighted by Mepsted (1988), who found that teachers' attitudes depended upon their degree of knowledge, understanding and experience of the children and their particular condition. Lack of knowledge and contact related to anxiety and opposition, with the disability taking precedence over the child's needs. This concurs with earlier findings that 'The major handicap of disabled people remains not so much their specific disability as the attitude towards them' (Furnham and Gibbs, 1984). Given such factors, the early contact and the hospital teacher's visit to school may be of singular importance to the head injured child's return. Hospital teachers or clinical staff are potentially the best sources of immediate information, as they have worked with the child throughout his early recovery. If he has also suffered peripheral and more obvious physical injuries in the accident, it may be these which are used to explain the absence, so avoiding the negative stigmata of brain injury. Following this initial contact, the receiving schools would need only a short, informal session for the hospital teacher or neuropsychologist to explain the basis of head injury, the child's particular difficulties, and offer collaborative suggestions for effective management. There may be some uncertainty in the relationship between schools and teachers, and the specialist advisory services in the implementation of the 1981 Education Act, but such interactions may be crucial for the effective management of head injury. The full rehabilitation team must persist in acting as child advocates in the process of educational planning and placement. Failure to do so will only result in delay and frustration for all concerned yet, as Telzrow (1987) suggests, militant attitudes without adequate understanding of other professionals' policies can only exacerbate this delay.

There are a number of factors which may influence a reintegration to school. The mechanisms of head injury typically produce relative degrees of cognitive, emotional, physical and social difficulties in coping with the normal demands of school organization, mixing with peers and generally functioning as a member of a large, active group of children. The child's return to school should generally be on a gradual basis, to increase both mental and physical stamina, and begin with familiar subjects to demonstrate success and build confidence in learning. In secondary school this may entail attending at different times of day, as subjects are seldom scheduled conveniently at the same time each day. As the child learns to cope with the physical and mental demands of school, a gradual increase to full-time attendance may be possible. The home tutor may be retained during this transitional period to give individual attention when not at school, particularly with any elements of the curriculum that the pupil has missed, or finds particularly difficult, and to provide top-up sessions out of term time. Most LEAs employ advisory teachers for special needs, or full-time hospital teachers, who could take responsibility for head-injured children's educational reintegration. They could ensure that all those involved are given appropriate advice, that information is passed between hospitals, schools and parents. Out-patient appointments for hospital follow-ups could be co-ordinated to minimize further disruption to schooling. It is also important for the child to understand that problems arising from the head injury are not his fault but, equally, this does not excuse him from working, or overcoming the difficult areas, or from behaving badly.

Classroom learning abilities are multifactoral and include motor skills, visual perception, sensorimotor integration, verbal and non-verbal memory, language, verbal and non-verbal reasoning, and social adaptability. Complex behaviours possess a serial order component (sensory input, integration and output) organized in time and space, which may be disrupted after head injury and misperceived by the teacher simply as careless inattention, distractibility, laziness or uncooperation. For example, if the child cannot follow what is being said because of slow information processing, he may be able to do little other than 'switch off'. When reprimanded accordingly, he is likely to be less willing to try and do well in class and so establish a pattern of failure. The most important part of any lesson is probably the initial ten minutes or so, when topics are introduced and instructions given, but this may be when the head-injured child encounters most difficulties. The teacher's instructions may not be sufficiently slow, clear and concise for the child to follow. Asking children to 'enter the room quietly, sit down, find page forty-three in the green book and read the first paragraph' may seem first paragraph' may seem straightforward, but it entails a sequential series of multiple instructions which the head-injured child may need to receive separately, to facilitate his comprehension, avoid confusion, embarrassment, or failure. Head-injured children may not only have difficulty in recalling particular information, procedure or technique, but they may not even recall the event in which that particular learning experience occurred. Similarly, lessons delivered in different classrooms entail moving around the school between periods, which may be both mentally difficult and physically tiring for the head-injured child who must remember what topic is next, which items to take with him, collect and carry them to the next room. Such routine activities may be easily disrupted by distraction, or difficulties in memory, organization and planning, whilst creating disproportionate fatigue which further restricts performance in the next class. The general ambience of each class may be quite unique, so creating different demands of the child. A purpose-built art room may provide a quiet, warm, welcoming and visually stimulating environment with individual attention, whilst a general classroom used for teaching a number of different subjects may have bare walls and rows of desks trained on the teacher and blackboard. Curricula subjects are often taught with idiosyncratic styles, expectations and tolerance. The group of pupils in any class may change between lessons, creating groups of differing ability, social and sexual configurations with whom the child must interact. The head-injured child may find it increasingly difficult to adapt to such frequent changes as the day proceeds and the level of noise and fatigue increases. Irrespective of premorbid abilities, initial post-injury classroom performance is likely to be well below premorbid levels and current peer levels which adds to the child's frustration and easily results in a progressive deterioration in motivation and performance. These problems may be equally disruptive for both the child in junior school, with its greater reliance on group work, and for the secondary school child who is typically confronted with a more disjointed day, requiring him to focus on each topic quickly, then change to another subject at the end of the period.

Social behaviour

Successful school performance helps the child to develop self-esteem and confidence in learning. Conversely, school failure may trigger secondary emotional problems, particularly in youngsters who are at risk for maladaptive behaviour as a direct consequence of the head-injury. For adequate social development a child should possess insight and the ability to infer subtleties in communication, such as body language, facial expression, and tone of voice. The extent of personal and social skills will depend upon the pre-morbid stage of personality development (Bromley, 1977) but, head-injured children may lack the confidence as well as the skills necessary to initiate interaction and participate in social situations (Newton and Johnson, 1986). Their approach may be inappropriate, dominating a conversation, not knowing when or how to terminate an exchange. Post-traumatic cognitive difficulties may interact with the stage of personality development to produce an overall poor social adjustment and restrict social development. Inflexible thinking may create particular difficulties which readily lead to arguments and confrontation, whilst difficulties in recall and discrimination of previous experiences and appropriate behaviour play a partial role in poor social judgement and behaviour. The rules of social behaviour are far less clear during unstructured free periods, such as lunch, room transitions, or holidays. Some head-injured children who behave impulsively or irrationally may show much greater control and hence better performance in the classroom, with its familiar associations of habitual, overlearned behaviours and clearly defined external structure to facilitate and guide behaviour that would otherwise be internally controlled and directed (Telzrow, 1987). The structure of a small classroom provides ideal training in group interaction, and may well be the child's first exposure to the novelty, noise and complexity of group situations.

Return to school may be stressful for the child and, in the presence of reduced neurological capacity, result in behaviour which is easily misinterpreted. Individuals who have incurred brain injury are often painfully aware of their intellectual and memory deficits, and will likely be afraid of being considered stupid or retarded. The head-injured child may find that it is particularly difficult to resume friendships. Many previous friends may have moved on to form different groups. He may feel different from other children in some ways, but be unable to express this verbally, and may show avoidance behaviours to disguise his fears. Teachers should remember that how children process information may be more important than simply demanding correct responses. An absent, incorrect, impulsive, or resistant answer should never be taken at face value. Such overt manifestations of 'problem behaviours' may primarily reflect axiomatic disorders of attention for example. Acting out, non-compliance and other avoidance behaviours, such as yawning, asking irrelevant questions, disrupting peers, humming or displacement activity may represent efforts to divert attention from their classroom activity and can indicate anxiety, confusion, lack of confidence, or true performance difficulties (Rutter, 1981). Memory and language problems will restrict their ability to make quick, accurate replies to questions, or to express themselves clearly. This often sets the stage for ridicule and the child rapidly learns to remain quiet under such potent reinforcers. Psychiatric problems are not uncommon following head injury (see Hill, this volume) and are often difficult for teachers to manage in the classroom, if only because of the head-injured child's unpredictably. Referral to an appropriately skilled psychologist or psychiatrist, preferably at a tertiary level, is an important early step.

Special education

In many cases the head-injured child may be unable to meet the demands of a mainstream school and would be better placed elsewhere. Specific educational policies do exist for children who constitute formally identifiable groups, such as the blind and partially sighted, but there appear to be no such policies for head-injured children. Within mainstream schools the pupil:teacher ratio depends upon the LEA, but usually means between twenty and thirty pupils, and over thirty in junior schools. It is impossible for a class teacher in these circumstances to give sufficient individual attention to any one pupil without depriving the remainder of the class. Consequently, if the head-injured child has special needs these must be formally recognized, extra staffing allocated, and specific cognitive needs met.

Special schools have the advantage that they are much smaller than mainstream schools, with higher staffing ratios, and experience in teaching children with learning difficulties. A major disadvantage is that pupils mix only with a population of children with other disabilities, against whom the head-injured child may rebel in fear of being stigmatized. The narrow range of pupil categories which are catered for by special schools include

(a) Blind or partially sighted
(b) Deaf or partially hearing
(c) Physically disabled
(d) Delicate
(e) Moderate or severe learning difficulties
(f) Emotionally and behaviourally disturbed
(g) Autistic

There may appear to be adequate resources only for those who fall into the traditional categories of handicap. It is not clear, however, into which group head-injured children might reasonably fit (Telzrow, 1987). For example, in their recent survey of children with special education needs, Croll and Moses (1985) found that 21.6 per cent of health problem children did not have learning or behaviour difficulties. Similarly, it is unlikely that many head-injured children have substantial physical handicaps, nor sensory impairment. In a school for the physically disabled, the head-injured child may be more mobile than many of the children, but have far greater problems with memory and concentration. None of these formal classifications are suitable for the unique needs of the head-injured child. It might be argued that all special groups cannot possibly be listed by name and that there are innumerable diagnostic categories for whom special educational provision is not adequate. Head-injured children, however, cannot be regarded as a minority group in any sense, and their omission can only reflect our ignorance of the problems they face and their often desperate need for help. Although there are terms under the general umbrella of special educational provision, these are considerably restrictive. This provision is allocated to those children who are deemed to have 'Special Educational Needs', defined as arising from learning difficulties and limitations of access to the educational provision made for all. Such a general definition clearly applies to head-injured children who encounter problems both with learning and participating in the social organization of the school, where teachers are responsible for large groups of individuals each with their own needs. Yet the needs of head-injured children are not adequately met by this provision, if only because of the generality of its definition and resources.

There have been many changes in Special Education since the 1981 Education Act. This implemented the Warnock Report's (Warnock, 1978) recommendations defining a pupil with special educational needs as having significantly greater difficulty in learning than the majority of children of his age, or a disability which either prevents or hinders him from making use of education facilities of a kind generally provided in schools. Warnock's argument that special educational needs should be regarded as a continuum, parallels the nature and severity of head-injured children's needs. The notion of one-in-five children having special educational needs (Croll and Moses, 1985) has lead to the involvement of greater numbers of ordinary classroom teachers becoming intimately involved with these children (Mepsted, 1988). There is now greater emphasis on keeping children with special needs within mainstream schools to facilitate peer group contact and offer the wide range of mainstream subjects. Yet this may in itself limit the head-injured child's opportunities for success, as his restricted capacities will be overstretched. Extra provision is allocated on the basis of a Statement of Special Needs, which is a report of the child's learning difficulties, compiled by teachers, educational psychologists, social workers, medical staff and parents. It allows a more objective, professional approach to the child's placement, with more parental involvement. The procedure of Statementing, its formulation, agreement and implementation, is an extremely lengthy process which may take a year or more. This presents problems for the head-injured child, not only because the family see it as yet one more bureaucratic inefficiency to obstruct their child's rehabilitation, but also because extra provision is needed in the early stages of recovery and, at least, on his initial return to school. His needs may change rapidly as recovery proceeds, and so placements need to remain. If a child is to be placed in a different school than his pre-accident one, then placement needs to be agreed before the child is ready to return, to allow adequate preparation. If Statementing is delayed for whatever reason, the child remains at home, with or without a tutor, when otherwise able to attend school and is thus not optimizing his recovery. The decision as to who initiates the statementing procedure is most likely to be taken by an Education Officer. There appear to be no formal mechanisms involving Health and Social Services staff so there is little if any joint planning. Although assessments of the children's needs should be independent of cash and political considerations, the final decision is largely affected by the prevailing lack of knowledge and misinformation surrounding paediatric head injury. Many Statemented pupils are able to remain in their mainstream schools with allocation of a support teacher, who may be a part-time special needs teacher or full-time ordinary teacher with part of their work allocated to remedial teaching.[1] It is unclear whether the amount of time that the child spends out of regular class receiving special help, is relevant to the amount or nature of such help, and how it integrates with the education offered in the ordinary classroom (Croll and Moses 1985). In this respect, a most urgent need appears to be educating the educators; no time is currently allocated in teacher training programmes for the needs of head-injured children, neither are there any inservice programmes to help teachers, although Manchester appears to be an exception (Stranack and Elliot, undated). The support teacher is typically employed to help the pupil only for part of the school day, which may vary from one to five hours a day, depending upon the severity of the child's difficulties and the LEA's financial allocation for support teachers. It may be argued that the more help and support given to head-injured children in the early stages, the more likely their successful reintegration and subsequent progress without additional help. The less support a child receives at this early and crucial time, the more likely problems are to arise in the future, and the more costly this will prove in terms of staff time, scarcity of resources, and the child's ultimate level of attainment.

Specialized teaching units

It has been noted that local authorities are responsible for organizing education but, the number of head-injured children may not be sufficient to justify special schools along the lines of those provided for other disability groups. The existing special schools do not adequately meet the head-injured child's needs, yet they face innumerable difficulties in returning to a mainstream school. Mepsted (1988) suggests a half-way house between the segregation of a special school and full-time provision within mainstream education and thence into the community. This appears to be a profitable avenue for exploration in this country. One further approach may be to establish specialized units for head-injured children, serving several LEAs, staffed with experienced and highly trained professionals. Attending such a unit on leaving hospital would provide the opportunity to take early advantage of individually tailored education and, with good subsequent progress, reintegration into mainstream school. Similar proposals have been made (Cohen, Joyce and Rhoades, 1985; Telzrow, 1987) to extend cognitive stimulation and development in students from pre-school through high school. Children are eased gradually and systematically from individual learning, to being part of a small group, than a larger class. In the school, students are expected to integrate cognitive skills that may be worked on separately in therapy. Observing problems which they have in the more normal school environment allows therapists and teachers alike to plan realistic and individually tailored treatment programmes. The existence of a special educational unit would allow staff to become highly skilled in dealing with the specific behavioural and learning problems after head injury, including emotional and behavioural immaturity, and slow cognitive development. The unit would also be able to take account of physical fatigue and impaired mobility by design of layout and class timetables. Furthermore, the entire school calendar could be designed to facilitate the learning process, omitting the long, unstructured summer holidays, for example.

We must ensure that the head-injured child is ideally placed to obtain maximal benefit from the educational system and that their needs are both recognized and adequately met, given reasonable constraints on the system as it exists. Individuals in both the educational and health care systems should identify an appropriate contact person and develop cooperative working relationships as a matter of priority (Telzrow 1987). It is very distressing that the present schooling system is woefully inadequate in meeting the special requirements of this very needy and large population. There follow two case histories, indicating the varied needs of head-injured children returning to school.

Case histories

Simon

A twelve year old boy sustained a serious head injury as a result of a playground accident. He ran against a wall, striking the left side of his head. Although he was only briefly concussed, his level of consciousness deteriorated over the next twenty-four hours. He sustained a left temporoparietal skull fracture and underlying epidural haematoma, mild left hemipareisis and brainstem oculomotor problems. He spent approximately two months in a general hospital, attending the on-site hospital school, but found difficulty in mixing with the older and more boisterous boys. Despite achieving IQ scores in the average and above range, his persisting difficulties were in visual attention, tracking and organization. He was also distractible and mildly disinhibited. He was placed in a mixed mainstream comprehensive school but, despite having missed a school term, he received no support in this transition. He was unable to cope with comments made by other children, felt very insecure, and found it difficult to make new friends. He left after three weeks, and received no further teaching for another two months. He was subsequently sent to a smaller middle school, where he found it easier to mix with his peers. A home tutor was assigned to his case over the following holidays and Simon felt more confident when beginning at a mixed secondary comprehensive the following September. This sequence of events put his education back at least one year. Unfortunately, nineteen months later, his family moved and he was sent to another large comprehensive which did not receive reports from his old school for nine weeks. In the meantime he was put into the remedial group, about which he felt very bitter, as he had always been in average ability classes both before and after the accident, despite the difficulties he encountered. The school were unaware of Simon's difficulties and he felt he was regarded as slow very quickly lost interest, motivation and progress. He then lost another term's schooling due to a back injury, followed by an eye operation to correct a sight defect resulting from the original head injury. As he was sixteen the following Easter, he decided to leave school and commence a Certificate of Pre-vocational Education course at a further education college. This covered basic education with practical elements and the flexibility to take GCSE if he did well academically. Hopefully he will be able to achieve his maximum potential here.

This case is just one of literally hundreds in this Health Region alone, all with similar problems. His return to school was complicated by the family moving house, and then further hospitalization. There is no guarantee that the head-injured child returning to school will not have other setbacks such as these to contend with, independent of the original injury. The main problem was that his difficulties were never fully recognized by the teachers. His eyesight was affected by the accident, making it very difficult to copy notes from the board and to scan pages in his books. If he lost his place it would take him some time to relocate it and this, coupled with the fact that his handwriting was very untidy unless he wrote slowly, meant that he was much slower in class than his peers, often missed what the teacher said, and was consequently labelled as slow and considered of low ability. He refused to use a typewriter, feeling that it would set him apart from the others in class. Even in lessons which required no handwriting, such as mathematics, Simon would only be able to complete half of the work because of his slowness in scanning the blackboard and book. He actually found mathematics particularly difficult, having missed so much through absence and the gaps in his knowledge had never been filled. Although his basic calculation was good, he had never learned some of the mathematical strategies for problem solving. Additionally, his poor eyesight made it difficult to read signs, fractions and powers in mathematical texts. Simon had difficulty in following verbal instructions and needed more time to assimilate information. He was able to understand and remember things, but only if they were explained carefully. If he had missed an explanation, either because of absence or because he was writing at the time, he would have been unable to pick this up. Teachers may expect pupils to be able to listen and to take notes simultaneously but this requires a division of attention at a high level and the head-injured child may be quite unable to do this. Simon did well to survive in so many schools with no additional help, yet still want to achieve more at college. One may reasonably ask just how much better he would have done, had he received the necessary help and support at the early stages of recovery. The absence of extra help may be partly attributed to his appearing to have physically recovered remarkably well from the injury, and looking normal to all intents and purposes. He looked older than his years and one would normally have expected a more mature level of behaviour than was evident. The effects of the head-injury merely exacerbated this discrepancy. Above all else, Simon wanted desparately to be treated as normal and has gone to great pains in his attempts to cover up any residual difficulties. It is easy to see from this case how head-injured children's difficulties may not be recognized. Realizing how important it is for adolescents to conform with their peer group and not appear different in any way, it is unreasonable to expect the pupil to explain to his teachers the nature and extent of his difficulties, even if capable of doing so. Reports from those who have worked with Simon should have promptly been communicated prior to the actual change of schools. Although the clinical psychologist reported that Simon should not return to normal schooling, he did not pursue the matter with the educational authorities. More individual tuition could have been given during his absence from school. Simon agreed that it would have been possible and useful from his point of view to take a small tape recorder into lessons to record what the teacher was saying so that if he missed something he could later replay it. If his teachers had been aware of why he was slow they would have probably treated him differently and may have been willing to give typewritten copies of notes written on the blackboard. All of this could have been provided without having to invoke the formal procedure of Educational Statementing. Given his high motivation and basic academic ability he would have been able to take greater advantage of his education and achieve according to his ability, instead of leaving school at sixteen with no qualifications and a bleak future.

Ann

A thirteen year old girl was struck by a motor car. She sustained a severe diffuse head injury, causing immediate unconsciousness; she remained in this state for two weeks. Her persisting difficulties were primarily an all pervasive slowness, poor memory, moderate right-sided hemiparesis, and difficulties in visual perception. Ann had been a high achiever in a mixed, mainstream comprehensive school and expected to do well in public examinations, progressing to higher education. Her school absence totalled seven months, during which time no education was provided from the local education authority and there was no resident hospital teacher. The failure of the LEA to provide a home tutor meant that the Statementing procedure was very slow in starting, took six months longer than it should have done and a full year to complete. The statement recommended that Ann should use a microwriter, because of her poor handwriting due to neuromuscular dysfunction and fatigue. A recurrent remark on all her subject reports was that she was very slow in completing tasks, including homework, and that work was poorly presented. Other difficulties outwith the handwriting, included mental fatigue, resulting in Physics and French being dropped and fewer subjects taken. Further, a loss of mobility and tiredness curtailed social activities generally, and made it more difficult to maintain friendships. The summer examinations, almost all written papers, caused her both physical and mental exhaustion. The concession of twenty minutes extra time for her difficulties was of very limited help. It took a year to obtain the microwriter mentioned on the statement but, if that had been available when Ann first returned to school, it would have made her progress much easier and helped considerably in her examinations. Fortunately she was very determined to succeed and had a great deal of support from her mother, but it would have been very easy for a pupil in such circumstances to have become disillusioned and to give up. On the positive side, Ann returned to her original school and, despite her difficulties, managed to take advantage of a limited curriculum and achieve academically, albeit to a much reduced extent. The school were extremely supportive and understanding of her difficulties, with the teachers prepared to make extra efforts to include her in their classes, and problems only arose when a supply teacher was covering a staff absence. It is regrettable that all schools are not as well organized. This case illustrates that although Ann was seriously injured and her academic performance declined, she continued to benefit from mainstream schooling to an extent that would not have been possible elsewhere.

Note
[1]Support teachers are often hourly-paid, not in full-time employment, and so their time is more rigidly fixed by the financial provisions of the LEA.

Chapter 13

The parent's perspective: through the glass darkly

Judith Wardle, Don Clarke and Anne Glenconner

Introduction

In this chapter three parents give their personal and unique experience of children's
head injury. It is evident that, despite the differences of each case, consistent and persistent difficulties related to the health care of the children emerged. Each of the
children sustained severe head injuries and continue to suffer disabilities, irrespective of
their age differences and the varying time since injury.

Parents contributing to a book about children's head injury in which all the other
contributors are specialists may appear, at first sight, to be at a disadvantage. No matter
how tentative the professionals' conclusions and to what extent they acknowledge the
limitations in their experience and knowledge, they present an objective and scientifically researched view of their field. In contrast, the traumatic experiences suffered by the
parents of the head-injured child prevent such subjectivity, their view remains objective and heavily coloured by emotion. From their contact with the various professionals involved with caring for the head-injured child, however, the parents do
have a unique view of how the concept of multidisciplinary rehabilitation actually
works. The parents' view is, therefore, central to the child's recovery, in that it represents an attempt to reconcile the disparate professional approaches. Parents confide in
each other about the appalling gaps in the system and the miseries suffered by themselves and their children, but seldom feel able to justifiably complain, for instance, that
a specialist was approached rather late, or else that he is not the appropriate person for
the child's needs. The doctor's attitude seldom encourages such confidences and
parents frequently feel guilty of being oversensitive and critical. When treatment and
support services are so woefully inadequate however, parents may justifiably offer con-
structive comment. Individual anecdotes related by parents tell of moments when a
doctor has shown uncompassionate attitudes, made errors or failed to provide adequate
facilities for both patient and relatives. There are also reports of poor co-ordination of
services, and a general lack of information made available to the parents.

The attitudes of the doctors and teachers toward a head-injured child and his parents vary widely at different times. There are a few who attempt to explain and assist but, more often, the parents are treated as inept persons to whom minimal information is provided because of their tendency to exaggerate the child's disabilities. The rare contact parents have with medical staff is frequently most unhelpful. To be told by a consultant that 'Your son is going to be a vegetable and I would suggest you go home and forget about him', is a pitiless and frequently ill-founded statement. Even if the neurological opinion about the outcome is fairly certain, there are more humane ways of communicating it to the already distressed parents; the place, time and manner of its delivery needs selecting with the greatest of care. In the current state of professional uncertainty and ignorance about recovery after head injury, medical staff may simply be afraid of not knowing, of being wrong and giving false hope, or feeling guilty about their task. Too often, the attitude taken by doctors is pessimistic and, in many instances, if parents were to take doctors at their word and give up, there is no doubt that the predictions would be self-fulfilling. Many parents have believed a sentence of doom, collapsed from grief, and abandoned a child who otherwise might have made a better recovery. Conversely, parents may be told that their child will make a good recovery, which they naturally assume to mean a resumption of near normal functioning. Yet they are not told of the differences between gross physical outcome (walking and talking) and the more subtle but pervasive and all-important difficulties in memory and mood control, for example. There is at present no information available which can help parents to understand these problems and reassure them. Consequently, if the doctors do not attempt to explain in simple terms the severity and nature of the injury, then we are left in the dark. Furthermore, if the parent attempts to seek out the small amount of literature that does exist about children's head-injury, this may be regarded by many as an unwelcome intrusion. Yet, when the child is discharged from hospital, the same parents are expected to have a whole battery of expertise to care for and rehabilitate the child. A head-injured child may be incontinent, unable to feed himself, have language, speech and motor difficulties, suffer from epileptic fits, unpredictable moods and uncontrollable behaviour. Regrettably, similar attitudes and states of affairs also affects the educational system. For example, the LEA or school appear to under-perform the Health Service, in terms of listening to the parents, taking advice from other health care professionals and, more importantly, simply acknowledging that the child has not yet 'got over' the effects of the head injury. It is an endless, heartbreaking account for those who have suffered at the often merciless hands of bureaucratic systems which appear to care little and know less, and are indifferent to initiating changes. Only by acknowledging that full extent of that suffering can such an appalling situation begin to be changed.

Early stages

In the immediate crisis of an accident the first people on the scene are usually the ambulance crew, about whom there is little evident criticism. Of course, the ambulance service is frequently restricted and, in any one case, they may have to travel a long distance to the accident but if they do get there in time they are efficient and caring. When the child is admitted to casualty, however, the parent is virtually forgotten, sometimes for hours, and left to their own devices in an alien and very stressful environment. The injured child must of course receive maximum attention as a priority but, even if the parents are not in need of medical attention, they do need emotional support and frequent information about what is happening. One parent described her experience as: 'We slept on benches, we had nothing to eat, we drank from those awful machines'. Another described the agonies of constantly being told that there was a three-hour wait before her son would be seen by the Casualty doctor, despite the fact that he was visibly becoming more drowsy and unresponsive due, it transpired, to the rapidly expanding extradural haematoma. Who cares that such mundane factors serve only to exacerbate the already high levels of stress affecting the parents?

If the child is transferred to Intensive Care the immediate task of sustaining life will be adequately catered for in most hospitals but, although the present regimes of drugs and life-support technology do keep the child alive, this is not enough. Little, if any, thought is given to how we may optimize the child's recovery, reducing the period of unconsciousness and beginning active rehabilitation early. No such possibilities are ever communicated to the parents; instead they are left to come across them indirectly in the form of generally inaccurate and misrepresentative press reports. The odds are heavily against a head-injured child arriving at a specialized neurological unit, partly because they are relatively few and widely dispersed but also because they tend to accept only the more severe injuries. It is also evident that many general hospitals simply do not refer head-injured children for specialist assessment, again perhaps because of lack of knowledge, or facilities. Even in the specialist unit, however, there may not be a comprehensive and co-ordinated tean approach involving the various specialists, such as paediatric neurologist, psychologists, therapists, nutritionists and hospital teachers. It is more likely that the head-injured child will spend a greater proportion of time in a local general hospital where medical staff may not even be resident or, indeed, fully understand the unique needs of the head-injured child and his family. Many children with head-injuries go to orthopaedic wards, where the staff have no specialized knowledge of head injury. Junior doctors doing a few months of orthopaedic specialization for example, may be left to supervise the progress of a head-injured child, visiting once or twice a day. This may lead to difficulties and delay in recognizing the symptoms of post-traumatic complications, such as raised intracranial pressure or haematoma. This kind of delay does, regrettably, occur and the consequences may be incalculable.

Despite the evidence which suggests that rehabilitation must begin early, as soon as the child is medically stable, many programmes begin only after discharge from hospital and have little, if anything, to recommend them. Whilst great attention is spent on maintaining the child's physiological stability, a major problem continues to be the absence of any effective treatment for head injury, a situation which appears not to have changed much in the last forty years. The head-injured child, more so than the adult, is almost the last person still subjected to a regime typified by allowing nature to take its course; bed-rest and peace and quiet; treat the body, let the mind heal itself. Such practices are perpetuated by the prevalent and indiscriminate belief in the notion that a child recovers spontaneously, more quickly and to a greater extent than an adult victim. If those who cared for the child in the acute stages after injury worked together as participating members of a team and listened to both professionals and parents, then they would be only too aware of the glaring fallacies inherent in that line of thinking. Doctors frequently regard alternative approaches to care with hostility or, at best, indifference. Yet, if one compares the situation with that of the AIDS virus, one may see an eager willingness by diverse groups of clinicians, scientists and lay people alike to explore the most unlikely approaches in the search for a cure. Even in the situation where the known consequences of non-intervention is death, where anything is better than nothing, people are reluctant to get involved. With head-injured children in coma, even if the attempted treatment is unsuccessful, it may be better to try than to do nothing. The surgeon who gallantly saves the child's life is generally worlds away from the reality of those of us who must live with the effects of head injury for the remainder of our lives. Tackling this problem and attempting a solution has at least three main requirements: the development of knowledge and skills by clinical research; a change in attitude by health professionals so that available knowledge can be applied more rigorously; and a way of increasing public knowledge and awareness of head injury, particularly through the media with its desire for stories with a happy ending, and the educational system with its blatant denial of the effects of head injury upon the child.

One of the authors (DC) has been intimately involved with the use of sensory stimulation of comatosed patients. As Johnson (this volume) suggests, it is only one of many possible approaches. Unfortunately, the evidence for sensory stimulation programmes as a means of early intervention with the unconscious patient is anecdotal, insofar as there is not yet the hard, objective data that comes from controlled trials. It is doubtful, however, whether such data could be obtained without considerable practical ethical and methodological difficulties. Head injuries are so heterogeneous in nature that it would be impossible to ensure that any two children were exactly comparable, or to obtain adequate numbers of children for statistical analyses without multicentre co-operation. From our experience with sensory stimulation to date, there is nothing to indicate which sense is likely to give the best result but the sense of smell may be the least effective. The most common form of stimulation is to play cassette tapes of currently favourite pop songs or messages from idolized TV or pop person-alities but, since most recent events are the ones likely to be most difficult for the child to recall, it may be best to try and evoke responses to voices and events that have been a constant factor in the child's life, or to sounds that were really important to the child six months or more before the accident. A parallel situation may occur with the elderly, who frequently cannot remember recent events but can recall those from the distant past. The work cannot be carried out by the nursing staff alone, although they certainly need to allocate more time to the unconscious child. It is essential that rela-tives and close friends are involved as, with their detailed knowledge of the child's interests and personality, they can provide the essential continuity of care at all stages of recovery. This means that an effective support system for the family is essential both in and out of hospital. The necessity of involving those intimately concerned with the child prior to the accident makes it all the more important to educate the general public in the nature and effects of head injury, so that friends do not suddenly retreat in emo-tional embarrassment on news of the tragedy.

The emergence of the child from coma is not by any means the end of the story. Indeed, it is the beginning of a further period of worry and great concern when the child may fluctuate between periods of normality and times when he is far from being his usual self. The more fortunate ones may have economic resources or attract media attention, both of which could ensure the involvement of many specialists and the availability of detailed information about possible treatments. Public attention, however short lived, also acts as a focal point for relatives to contact each other. As a result of publicity, the child's plight becomes widely known and the family feel less isolated. When some recovery is apparent, it is abundantly clear that a carefully planned, structured and sequenced programme of increasing task difficulty, provided by a multidisciplinary team is necessary to achieve the best results. Regrettably, this systematic approach is far distant from the reality of the head-injured child's care. Typically, there is no team, no programme of stimulation and essentially no rehabili-tation. In most hospitals, physiotherapists are the most likely to become directly involved with the child's care and, generally they seem more aware of the needs of head-injured children than other members of hospital staff. This is perhaps because of their early and frequent contact with the child. Speech therapists are often ignored by medical staff, despite having a potentially important contribution in the early stages of care. Similarly, in spite of the fact that Occupational Therapists' training makes them ideal for working with head-injured children, particularly in the acute stages, it is equally unlikely for them to be involved (Johnson and Roethig-Johnston, 1988). In most cases it falls to the parents to try to find out what they could be doing for their child and from whom they could obtain advice. The parents are subjected to persistent stress, whether spending hours at the bedside of the child in coma, or facing the problem of a child who cannot return to his old school.

The general public may well view recovery from coma as little short of a miracle, and the press perpetuate this notion. It is exasperating to be told that this has occurred, however, when it is blatantly obvious that regaining consciousness does not imply a full neurological recovery, nor that the child will be normal again. The parents will undoubtedly have physically and emotionally exhausted themselves by attempting every possibility for their child. The miracle is indeed that of the parents' fortitude and love in never giving up the struggle to improve their child's condition. One mother rejected the notion that her son's recovery came about as a result of a miracle: 'Other mothers whom I have contacted confirm that one has to fight for the right treatment but, when recovery does commence, it is erroneously pronounced as a miracle, disregarding all the hard work one has put in'.

There is a great deal that a family could do for the injured child, if only they could be given encouragement and advice, rather than be treated as hapless fools. The average parent must struggle along, drained of physical and emotional energy, and often short of money because of giving up many hours of work and the cost of travelling to and from the hospital and eating in its canteen. These are the people upon whom the child depends for future recovery and care; everybody praises the parents' devotion but little is done to help them.

Later stages

Why are the questions of longer-term rehabilitation practices and facilities for head-injured children virtually neglected? Parents are rarely told about the few available units that do accept children, perhaps because the local health or education authority would have to fund the child's stay. If there is a deliberate policy of sending children home because they need their families, then the families need advice and support about their management. It is more likely, however, that the present situation results from an absence of policy, based on misconceptions and ignorance surrounding head injury in children. The level of therapy provision in the community is totally inadequate for supporting the families of head-injured children. For example, in the case of a hospital which could not provide any facilities for rehabilitation, the head-injured child remained in hospital for six weeks longer than was medically necessary, simply because it was the only way of providing the daily physiotherapy he needed. When he was discharged from hospital, the physiotherapy was reduced to two sessions a week, the second of which was in the physiotherapist's own time. In addition, he had two sessions with a speech therapist but, unfortunately, she knew little of the effects of head injury. Two sessions with a home tutor were also provided, who similarly knew nothing about the special needs of head-injured children. The level of provision of all kinds seemed to be clouded by ignorance, misconceptions over recovery and, of course, staffing levels, and little according to actual need. The haphazard provision of available resources for a head-injured child at home does not constitute an adequate rehabilitation programme. Facilities for assessing the needs of a handicapped child do exist at Paediatric Assessment Centres but, even there, the specialist knowledge of head injury may be sadly lacking and there is no guarantee of provision. Entry to a special school does not improve provision or therapy because staff are still part of the limited resources of the community services. The district therapist, for example, works for the Health Authority and has nothing to do with the educational system. It is the parent who must be prepared to fight to obtain adequate therapy guidance. Many forms of therapy are virtually non-existant. Similarly the dearth of speech therapists has most recently brought to public attention the absurdity of the rigid division between health authority and education authority, which allows both to disclaim responsibility thus denying the child opportunities for better recovery and education. Indeed, but for a late amendment to the new Education Bill, it would remain illegal for LEA's to fund any therapy provision. The health authorities declare themselves unable to provide adequate levels of therapy because they are short of money and staff. In this country, unlike the United States, no head-injured child has a right to any kind of therapy, so there is no redress. Furthermore, since appropriate educational facilities are not available for head-injured children, even maximum provision of therapies would not be sufficient for a full rehabilitation programme. Moreover, as educational Statements are evasive as regards the quantity of therapy that a child needs, it would be very difficult to prove the inadequacy of provision in any one case.

Some long overdue improvements are now being made in assessing the needs of head-injured children, with obvious implications for their education, but it is early days yet and the educational system appears not keen to change. As suggested by Furlonger and Johnson (this volume), the more severely head-injured child may be inappropriately placed in a school for the physically handicapped, where the teachers are likely to have no experience of traumatic brain-injury and the associated cognitive and behavioural difficulties as opposed to congenital neurological handicap. Again, it is the parent who must try to find out what is known about educating head-injured children as teachers are often too busy coping with everyday problems to undertake special research for the sake of one child. Moreover, the specific nature of post-traumatic difficulties experienced by the child are likely to make individual tuition essential. This places a strain on staffing levels even in special schools. Until education authorities and, indeed, the Departments of Education and Health become aware of the unique needs of head-injured children, the education they so desperately need is not going to be made available. At the other extreme, the child who outwardly appears to have made a good recovery is equally disadvantaged in school, since the teachers may not even realize there could be problems extending beyond the period of acute recovery. For example, one child was told that he could no longer use his accident as an excuse for poor school work and behaviour because, the accident had occurred four years previously and he should have his memory back by now. Children are similarly reported by their teachers as lazy, delinquent, and their problems attributed to lack of parental control. Such subjective and misinformed comments pass ill judgment upon the parents who are likely to have done their best to help the child's recovery and their return to school, yet receive no acknowledgment, support or direct help from the teachers who are, after all, in *locum parentis* and responsible for helping determine the child's future.

Concluding remarks

From the day of the accident, through the coma, the period at home and the return to schooling of whatever kind, the parents' energy is constantly sapped by the ever-demanding routine care of the child and family, the need to seek information and fight for provision for the head-injured child. If the child is to attain the best possible level of recovery, he needs parents who are as physically fit and mentally acute as possible when caring for him, not worn out by battles with those who should be assisting. As parents we would ask that you help us to help our children.

Chapter 14

Understanding parents

David Hall

Introduction

Perhaps the title of this chapter should be 'Trying to Understand Parents'. Although one may empathize with parents who have a head-injured child, it may be that only those who have been through such trauma can really understand. For professionals who treat head-injured children and have to respond to the grief of the families, compassion and technical or therapeutic skill are necessary but insufficient attributes. A conceptual framework is required, to help them make sense of the intense and often distressing emotions which they encounter (Quine and Pahl, 1987). One of the most profitable lines of enquiry has been based on the investigations into bereavement. The study of the way in which an individual or his loved ones react to approaching death has a wider relevance. It is now acknowledged that these emotional and intellectual responses are similar to those experienced by parents whose child is either born handicapped or acquires some form of handicap during infancy or childhood (Bicknell, 1983). Although the child is not dead, it is to the parents the death of the perfect child they had hoped for and expected to have. The idealized child of their dreams is replaced by one who is imperfect or damaged.

This chapter begins with an outline of the classic bereavement reaction. Each stage is described in detail, with illustrations and examples related to the special problems of head injury. The next section considers the ways in which the parental response to head injury differs from that to a handicap diagnosed in infancy, and the reasons for these differences. Comparisons are also made between head injury and other forms of damage to the nervous system. Finally, the implications of these emotional responses for the care of the child and family are reviewed, both with regard to the immediate post-injury phase and over the succeeding months and years.

The bereavement reaction

The classic stages of the grief reaction are summarized in Figure 14.1. Although some may find it disturbing and even macabre to describe human emotions in these rather rigid and artificial terms, this work has been invaluable to professionals who deal frequently with grief-stricken relatives (Barin, Leger and Backman, 1985). It has been particularly relevant in helping young people to deal with distressing situations, for which their life experiences have not yet prepared them. It is important to realize that people rarely experience the emotions of bereavement in this orderly and logical sequence (Hock, 1984). Figure 14.1 is only intended as a schematic illustration of a helpful concept. Individuals may experience any or all of these emotions simultaneously or in any order. It is not uncommon for a parent who one thought had come to terms with the situation to revert to an acute grief reaction with all the freshness of the original occasion, perhaps on an anniversary or when some incident reminds them of the past or of what might have been. Each member of the family grieves in his or her own way; if they fail to appreciate this, communication in the family may break down at the time when mutual support is most vital.

Figure 14.1

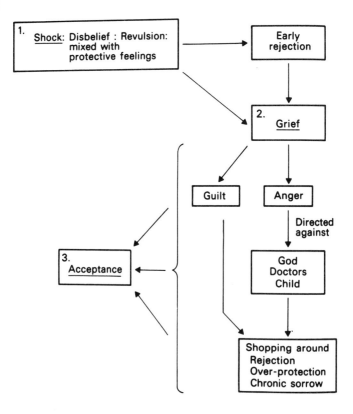

Shock

The immediate response after the accident is that of stunned shock. The parent may be powerless to act, or alternatively may become surprisingly calm and efficient, only to react a little later. There are few incidents more sudden and devastating than a road traffic accident. There may be a mixture of protective instincts towards the child and a desire to stay with him and nurse him. This instinct can seldom be fulfilled while the child is in the intensive care unit, because of the technical skill required to ensure his survival. The protective instinct may be coupled with an opposite emotion, a revulsion for the damaged individual surrounded by all the equipment required to maintain life. This conflict may lead to behaviour that seems irrational to the nursing staff, for instance over-reaction to minor incidents and unpredictable patterns of visiting and involvement. In the phase of shock, parents may find it all but impossible to take in the information that is given to them. There is evidence from systematic studies, clinical experience and parents' accounts, that less than a third of what is said (even in less stressful circumstances) is absorbed. This finding highlights the importance of good communication and of frequent repetition. It will be necessary to repeat, perhaps many times, the facts and predictions that have to be conveyed (Fletcher, 1973).

Denial

There is an element of denial which runs through these early stages and indeed may persist for months or years. Whatever parents may be told, they will not hear it until ready to cope with the information offered to them. The parents' apparent reluctance to absorb the full extent of the child's injuries and their likely sequelae may be a protective mechanism that professionals should not try to destroy. This respect for people's feelings must not be confused with deliberately giving a falsely optimistic prognosis, a kindness which in the long run will prove to be false and will not be appreciated, either by the parents or those caring for the child.

Grief

As the phase of shock passes, the full intensity of grief strikes the parents and also other close family members, particularly grandparents and siblings. Other relatives, friends and school teachers will also be affected. Not knowing how to respond to the parents' grief at this time, relatives and friends may avoid them and add to their isolation. Grief can be projected inwards, with thoughts of guilt and blame. Guilt sometimes has a basis that is wholly or partially rational. For instance, the child was sent on an errand that involved crossing a busy road or was left in the care of a young sibling. Frequently the self-blaming tendency has more to do with the search for an answer or explanation — 'why should this happen to our family?' — than with any legitimate feeling of responsibility. Grief may be accompanied by episodes of panic. The parents may suddenly feel that they have lost control of their emotions and that they are losing their sanity. Sleeplessness and somatic symptoms may occur and it is important to recognize them for what they are. Denial continues to be a prominent feature. This can be regarded as a coping strategy which reflects the need to shut out the intolerable events that have occurred. The parents behave as if the child has only suffered some trivial illness that will soon be better. There may alternatively be outward projections of the grief which may be turned to anger. One obvious focus may be the driver who caused the child's head injury, but there may be other less direct targets. For instance, a spouse or relative may be held to blame, whether rightly or wrongly. It is important to distinguish between this anger which is a natural part of the bereavement response, and anger which is justifiably directed, for example, at the health care system (see below). The one may merge into the other and sometimes parental anger becomes a powerful means of improving the care provided for a particular group of children.

Death

Parents are likely to question whether the child would be better off dead if severe brain damage is anticipated. Such thoughts are only likely to be expressed if parents are given the opportunity to discuss them. This presents particular problems for the neurosurgeon who is aware of the immense difficulties in giving an accurate prognosis at the time when the child's life is still dependent on mechanical ventilation and intensive care. He knows that withdrawal of ventilator support would not usually be practical or ethical, and may result in even worse brain damage, rather than death. Neurosurgeons may differ in the extent to which they can discuss this dilemma with parents, but few would be willing to discontinue treatment, whatever the views of the family.

Bargaining

Another phenomenon of the grief phase is bargaining. Parents begin to recognize that there may be permanent damage, but at this time their main preoccupation is with survival. 'Please God let my child survive, if you let him survive I don't mind how handicapped he is, I'll look after him'. Parents may also undertake various actions in a desperate effort to restore the child to his previous state; for example, they use tapes or special coma-kits to provide 'brain stimulation'.

Adjustment and acceptance

As the child recovers consciousness and it becomes clear that survival rather than death is the likely outcome, the parents have to start coming to terms with what has happened. Acceptance is the word often used to describe this phase. It has been defined as the death of the imaginary perfect child and the redirection of parental love to the newly perceived child as he is in reality. It is difficult to describe what happens at this stage, or to understand why there are such differences between individuals. Parents learn to live again, to pick up the threads, and perhaps to enjoy happiness again. The anguish may become bearable but it never goes away. There are many small crises to be survived before the family can be said to have adjusted: the child's first birthday after the accident; the first outing or holiday without the handicapped child being present, or with him sharing the activities in a restricted way; the first time the child is left with the minder or carer so that the parents can have some time for themselves.

In practical terms, there may be serious difficulties to overcome: one parent may have to give up work and this can cause financial problems as well as the end of a valued career; adaptations may be needed, such as building works to permit wheelchair access. If any of these are to be financed by the proceeds of litigation, which can take five years or longer, it is difficult for adjustment to be completed even from the practical point of view, let alone from the emotional angle.

Siblings have to carry on with their own lives and activities and this may be difficult because of the demands of the now injured child. They may experience feelings of guilt because they have survived intact; resentment and hostility because of the care needs of the handicapped child; adjustment problems at school, perhaps related to ridicule or cruel remarks from peers about their head-injured sibling. Concern about the burden of responsibility which may fall on them in adult life beomes an issue for teenager siblings.

Adjustment may proceed in stages, often interrupted by episodes of fresh grief and anxiety. There may be times when the parents feel a sense of rejection for the damaged child and question whether they can carry on caring for him; yet often, if one gently raises the suggestion of residential care or even of respite care, they may be angry that one doubts their commitment. Perhaps the apparent rejection is again a means of distancing themselves from the pain of knowing that this damaged person is their own offspring; it would be easier to care for such a person if there were not that sense of personal loss. A well recognized form of rejection or avoidance is seen in the parent who becomes an active campaigner for the relevant voluntary organization, develops an expertise in technological aids for the handicapped, or engages diligently in legal battles to obtain compensation. All of these activities are of course valuable both for the child and for society, but they can at the same time be a means of spending as little time as possible with the child who is the cause of the grief. This may lead in turn to resentment on the part of the other parent if they do not share the same aims.

There may also be periods of over-protection which can become a serious problem for the child who retains the capability for independence, or is not allowed to develop it. It is quite understandable that parents should be anxious about allowing any freedom or independence to a child who has sustained serious brain injury, yet this step is a crucial part of the rehabilitation process.

Searching for answers

A more worrying reaction to the handicapped child is the endless search for 'second' opinions, the so-called 'shopping around syndrome'. In the case of the head-injured child, this is not in search of a diagnosis, as one may see in children whose handicap has unknown causes. It more often represents a need for better information about the nature of brain injury and its sequelae.

Not surprisingly, parents seek some means of curing or repairing the injured brain. They may become obsessed with a supposed miracle form of treatment, such as that offered by some private organizations. The layman finds it hard to evaluate claims such as 'we only use one tenth of our brains, so the brain damaged child can make up for his damaged brain cells by bringing others in to action'. Easy access to comprehensible professional advice helps to reduce the search for endless opinions, although the prevalent negative attitudes to rehabilitation may drive parents to seek other less orthodox solutions.

The Peto method of Conductive Education, which has received much publicity recently, has also been seen as a means of bringing about great improvements in head-injured children. It may well have its place in the management of cerebral palsy, but it has not been evaluated with head-injured children. The approach of those who provide this service in Budapest is professional yet compassionate, but its promotion on British television has given some parents the idea that miracles can be achieved by this method.

Yet another area which has attracted disproportionate interest is the role of food additives, minerals and special diets in the function of the nervous system. Many parents feel compelled to test some or all of these treatment methods. Professionals must recognize that what we think of these systems in scientific terms is immaterial; the parents' need to examine them is part of the healing process and should be acknowledged.

Perhaps there is an element of pilgrimage about many of these searches. There is some primitive belief in all of us that suffering is good for us and may bring its own reward. Thus, searching for cures at considerable expense and inconvenience, is thought to be a meritorious act and one which may be rewarded with improvement. Sometimes parents feel obliged to explore unorthodox methods because of pressure from friends or relatives, even though they themselves have little expectation that there will be any benefits. Almost any form of treatment may seem preferable to inactivity, which may be interpreted by those outside the family as evidence of hopeless-ness or of lack of care.

It is hard for anyone to believe that nothing can be done to repair the injured brain and restore the child who has been lost. This is particularly so in the modern era when science and medicine are perceived to have all but conquered death and disease. Our lives are more ordered and predictable than those of any generation before us. This is not to suggest that pilgrimages are necessarily undesirable. It may be necessary for some families to test all the various systems on offer, before they can relax secure in the knowledge that they have done everything possible. Certainly, it is not for us to criti-cize them for investigating unorthodox treatments. One should simply explain that they are not accepted by most professionals, because they lack both scientific plausi-bility and adequate evaluation. Alternative approaches may be suggested, but the parents should be supported in their eventual decision, even if one does not agree with the course of action they have taken.

Religious pilgrimages do not come in quite the same category as other 'shopping-around' searches for a miraculous cure. They often represent, paradoxically, the reaching of the stage of acceptance. By going on a religious pilgrimage, the parents are saying 'I hope very much for a cure but if that is not God's will, I will accept it'.

Pathological grief

Some parents sink into a state of pathological grief, from which they do not seem able to recover. They become profoundly depressed and are unable to take any pleasure in life again. Home life and marriage may suffer, and other siblings inevitably feel the effects. This is not merely a state of continued sadness, which is normal, but a problem that needs expert help. It cannot be diagnosed purely on the basis of how long the parents have continued to feel sad or to have episodes of weeping or despair.

Adjustment is a continuous process

Acceptance is not a static phase; it has to change and develop as the handicapped child grows, reaches puberty and becomes an adult. Life does not become easier for the parents of a brain-injured child, whatever the nature of the disability. They have anxieties about increasing physical strength and sexuality. When the brain injury has had more effect on the psyche and intellect than on motor functions, there will perhaps be concerns about disinhibition, so that boys are perceived as potential sexual delinquents or rapists and girls as being likely to fall prey to any passing male. Physical violence and outbursts of rage may also become a problem (see Hill, this volume).

The parents not only have to work out their own acceptance, but also that of grandparents and siblings. Not least, they must cope with the depression of the injured individual if he has sufficient insight to realize what he has lost, or to appreciate the changed attitudes of others. Grandparents are often a source of continued sadness and tension since they may find it harder to come to terms with their loss than the parents.

Some people seem ultimately to accept what has happened to their child more completely than others and they are able not only to continue with their lives but even to enrich their lives as a result of the experience. Such people often make a great contribution to the welfare of other handicapped children or adults, both by supporting parents individually and by campaigning for and organizing better services and legislation. It is difficult to know what factors determine the outcome for each family; a sound and creative marriage, positive personality traits, social and family support networks, religious beliefs may all contribute. Nevertheless, one is often surprised by the way in which young and even apparently feckless parents adapt and respond to the stress of having a brain-injured child.

What is different about head injury?

Most health professionals have acquired an understanding of the bereavement response of parents through work with disabling conditions such as cerebral palsy, mental handicap, deafness, blindness, autism or dysphasia. The same principles can be applied to the counselling and support of parents with a head-injured child, but it is important to be aware of certain quantitative differences. While there is no systematic study on the point, it is our impression that the intensity of shock, anger and grief is more profound following head injury than after the discovery of a handicapping condition in infancy. The reasons for these observations deserve further consideration.

It is reasonable to speculate that the age at which the child becomes or is found to be handicapped has a profound influence on the response of the parents. Parents develop an image of the child they hope to have during, and sometimes before, the pregnancy. By the time the baby is born, he or she is the focus of many complex hopes, dreams and expectations on the part of the whole family. Thus the first concern of most parents when the baby is born is to be assured that all is well and that the baby is perfect.

Parents realize however that things can go wrong with a pregnancy or birth and most people would wish to be informed of the possibility of handicap as soon as the physician suspects it. There is evidence that the level of parental satisfaction and acceptance is higher when this is done. Although professionals might reason that early diagnosis is desirable in order to facilitate genetic counselling or treatment, it seems to be just as important in cases where neither consideration is relevant.

Parents probably try to protect themselves against grief and distress by determining that the child is normal before they have made too profound an attachment. This is an experience vividly described by the parents of premature infants whose survival is uncertain; they withhold the full measure of parental love because they doubt their ability to cope with the infant's death. When a baby is found to have some handicapping condition, either at birth or in the first few years of life, it is largely the future dreams that are shattered. The older the child is when the problem is discovered, the longer they have had to develop their dreams and plans. However, not all serious handicapping conditions are discovered suddenly; many are first suspected by parents, and there is a gradual dawning realization that something is wrong. In these circumstances, by the time a diagnosis is made, it may actually be a relief to know the nature of the problem, so that the stages of bereavement described above are attenuated or foreshortened.

Contrast this situation with the occurrence of a sudden catastrophic injury to the brain, whether caused by trauma, asphyxia, meningitis, encephalitis or encephalopathy. Whilst the mechanism of brain injury in cases of trauma is of course different from that seen in cases of infection or encephalopathy, to the parents, the impact of sudden brain injury is similar, whatever the precise cause may be. The parents have become attached to a normal child and have no reason to be concerned about his or her health or development. He is acquiring a personal life history unique to himself and intertwined with the lives of the parents. The parents have built up an immense investment in that child. For years they have nurtured the development of his skills, abilities and temperament. The incident which changes all that comes out of the blue, with no warning or time to prepare. What is lost is not merely a dream of what might have been but an actual loss of the personality.

It is useful to consider another group of patients, those who have lesions or diseases affecting the peripheral nervous system. Two good examples are muscular dystrophy and traumatic paraplegia. Terrible though it is to see a young person disabled, losing the ability to move, control the sphincters or enjoy normal sexuality, the person is still there and it is possible to communicate and respond. The brain and, therefore, the intellect and personality, remain intact, although there may of course be various psychological effects of the disability.

The unique tragedy of brain injury, as compared to other terrible illnesses or accidents, is the loss of the person and their replacement by someone different. This new person is not totally different but is a pale shadow of the former self, a constant reminder of the lost child. Often it is the person's less desirable characteristics which are prominent. This situation is unlike the death of a child. The parents have no chance to finally accept and adjust; each day they have to deal with their grief again.

The professional response

In the case of acquired brain injury it is rare that either parents or professionals seem to question whether the child should have been allowed to die. Many professionals might feel that death would sometimes have been a better outcome, and that if it had been their child they would have wanted to withdraw life support and discontinue ventilation. In clinical practice, however, this option is not often considered. The outcome of head injury in the early stages is so unpredictable that few neurosurgeons would feel this was a legitimate course of action. Those who have dealt with this situation in cases of meningitis or encephalopathy are perhaps more likely to have withdrawn life support when the only possible outcome would be profound handicap; but they may also have been asked by the parents to continue treatment in such circumstances, whatever the predicted outcome may be. There can be no single right answer to this dilemma.

One must not neglect the effect on the professionals of having to deal with such distressing decisions. They may sometimes be reluctant to become involved in the rehabilitation of seriously damaged children, whatever the cause, because they feel instinctively that the medical care that kept the child alive was meddlesome and a misuse of technology. This criticism is seldom expressed or even admitted to themselves, because they also know that given the same clinical situation they and most other doctors would have had no choice but to follow the same treatment regime.

This insoluble conflict makes it very difficult to continue contact with, and work for, the child. A common response is to treat rehabilitation as an unimportant 'Cinderella' speciality, and to question and undermine the possible benefits of therapy. A negative attitude is therefore conveyed to the parents and therapists in a subtle way and contributes to low morale in all those concerned for the child's progress. Such negative attitudes are in striking contrast to the very positive and enthusiastic view put to parents when they visit rehabilitation units which are privately funded, or with charismatic leadership and dedicated staff. There are lessons from parents' reactions to such organizations which must be heeded in the planning of rehabilitation facilities for head-injured children.

The parents' anger

It is easy to dismiss the anger of parents with a head-injured child as part of their natural response to grief, but the focus of their anger should be investigated. In the case of children with handicaps discovered at birth, there may be an obvious direction of their anger at the unfortunate obstetrician. Although this is often inappropriate from a medical point of view, it is understandable that parents should feel that a badly supervised birth was the cause of the problem. When a child has become handicapped as a result of extreme prematurity, anger may be directed against the neonatal team who saved the child's life against enormous odds, but left them to care for a handicapped child. This anger is not readily expressed and, indeed, is sometimes felt more by other professionals, than by the parents, who do not always understand the nature of the decisions that were made and the alternatives that could have been adopted. For the reasons discussed above, it seems quite unusual for parents to direct anger at the neurosurgeon or intensive care team in cases of head injury. They may nevertheless feel and perhaps express intense anger at other aspects of care, such as lack of communication by medical staff, inadequate information about the nature of the head injury, mediocre or non-existent rehabilitation services. The poor liaison between the neurosurgical unit, the referring hospital and the education authorities in the child's home town is a recurring theme and a source of particular irritation. Anger that is directed against such unnecessary problems is legitimate and must be acknowledged.

Counselling

The principles of counselling apply to the care and support of the parents and siblings of a head-injured child as they do with other handicapping conditions. Doctors are often too eager to talk and explain, and do not listen carefully enough to what the parents are saying or wanting to say. Information is vital but it must be given slowly and in easily digested amounts. It is known that distraught parents do not take in much of what is said and that certain procedures are helpful. These include giving important items of news to both parents together whenever possible, in a quiet place rather than in the open ward; allowing ample time for questions; suggesting someone else is with them, either a friend, relative or nurse, who can repeat what is said after the doctor has gone; repeating the same information a few days later so that parents can recap, clarify and ask further questions. Perhaps the most important service one can render the parents and the child is to listen to what they are saying; to respond positively; and above all, to share with them the emotional trauma and distress. This does not mean that one should become deeply involved in their grief; that is not helpful to either party. The important need is for them to know that the professionals are not running away from the problems they face, but have seen the same situations before and have been able to cope with them.

The interminable chronic stress of caring for a head-injured child may well destroy the parents' marriage, their physical health and their careers. Furthermore, they live with the constant worry of not knowing who will take up this burden of care when they fall ill or die. These are issues that might the addressed as part of a long-term counselling and therapy programme.

Hope and realism

An important issue in dealing with the parents of handicapped children is the question of hope versus realism. Professionals are commonly accused of being either too optimistic, not telling the truth because it is too painful; or too gloomy, refusing to give any hope at all. It is not easy to avoid these two pitfalls. When dealing with head injuries, one hopes that the child will continue to improve for many years, although the rate of improvement may decline each year. Thus there is always some reason for hope.

At the same time, as the acute crisis phase recedes into the distant memory, the fact that the original personality is not going to be restored becomes increasingly obvious. The gap between the child and his peers becomes wider in all areas of development. There is always both good news and bad news.

To what extent should professionals promote the idea of rehabilitation and therapy? There is no doubt that parents expect doctors to take active measures to promote recovery and few people doubt that these are beneficial. Although no amount of therapy can repair damaged nerve cells or pathways, therapy programmes help to unlock whatever potential is available and give structure and motivation to the individual who may otherwise give up and sink into apathy and despair. At the same time, one must be careful that parents do not get the impression that the experts can work miracles. This is an unprofessional approach for which some unorthodox intensive treatment regimes have been condemned. Yet these programmes become popular because they are presented with the enthusiasm and commitment which are sometimes lacking in the statutory services.

Conclusion

Human behaviour in the face of intense grief is as legitimate a subject for scientific study as the methodology of intensive care. When the findings of this research are interpreted and used with compassion and common sense both parents and professionals will benefit.

Chapter 15

The incidence and prevention of head injuries

H. R. M. Hayes and R. H. Jackson

Introduction

Accidents represent a major cause of mortality and morbidity in childhood. This chapter reviews the available data on children's accidents and, more particularly, on head injuries, setting the latter in the context of the overall spectrum. The nature of the head injuries resulting in death and admission to hospital are also examined. Following consideration of the types of accidents which most frequently give rise to head injuries, possible preventive approaches are discussed.

The incidence of fatal head injuries

Numerical considerations

In 1984 in England and Wales, 990 children aged under 15 years died following accidents. These deaths represented almost one in eight of all deaths in this age group. The role that accidents play in childhood mortality becomes significantly more dramatic if children under 1 year old are excluded. In this age group, the majority of deaths are associated with birth complications and congenital anomalies. For the 1 to 14 year olds, accidents are the leading cause of death with over one third of the 2,475 deaths being so caused (Office of Population Censuses and Surveys, 1985). Tables 15.1 and 15.2 illustrate, in numerical and percentage terms respectively, the contribution of accidental deaths, together with the part played by head injuries.

Official statistics for England and Wales for 1984 reveal that 403 children died as a result of head injuries. Some may have been caused by assaults on the children or through suicides; the proportions of these cannot be readily determined from the published figures as the details of the injuries and their causes are not cross-tabulated. The consequence of this is that, where head injuries have been expressed as a percentage of

Table 15.1: Causes of mortality in childhood, England and Wales, 1984.

Cause of death	Under 1	1–4	Age (years) 5–9	10–14	0–14
All causes	6037	1064	608	803	8512
Accidents	125	276	255	334	990
Head injuries	24	88	123	168	403

Source: Office of Population Censuses and Surveys, 1985.

Table 15.2: Proportions of childhood deaths resulting from accidents and head injuries, England and Wales, 1984.

Cause of death	Under 1	1–4	Age (years) 5–9	10–14	0–14
Accidents					
% of all causes	2.1%	25.9%	41.9%	41.6%	11.6%
Head injuries					
% of all causes	0.4%	8.3%	20.2%	20.9%	4.7%
% of accidents	19.2%	31.9%	48.2%	50.3%	40.7%

accidental deaths in Table 15.2, the figures may be slightly exaggerated. The error, however, is not thought to be large. Table 15.2 shows that less than one death in twenty overall is caused by a head injury, but the proportion rises to over one in six for children aged 1 to 14 years. This is largely a reflection of the substantial role of accidents among this age group noted above.

The contribution of head injuries to traumatic deaths is high in all age groups, ranging from 19 per cent among babies to almost 50 per cent for the over 4 year olds. This gradient is linked to the changing nature of children's accidents with age. Babies most frequently die from choking and suffocation, house fires, drowning and falls from furniture or their carers' grasp. Only the final type of accident results in head injuries. With increasing mobility, the hazards change. Toddlers regularly die from poisoning, fires and from causes resulting in head injuries, most notably falls on stairs or from windows and, to a small extent, as pedestrian casualties. Not only does mobility and the nature of their activity change as they become older but their environment expands. Those children older than 4 years go to school and playgrounds, increasingly facing the dangers of traffic, initially as pedestrians but also as pedal cyclists as they reach 9 or 10 years. Play is more adventurous and boisterous at this age. Deaths caused by falls from trees, walls and other natural features are frequent, as well as from causes not producing head injury, such as drownings. Throughout childhood, deaths as car passengers are observed, totalling about seventy per annum, many of which are associated with head injuries. The relationship between accident type and the associated injuries clearly has a bearing on the prevention aspects and this is considered more fully later in this chapter.

With the exception of the types of accidents in which the child may be regarded as a passive party, being dropped, caught in a house fire, or travelling as a car passenger for example, many are linked with adventurousness and the freedom to explore one's own world. These traits are, for various reasons, more characteristic of boys than girls. Consequently, it is not surprising that, among children dying from head injuries, boys outnumber girls in all age groups. The lowest boy:girl ratio is 1.4:1, and is among babies, while for all other ages it is at least 2.2:1. The latter ratio is above the average for all fatal accidents, which is more typically in the range 1.5:1 to 2:1.

To complete the numerical consideration of head injury deaths their numbers per unit population are examined. Each year approximately one child in 1,000 aged 1 to 14 years dies due to injury and poisoning. Head injuries claim the lives of about one child in 2,400 annually (Table 15.3). Expressed another way and taking into account the different involvement rates of boys and girls, in the same age period, boys have a one in 137 chance of dying due to a head injury and girls a one in 285 chance.

Table 15.3: Annual death rates among children aged 1–14 years, England and Wales.

Causes of death	Deaths per 10,000 population per annum
All causes	27.6
Injury and poisoning	9.7
Head injuries	4.2

The nature of head injury

The head injuries are divided into two groups in the source of official statistics, Mortality Statistics (Office of Population Censuses and Surveys, 1985): fractures of the skull (ICD codes 800–804) and intracranial injuries excluding those with skull fractures (ICD codes 850–854). Because of the way in which the data are presented therein, it is only possible to identify the numbers of children suffering lesions that were considered to have been the cause of their death. These numbers will be different from those who actually received such injuries since in some cases the death may have been caused by a separate lesion. For example, a child pedestrian may have suffered a skull fracture and a ruptured aorta, the latter being the cause of death and thus the presence of the former not being officially tabulated. The lesions described in the section are only those causing death. The numbers of children suffering different fatal head injuries are given in Tables 15.4 and 15.5.

Table 15.4: Fatal skull fractures, England and Wales, 1984.

ICD Code	Injury	Under 1	1–4	5–9	10–14	0–14
				Age (years)		
800	Fracture of vault of skull	1	3	0	1	5
801	Fracture of base of skull	1	4	8	15	28
802	Fracture of face bones	0	3	4	8	15
803	Other and unqualified skull fractures	8	50	67	87	188
804	Multiple fractures involving skull or face with other bones	0	7	7	19	33
800–804	Fracture of skull	10	64	83	124	281

Source: Office of Population Censuses and Surveys, 1985. (Table 2).

Table 15.5: Fatal intracranial injuries, England and Wales, 1984.

ICD Code	Injury	Under 1	1–4	5–9	10–14	0–14
				Age (years)		
850	Concussion	1	0	1	2	4
851	Cerebral laceration and contusion	0	6	12	15	33
852	Subarachnoid, subdural and extradural haemorrhage following injury	7	9	5	3	24
853	Other and unspecified intracranial haemorrhage following injury	1	2	1	6	10
854	Intracranial injury of other and unspecified nature	5	7	21	18	51
850–854	Intracranial injury, excluding those with skull fracture	14	24	40	44	122

Source: Office of Population Censuses and Surveys, 1985 (Table 2).

The epidemiology of non-fatal head injuries

Numerical considerations

The incompatibility of sources of fatal and non-fatal data necessitates the information presented in this section being based upon a different year and a different geographical catchment area from that dealing with fatalities. The basis of this section is data derived from the Hospital In-Patient Enquiry (HIPE) for England covering 1985 (Department of Health and Social Security, 1987). This publication gives details of the numbers of deaths in and discharges from NHS hospitals, based upon a random 10 per cent sample provided by regional health authorities. These figures can be regarded as closely equating with the number of children suffering accidents and requiring admission to hospital. Of the 818,610 children under 15 years admitted to hospital in England in 1985, 119,550 (14.6 per cent) were accident victims. Just over one third of these casualties were admitted because of head injuries (see Tables 15.6 and 15.7). The rates of admission per unit population for different causes are given in Table 15.8.

Table 15.6: Hospital admission in childhood, England, 1985.

Cause of admission	Age (years) 0–4	5–14	0–14
All causes	446200	372410	818610
Accidents	47320	72230	119550
Head injuries	14590	25780	40370

Source: Department of Health and Social Security, 1987 (Table 14).

Table 15.7: Proportions of hospital admissions resulting from accidents and head injuries, England, 1985.

Cause of admission	Age (years) 0–4	5–14	0–14
Accidents			
% of all causes	10.6%	19.4%	14.6%
Head injuries			
% of all causes	3.3%	6.9%	4.9%
% of accidents	30.8%	35.7%	33.8%

Table 15.8: Annual admission rates per 10,000 population among children, England, 1985.

Cause of admission	Age (years) 0–4	5–14	0–14
All causes	1509	613	904
Injuries	160	119	132
Head injuries	49	42	47

While in absolute terms the numbers of head injuries caused by accidents are high, with any child having a 1 in 15 chance of being admitted to hospital during the first 14 years of life with such an injury, the data in Tables 15.6 to 15.8 can give no indication of the severity of the injuries nor of their consumption of health service resources. It is beyond the scope of this paper to go into admission policies following head injuries but the reader should bear in mind that admission *per se* should only be regarded with caution as an indicator of injury severity. Local policies on whether to admit or not vary; decisions will of necessity reflect the casualty officer's awareness and experience in paediatric head injury, as well as the parents' ability to monitor the condition of the head-injured child in safety at home, taking into account social and other factors. Many of the admissions are only for observation and are usually for less than forty-eight hours.

Just as with fatal head injuries, there are marked differences between the numbers of boys and girls involved. In the 0 to 4 years age group, the boy:girl ratio is 1.33:1, while among 5 to 14 year olds it is 2.19:1.

The nature of the head injuries

Examination of Tables 15.9 and 15.10 shows that the great majority of head injuries necessitating admission are intracranial injuries as opposed to skull fractures, the reverse of the situation for fatal cases.

Table 15.9: Non-fatal skull fractures, England, 1985. 10 per cent sample only.

ICD Code	Injury	Age (years)		
		0–4	5–14	0–14
800	Fracture of vault of skull	97	49	146
801	Fracture of base of skull	35	47	82
802	Fracture of face bones	11	128	139
803	Other and unqualified skull fractures	38	20	58
804	Multiple fractures involving skull or face with other bones	0	2	2
800–804	Fracture of skull	181	246	427

Source: Department of Health and Social Security, 1987 (Table 14).

Note: The above table is extracted from HIPE. It gives only 10 per cent of admissions. It is unsafe to extrapolate these figures to a 100 per cent base due to possible errors associated with small samples.

Table 15.10: Non-fatal intracranial injuries, England, 1985. 10 per cent sample only.

ICD Code	Injury	Age (years) 0–4	5–14	0–14
850	Concussion	92	313	405
851	Cerebral laceration and contusion	1	5	6
852	Subarachnoid, subdural and extradural haemorrhage following injury	1	15	16
853	Other and unspecified intracranial haemorrhage following injury	3	2	5
854	Intracranial injury of other and unspecified nature	1181	1997	3178
850–854	Intracranial injury, excluding those with skull fracture	1278	2332	3610

Source: Department of Health and Social Security, 1987 (Table 14).

Note: See note to Table 15.9.

Head injuries presenting at accident and emergency departments

There is an absence of information on head injuries which present at accident and emergency departments of hospitals nationally as there is no uniform data collection system. It is therefore necessary to rely on local studies undertaken at different hospitals. The results from such studies, however, cannot be reliably extrapolated to produce nationally representative data, either of the numbers of children presenting or of their injuries. This deficiency in the data collection system has consequences for the identification of suitable preventive measures and for the evaluation of their effectiveness. There are exceptions to this shortcoming which must be recognized and used to their maximum benefit.

Most notable is the Home Accident Surveillance System (HASS) managed by the Department of Trade and Industry. Established in 1976, data on accidents in the home have been collected by specially trained clerks at a rolling sampling of twenty hospitals in England and Wales. The system is aimed primarily at monitoring product-related accidents but can provide a useful basis of any type of home accident or its consequence. It has recently been extended to cover accidents outside the home (except accidents in the workplace and road traffic accidents) as a part of the European Home and Leisure Accident Surveillance System, operating eventually in all member states of the European Community. HASS publishes annual reports giving a broad overview of home accidents and is used as the starting point for in-depth investigations of particular types of accidents.

The second potentially even more valuable sources of data on head injuries are those accident and emergency departments with computerized record-keeping systems. A number of hospitals now operate such systems which nominally allow analyses of accident patterns and injury types to be undertaken easily. It is perhaps surprising that there appear to be few if any published studies based upon these systems. Equally sad is the absence of any initiative to collate and analyze centrally the mass of valuable data held within these departments.

Various small scale, usually manually based studies of children presenting to accident and emergency departments with head injuries have been published. Because of their scale and local nature, they are more useful in providing information on the types of accidents involving such injuries rather than being regarded as part of an epidemiological review. They are thus considered in the following section.

The types of accidents involved

The published databases used to describe the numbers and nature of the fatal and non-fatal head injuries reviewed above give little information on the types of accidents in which these injuries occur. Analyses of the records held by the Office of Population Censuses and Surveys would reveal useful information but this would require a special study. The data forming basis of HIPE are less useful as the cause of the injury, the ICD E-code, is not present in the records. (In Scotland, this code is used and thus the data can be usefully analyzed to examine injury causation).

There are a number of studies undertaken in the UK which give an indication of the nature of the accidents resulting in head injuries. Craft, Shaw and Cartlidge (1972) and Craft (1975) report that one third of the 200 children consecutively admitted to hospital in Newcastle-upon-Tyne with head injuries received them in road accidents, principally as pedestrians, and about one quarter were in the home, mostly falls. Similar causes, although in differing proportions, are reported in Field's (1976) extensive review. Field's work provides a thorough review of the literature for children's and adult's head injury epidemiology in the United Kingdom and elsewhere and includes data on children attending accident and emergency departments, not simply hospital admissions.

The prevention of head injuries

The prevention of accidents in childhood can be brought about by education, engineering and enforcement. This is an easy statement to make but a far more difficult one to execute. Of these three routes, perhaps education is the most important. However, education *per se* may only have a limited effect in accident, and hence injury, reduction terms but it can provide the basis for engineering measures and for the enactment and enforcement of legislative measures.

The educational process can be applied to the child at risk; to those well placed to transmit a safety message to the child (parent, carer, teacher) or to the parent (health visitor, GP, road safety officer, journalist, etc.). Equally, the attitude of each of those listed has to be modified and they in turn have to have knowledge to pass on. To implement an engineering countermeasure, for example, the planner, product designer or architect has to have an understanding of the nature of the problem, a recognition of the consequences of their action or inaction, authority to change a design and, of course, the skills to produce a safe solution. The politician at national and local level, the corporate decision-maker or the standards committee representative, each has to have the will and knowledge to take decisions to promote safety.

But who is best placed to educate this myriad of accident preventers? There is no single answer but high among those who are well placed are the practitioners who have access to the information about accidents and see the consequences of them at first hand — doctors, nurses, social workers, parents, etc.; in other words, those left to pick up the pieces after the event. These groups must accept the role and, through their professional organizations, ensure that necessary steps are set in train.

At a more specific level, what countermeasures can be implemented to prevent or reduce the severity of commonly occurring causes of head injury? Two broad groups of accidents have been identified as relevant — falls and road accidents.

Falls

The nature and location of falls in childhood vary with age. Babies are regularly dropped by adults and siblings (Nixon, Jackson and Hayes, 1987). The prevention of these accidents can only be brought about through education of parents to make them aware of the risk and consequences of such events. Closely linked with these are falls by adults on stairs while carrying a baby, sometimes precipitated by fainting fits in new mothers. In these circumstances with both adult and baby falling, the consequences can be tragic. Health visitors and GPs could play a key role in educating parents about these dangers. As previously noted, children explore their immediate environment and test their developing skills as part of growing up. Babies crawl up stairs and toddlers attempt to emulate parents or older siblings by going down stairs unaided. The logical countermeasure for the falls which result is the use of stairgates, ideally at the top and bottom of the flight. To ensure maximum effect, they should be self-closing gates so that there is no reliance on parents' remembering to close them correctly. Gates are preferred to fixed barriers as the latter can themselves cause accidents as parents climb over them. To minimize fixing problems, new houses could be built with wooden batons in place to accept their mountings. Gates may be beyond the financial means of many families and thus provision should be made for them by social service departments. Either financial help or loans of such equipment should be available when needed.

A particular danger in the home is falling from a window. Climbing routes to windows should be avoided by careful placement of furniture, and window locks and stops to prevent them from being opened more than 100 mm should be fitted. The highest risk rooms are the child's bedroom in a normal house and any room in a flat above the ground floor.

As the child gets older its range increases and play equipment either in the school or public playground can present a hazard. Climbing frames have long been recognized as a special risk, but slides also give the opportunity for falls. There are two possible countermeasures here. In some circumstances slides can be built into contoured land, thereby avoiding the danger of a fall completely. If this cannot be achieved, so as to avoid the loss of the challenge and excitement offered by such equipment, energy-absorbing surfacing can be installed around it. Clearly this does not prevent the fall, but it can minimize its adverse consequences.

Also associated with the freedom to play outdoors are the natural features of the environment: trees, quarries, cliffs, and so on. It is not possible to remove or guard all of these and society would find such moves unacceptable. One has to rely, therefore, on the educational process aimed directly at the child to warn them of their dangers. Skills training is relevant in such circumstances for the older child. It can be argued that by providing the child with the necessary skills and equipment to cope with a potentially hazardous situation, such as climbing a rock face, the risk of an accident through uncontrolled exploration is reduced. This argument no doubt has validity but it is essential to remember that children must be of an age to understand the reason for the skills training and to execute successfully what they are taught.

A final type of fall to be considered is the fall from a horse. It is exceptional as it is one of the very few examples of an accident that affects girls more than boys, due of course to differences in their exposure to the risk. Head protection is available and its use is essential. As with any protective helmet, the riding hat must be properly fitted and correctly fastened to be effective. The helmet used must offer clearly defined protection through compliance with current British Standards. In organized riding events, the use of such protective helmets must be made mandatory by those staging the event who have a responsibility to protect the children involved. Equally, leading riders do no service to their own safety, or that of others wishing to emulate them, by being seen with helmets not correctly worn.

Road accidents

These are the second major cause of head injuries. Children are injured principally as pedestrians and pedal cyclists with distinct age grouping for each class of road user.

Child pedestrian casualties peak at about 6 to 8 years while pedal cycle casualties reach a maximum in the 10 to 12 year age groups. There is, however, a need to be cautious in any examination of the officially published statistics on road accidents as they relate to these user groups (Department of Transport, 1987). Only those accidents reported to the police are contained therein. Hospital-based studies have shown that many more casualties present at accident and emergency departments with police under-reporting reaching 90 per cent for pedal cycle accidents producing slight injuries (Bull and Roberts, 1973; Hobbs, Grattan and Hobbs, 1979; Pedder, Hagues, Mackay *et al.*, 1981).

To prevent injuries to pedestrians and pedal cyclists, because of the forces involved when a relatively heavy and stiff object such as a car strikes a light, flexible creature (a human being), one has to try to stop the impact from happening rather then relying completely on mitigating its effect by energy-absorbing measures. There is a notable exception to this philosophy — the protective helmet for pedal cyclists. However, even this can only protect one, albeit highly vulnerable, body region and then only to a limited extent. It is, nevertheless, the only device available for the individual to adopt which can give some protection in a crash. Other safety devices such as high visibility sashes or spacers, or courses of action such as cycle training schemes are routes that cyclists themselves can choose to follow to reduce the likelihood of an accident occurring. Unlike helmets, however, they cease to be effective when metal or road surface violently contacts the rider.

Training in accident prevention should not only be aimed at the vulnerable road users. Drivers of motor vehicles also need to be aware of the dangers they present. It is difficult to demonstrate the effectiveness of driver training and education and one may thus be forced to modify driver behaviour by highway and traffic engineering schemes especially where pedestrians and pedal cyclists are particularly at risk. It is beyond the scope of this paper to go into this subject in detail but examples of this approach include the segregation of vehicles and vulnerable road users, reductions of vehicle speeds by the redesign of residential roads and use of speed bumps and the provision of off-street parking in residential areas. In parallel with such measures, the provision of off-street and traffic-free facilities could reduce child road casualties, but one must ensure that they are sited where they can be reached in safety.

Head injuries also occur to child car occupants in crashes. They are less frequent than pedestrian and pedal cycle casualties but are far easier to prevent. Child restraints are highly effective in injury reduction terms and are readily available. The legislation requiring restraint of front seat car passengers reduced head injuries overall (Rutherford, Greenfield, Hayes *et al.*, 1985) and efforts must now be concentrated on restraint use in rear seats which are mistakenly regarded by the public as safe; 'less dangerous than the front seat' is the message which must be disseminated. The effects of the Motor Vehicles (Wearing of Seat Belts by Children in Rear Seats) Act 1988 must be monitored as was the front seat requirement.

Chapter 16

Children with a claim

Denise Kingsmill

Introduction

This chapter outlines some practical guidance for parents who are involved in, or who are considering embarking on a legal action for compensation on behalf of their injured child. It is not intended to be a learned academic exercise on the law, or a technical analysis of the strategies in cases of this kind. It is hoped that the principles and procedures involved in making a civil claim on behalf of a head-injured child will be easier to understand and the law made more accessible to those who need to use it.

First steps

The investigation and preparation of a claim for compensation on behalf of a head-injured child can be a long and complicated process. It can cause additional financial and emotional strain to parents who have already experienced the profound shock and distress of having a head-injured child. Only a very small proportion of accident victims who are entitled to make a claim in fact do so, or even consult a solicitor. Of those that do seek legal advice, relatively few are lucky enough to find a lawyer with the requisite specialist experience in personal injury which is essential to achieving the best possible result. The day of the general practitioner in the law is, or should be, over. The parent of a head-injured child claiming compensation on their behalf needs a specialist with extensive experience and a proven track record of successful cases in personal injury. A high street solicitor who may do an efficient job of conveying a house, drafting a will or guiding someone through a painful divorce, will not necessarily have the skills to handle a complex claim on behalf of a head-injured child. Even the large, highly efficient personal injury firms, geared to industrial accidents, tend to handle claims in a conveyor belt style, with an emphasis on standard letters and responses, and may not have the commitment and involvement needed for claims of this kind.

Access to the specialist lawyer

The Law Society will, of course, assist in providing a list of practitioners who specialize in this field, whilst charities such as Headway or the Children's Head Injury Trust will also provide the names and addresses of experienced solicitors from their own involvement in cases. Alternatively, many of the medical and psychological staff who care for the head-injured child will know of experienced and successful lawyers from their experiences with other patients. Similarly, the parents of other head-injured children can also tell of their experiences in tracking down a suitable lawyer and advise accordingly. Nevertheless, at the end of the day the parents must make their own choice. They should not hesitate to interview the solicitor and ensure that they are dealing with someone who is appropriately experienced and successful, who is sympathetic and understanding of their needs and those of their child. They will also be dealing with this solicitor for a long time, as compensation claims may take some years, and so it is important that they have confidence and trust in their lawyer. People are often intimidated by lawyers and do not seek sufficient information, relying only on what the lawyer volunteers. Parents should not hesitate, however, in demanding a good service from their solicitors; they should expect easy accessibility both in person and on the telephone, that their letters are answered expeditiously, and that they receive regular reports on the progress of their case. Such demands should not be unreasonable, however, as parents must also bear in mind that solicitors costs are based on the amount of time spent on a case. Profit margins in personal injury cases are slim compared to other kinds of legal work and solicitors often have to carry substantial caseloads. This means that clients do not always receive as much individual attention as they might like. In the United States where the lawyers operate on a contingency (no win, no fee) basis but where, in successful cases, they receive fees of between 20 and 30 per cent of the damages awarded to the injured persons, it is possible to deal more thoroughly with fewer cases. Most specialist personal injury practitioners would welcome the introduction of a form of contingency fee in this country, since it would enable them to provide a better service to their clients. It would also facilitate the development of more specialist knowledge of particular kinds of injury and particular groups of plaintiffs, such as children.

If not now, when?

When a child has an accident and sustains a head injury, most parents' primary concern is naturally with hospital treatment and the prospects of recovery, rather than with claiming compensation through the legal system. Whilst this is obviously an appropriate priority, it is also important to remember that the delay in pursuing legal claims can seriously hamper the investigation of the case and so prejudice a successful outcome. It is necessary, therefore, that parents seek advice as to whether or not their child has a claim at the earliest possible time.

In general terms, proceedings against the defendant must commence within three years of the date of the accident. In the case of children, this limitation period is extended to three years after reaching 18 years of age, the age of legal maturity. Up to the age of 18 years, the child must sue through a next friend, usually a parent, although it could be a grandparent or other relative, or even a social worker. For a three year period after the age of 18, children have the right to commence proceedings in their own name, in respect of a claim arising at any time in their period of legal infancy. If, by reason of their injuries, they are incapable of managing their own affairs then the appointed next friend may continue to act on their behalf. The same time limits apply to cases pursued through the Criminal Injuries Compensation Board, and in claims for medical negligence. In certain cases there may be grounds for the courts to exercise their discretion in extending the time limits further. Consequently, although it would appear that there is plenty of time within which to commence proceedings, in practical terms this is not so; the simple fact is the sooner the better. The memories of witnesses fade, road configurations change, defendants disappear; the police only keep records of road traffic accidents for three years after the date of the accident, at which time they are destroyed and no contemporaneous record will exist. It is important, therefore, that the circumstances of an accident are investigated by an experienced lawyer as soon after the accident as possible.

The bases of claim

At the scene of a road traffic accident, where a child has been seriously hurt, the focus of everyone's concern, including that of the police, it to get medical help for the victim and convey her to hospital as quickly as possible. The painstaking business of obtaining the names and addresses and statements of witnesses is not always given a high priority. It is important to remember that the role of the police in investigating road traffic accidents is primarily to determine whether a criminal offence has been committed. They are not concerned with whether a claim for compensation may exist but, rather whether they must pursue a conviction. Thus, a witness who did not see the accident itself, but did notice the child standing by the road waiting to cross, will be of no interest to the police but can give vital evidence in a civil claim for damages by showing that a vigilant motorist should have been aware of a young child about to cross the road, and so slowed down, stopped or sounded a warning by using his horn. The motorist's failure to do these things is unlikely to render him liable to prosecution for careless driving but can make him guilty of negligence in the eyes of a civil court. Furthermore, a motorist may be driving well within the speed limit and so quite legally from the point of view of the police, but this may be considered as too fast for the built-up streets around a school where children are likely to be playing. It is important to make absolutely clear that if the police do not prosecute a motorist, this does not mean that a good civil claim cannot be made against him. Parents should also be aware that it is possible to claim damages in cases where the defendant motorist is uninsured or where he cannot be traced, as occurs with hit and run drivers. In these circumstances, the claim will be dealt with by the Motor Insurers' Bureau. In the case of an uninsured or untraced driver, the Motor Insurers' Bureau will nominate an insurance company to deal with it on their behalf and the claim will proceed in the usual way.

In many accidents involving children, the question of contributory negligence arises. This refers to the extent to which the behaviour of the child may have contributed to the accident. In the case of very young children the Law Courts do not reduce awards because of the conduct of the child victim. A child up to the age of eight or nine is not expected to be able to predict the outcome of its behaviour to the extent of being held contributorily negligent for its consequences. As children become older and more experienced in traffic, however, they are expected to develop a sense of speed and distance, and an understanding of appropriate behaviour on the road. A failure to exercise this care on the part of an older child can lead to a finding of contributory negligence and a reduction in the amount of damages awarded. It is rare, however, that such a finding will wipe out a child's claim altogether. Some parents have been slow to pursue claims on behalf of their children, believing that the accident was the child's fault — 'he ran out in front of the car, what could the driver do?'. The fact is that a driver could and should do a great deal in these circumstances. In cases of severe accidental injury, even a finding of 75 per cent contributory fault on the part of a child still means that there is a substantial award payable by the defendant.

Damages

After a proper investigation has established that there are reasonable prospects of a successful claim on behalf of a head-injured child, parents should be aware of what can be claimed. Awards in personal injury cases are made up of several elements and it is important for parents to have a clear idea of what factors are taken into account. This will enable them to give their lawyers full instructions and to be in a better position to evaluate any offers that may be made during the course of a case. Damages are awarded for pain, suffering, and loss of amenity, which broadly means the loss of the ability to enjoy life and to do the things which uninjured people are able to do. Damages under this section are known as general damages. It must be emphasized that, in a serious head injury case, damages for pain and suffering will only form a relatively small element of the total claim. The amounts awarded under this heading are notoriously low in the United Kingdom. For example, in the late 1980's the Courts were making the following awards for pain and suffering:

	£
Severe brain damage with perception	75–80,000
Severe brain damage without perception	50–60,000
Grand mal epilepsy	55–60,000
Total blindness with loss of taste and smell	65,000
Paraplegia	(depending on age) 55–65,000
Tetraplegia	80–85,000
Loss of one eye	15,000
Loss of one leg	30–37,000

Such awards make a shameful contrast with those in defamation cases, such as those of Jeffrey Archer and Koo Stark, where damages are awarded by juries, rather than judges as in personal injury cases. It is especially poignant as the ordinary people comprising a jury are likely to have a better understanding of how lives can be devastated by accidents and by injury, than is a privileged and usually elderly judge far removed from the rigours of having to cope with a dependent and injured child, with little help, and whilst endeavouring to maintain a semblance of normal life for the rest of the family.

Expert reports

The amount of general damages awarded will be based on the severity of the injuries sustained and the effects on the child. The child's injuries need to be carefully and comprehensively described and recorded in a series of Medical Reports. These should provide sufficient information for the lawyer to submit a claim for any of the losses and expenses incurred as a result of the accident. It is important that the doctors, psychologists and therapists who examine the child should act together as an interdisciplinary team in order to provide the thorough, comprehensive reports which identify the particular needs of the head-injured child. It is part of the lawyer's role to co-ordinate the skills of the various specialists and collate their reports in such a way as to present a coherent and maximal claim on behalf of the head-injured child. These reports will be vital tools in instructing other experts who advise in relation to the cost of providing necessary services, appliances, therapies and other requirements of the child. Together, the reports should provide a judge with a clear picture of how the child's life has been affected, both in relation to the family and the future.

In the case of the head-injured child, the first report is usually obtained from a neurosurgeon, who should describe the precise nature of the brain injury with great accuracy, the likelihood and extent of recovery, the possibility of further deterioration or development of associated disorders such as epilepsy, and the effect on life-expectancy. Head injuries usually have severe emotional and behavioural consequences for children, which need to be described and recorded by the child psychiatrist. It is also important that the psychiatrist gives an opinion on the way in which the child's injury has affected the well being of the whole family (Lezak, 1988b). The neuropsychologist should accurately delineate problems in concentration, learning and memory, and other cognitive functions, indicating their impact upon the child's education and future. Each member of the team instructed by the lawyer should see each other's report so that agreement can be reached and a comprehensive, unified view of the child's disabilities established. Their reports should also contain specific recommendations for the child's independence and employment. For example, the lawyer needs to know whether the child will ever be capable of living independently in the future, or whether constant care and attention will be necessary. It will be important to establish whether that care and attention should be provided at home or within an institution. The extent to which the parents can assist in the provision of care and attention should also be recorded. If a child needs night time care, it will have a significant effect on the cost of nursing assistance and it is vital for this requirement to be included in the reports.

It is not sufficient for the experts' reports simply to describe and comment generally on the medical condition, or level of intelligence. The practical consequences of the injuries sustained and the persisting disabilities, however subtle, must also be discussed. Will the child be capable of work in the future? When and with what limitations? To what extent has the capacity of the injured child to form relationships been affected and what are the likely long-term consequences for marriage and parenthood? These are vital questions to which doctors, psychologists and therapists must address their minds when preparing reports, since the answers will make a profound difference to the preparation of the claim for compensation and, significantly effect the amounts and, therefore, the child's future.

The doctor who has treated the child is not always the best person to provide a medico-legal report. There is a somewhat arrogant, although possibly understandable, belief on the part of some doctors, especially neurosurgeons, that exercising their professional skills upon a patient will lead to the child making an excellent, or full recovery. This optimistic approach can mean that the report is not as useful as one produced by an independent expert who can assess the child's history, condition and recovery more objectively. Reports are also needed from specialists in other, non-medical fields, such as architects who can advise on accommodation and adaptation to homes, nursing specialists who can advise on the cost of care and financial experts who can provide advice on the most efficient management of compensation monies. Most experienced lawyers will have contact with many and varied experts who can produce comprehensive reports in their areas of specialization and who can be trusted to stick to their opinions even in the face of vigorous cross-examination by the opposing side in court. An injured child may have only one bite of the compensation cherry, so it is vital that a full and realistic picture of the child's disability is painted before being set before the judge.

One of the most poignant features of cases involving head-injured children is the loss of potential. No-one knows what the future would have held for a child if an accident had not happened. Yet, it is a picture of that future which must be established if the child is to be properly compensated for its loss. Perhaps the most difficult aspects of this is establishing what a child's future work pattern might have been. In a very young child, this is almost entirely speculative and the sums awarded are often low, which can only be to the total detriment of the child. The mythical notion of younger brains recovering more fully has permeated the legal system, perpetuated by inadequate medical reports, or incompetent 'experts' (sic). If the immature brain of an infant or young child is more vulnerable then awards of compensation should be correspondingly higher. With the older child it is often possible, with the help of school reports and by drawing parallels with the achievements of parents and siblings, to establish a realistic projection of lost potential earnings. This is likely to form a very significant part of any award if meticulously and realistically prepared.

Parents should be aware that they also can claim for their own loss of earnings directly attributable to their child's accident. The court will award compensation to parents for wages lost while taking care of their injured child; a non-wage earning parent may also be compensated for the provision of nursing and other services to the injured child. This is likely to be at the rate that would have been paid to a professional. As a matter of public policy, damages are not awarded for grief and sorrow, but where a parent has suffered a foreseeable psychiatric reaction to witnessing the child's accident or its consequences then it may be possible to make a separate claim for damages.

Head-injury in childhood has major implications for education, particularly in terms of the learning and recall of new information. It is important, therefore, that the educational needs of the injured child are properly and accurately assessed. In many cases injured children are transferred into the special school system which may not be the right place for them. Such schools tend to be geared towards the provision of education for children who have been handicapped since birth, which is not necessarily the right approach for the head-injured child. It may be that a small, private school which is able to meet the demands of a head-injured child by providing extra tuition and help with socialization is the best option. Alternatively, additional tuition and support may be provided within the context of the child's previous school. It is possible to claim for any additional educational expenses that have arisen as the result of the accident.

Time and interim payments

Claims for compensation can take many years to come to court. This is often because the long process of recovery and rehabilitation means that it is not possible to give an early, final opinion on the prospects and extent of recovery. The paucity of State provision for the rehabilitative care of head-injured children in Great Britain is a national disgrace. Facilities provided in the private sector are scarce and available only at great cost. Parents should ensure that their lawyers seek interim payments of damages at an early stage in order that such costs may be met. Not all cases will merit interim awards, but insufficient use is made of this litigation tool and parents must ensure that the possibility of obtaining an interim award has been fully explored by their lawyer. In order to obtain an interim payment the court must be satisfied that at the trial of the case the plaintiff child would obtain judgment for substantial damages against the defendant. In cases where there is doubt about liability of the defendant it will be difficult to persuade a court that an interim payment should be made even if the child is very severely injured. However, in cases where interim payment is appropriate this can be used to pay for additional nursing costs in order to relieve the stress on parents, or to make adaptations to the home in order to facilitate the care of the injured child. Voluntary interim payments can be negotiated with the insurance company without a court order, although many insurers are reluctant to agree because they believe that it slows down the litigation process and reduces the pressure on the plaintiff to get to trial. This should not deter the plaintiff's solicitors however, and if voluntary interim payments are not forthcoming they should make applications to the courts. Although it is obviously preferable for solicitors to make one application for a substantial sum, it is possible to go back more than once to the court for interim payments if further needs develop or expenses increase.

It is important that lawyers should act with expedition in prosecuting claims on behalf of head-injured children, but it is essential that these claims are not settled too early. Often it is not until adolescence or early adulthood that accurate assessment of disability and projected needs can be made. It is possible to seek a provisional award of damages, which enables the plaintiff to obtain an initial award of damages and then go back to the court should the position deteriorate in the future. There are, in fact, only very few cases where provisional awards are advantageous to plaintiffs. In cases where there has been exposure to a toxic substance, such as asbestos, and the full effects of such exposure are not yet known then provisional damages may be appropriate. However, the court is obliged to make an award in such cases on the assumption that the negative consequences will not occur. This means that the awards tend to be relatively low. Arguably, awards of provisional damages will give the infant plaintiff a second bite of the compensation cherry. On balance, however, it is probably preferable to obtain a once-and-for-all settlement, based on as accurate a presentation of the consequences of an accident as possible.

Settlement of a case

All settlement claims on behalf of children up to the age of 18 years must be approved by the court. The court has a special responsibility towards children and will require the parties to explain and justify the level of settlement agreed. When a case is settled on behalf of an infant, the money is not paid out immediately but must be controlled and protected. The Court of Protection should be consulted as to the administration and management of the plaintiff's affairs and the office of the Court of Protection should provide advice to both the solicitors and family of the injured plaintiff. There is a leaflet available from the Court of Protection setting out the current level of fees, which may be recovered by way of damages. The funds of child plaintiffs may be invested in the court, with the advantage that this is cost-free. The principal purpose of the investment, however, is to protect the fund and not to increase it. The range of investments may be regarded by some as rather conservative. It is arguable that a child plaintiff who has received a substantial sum of damages is entitled to more sophisticated financial advice than the Court is able to provide. However fund management and specialist accountancy advice is not usually regarded by the Courts as a recoverable item in damages. Nevertheless it is possible to set up a private trust and claim the costs of such a trust from the other side.

Concluding remarks

It is evident from other contributors to this volume that head injuries sustained by children are not uncommon and may have quite substantial and far reaching effects upon a child's life. It is likely that many claims for compensation are not pursued because those effects have been seriously underestimated, particularly in the case of the child who looks, to all intents and purposes, quite normal and unscathed from the accident. Parents of such children, who are glad to have their child in one piece and looking as he did before the accident, but who do not pursue a claim for compensation may be doing a grave disservice to their child in the long term.

References

ADAMS, G.H., GRAHAM, D.I. and GENNARELLI, T.A. (1981) 'Acceleration induced head injury in the monkey: the model, its mechanical and physiological correlates'. *Acta Neuropathologica*, 7, pp. 26–28.

ALAJOUNANINE, T. and LHERMITTE, F. (1965) 'Aquired aphasia in children'. *Brain*, 88, pp. 653–662.

ALEXANDER, M.P. (1987) 'The role of neurobehavioural syndromes in the rehabilitation and outcome of closed head-injury', in LEVIN, H.S., GRAFMAN, J. and EISENBERG, H.M. (eds.) *Neurobehavioural recovery from Head-injury*, New York, Oxford University Press.

ALMLI, C.R. and FINGER, S. (1984) *Early Brain Damage: Volume 1: Research Orientations and Clinical Observations*, New York, Academic Press.

ALTSCHULER, R.A. (1976) 'Changes in hippocampal synaptic density with increased learning experience in the rat' *Society for Neuroscience Abstracts*, 2, p. 438.

AMAN, M.G. (1984) 'Hyperactivity: nature of the syndrome and its natural history'. *Journal of Autism and Developmental Disabilities*, 14, pp. 39–56.

ANDERSON, G.H. (1981) 'Diet, neurotransmitters and brain function', *British Medical Bulletin*, 37, pp. 95–100.

ANDERSON, M. (1988) 'Inspection time, information processing and the development of intelligence'. *British Journal of Developmental Psychology*, 6, pp. 43–57.

ATKINS, R.M., TURNER, W.H., DUTHIE, R.B. and WILDE, B.R. (1988) 'Injuries to pedestrians in road traffic accidents'. *British Medical Journal*, 297, pp. 1431–1434.

BACH-Y-RITA, P. (1980) *Recovery of Function: theoretical considerations for brain-injury rehabilitation*, Bern, Huber.

BACKETT, E.M. and JOHNSTON, A.M. (1959) 'Social patterns of road accidents to children'. *British Medical Journal*, 1, pp. 409–413.

BADDELY, A. (1988) 'Cognitive psychology and human memory'. *Trends in Neuroscience*, 11, pp. 176–181.

BADDELY, A., and HITCH, G. (1974) Cited by BADDELLY, 1988.

BAKKER, D.J. (1984) 'Brain as a dependent variable'. *Journal of Clinical and Experimental Neuropsychology*, 6, pp. 1–16.

BAKKER, D.J. (1986) 'Scholastic effects of hemispheric-specific stimulation in sub-typed dyslexics' in FLEHMIG, I. and STERN, L. (eds.) *Child Development and Learning Behaviour*, Stuttgart, Fischer.

BAKKER, D.J. and VINKE, J. (1985) 'Effects of hemispheric specific stimulation on brain activity and reading in dyslexics'. *Journal of Clinical and Experimental Neuropsychology*, 7, pp. 505–525.

BANDURA, A. (1969) *Principles of Behaviour Modification*, New York, Holt, Rinehart, Winston.

BARAC, B. (1967) 'Vestibular influences upon the EEG of epileptics'. *Electroencephalography and Clinical Neurophysiology*, 22, pp. 245–252.

BARBEAU, A., GROWDON, J.H. and WURTMAN, R.J. (1979) *Nutrition and the Brain. Volume 5: Choline and Lecithin in Brain Disorders*, New York, Raven Press.

BAREGGI, S.R., PORTA, M. and SELENATI, A. (1975) 'Homovanillic acid and 5-hydroxyindole-acetic acid in the CSF of patients after a severe head injury. 1. Lumbar CSF concentration in chronic brain post-traumatic syndromes'. *European Neurology*, 13, pp. 528–544.

BARIN, J.J., LEGER, D. and BACKMAN, K.M. (1985) 'Working with the family', in YLVISAKER, M. (ed.) *Head Injury Rehabilitation: Children and Adolescents*. London, Taylor and Francis.

BARRETT, D.E. and FRANK, D.A. (1987) *The Effects of Undernutrition on Children's Behaviour*. New York, Gordon and Breach.

BARRETT, P. (1988) The Measurement of Inspection Time: *Personality and Individual Differences* (in press).

BARRIE-SHEVLIN, P. (1987) 'Maintaining sensory balance for the critically ill patient'. *Nursing*, 3, pp. 597–601.

BASKIN, D.S. and HOSOBUCHI, Y. (1981) 'Naloxone reversal of ischaemic deficits in man'. *Lancet*, 11, pp. 272–275.

BAWDEN, H.N., KNIGHTS, R.M. and WINOGREN, H.W. (1985) 'Speeded performance following head-injury in children', *Journal of Clinical and Experimental Neuropsychology*, 7, pp. 39–54.

BELL, R.W. (1975) 'Interactive effects of variable population density and dietary protein sufficiency upon selected morphological, neurochemical and behavioural attributes in the rat', in SERBAN, G. (ed.) *Nutrition and Mental Functions*, New York, Plenum Press.

BENDIXSON, T. (1976) *Instead of Cars*. Harmondsworth, Penguin Books.

BENEDICT, C.R. and LOACH, A.B. (1978) 'Clinical significance of plasma adrenaline and noradrenaline concentrations in patients with subarachnoid haemorrhage'. *Journal of Neurology, Neurosurgery and Psychiatry*, 41, pp. 113–117.

BENTON, A. (1986) 'Reaction time in brain disease, some reflections'. *Cortex,* 22, pp. 129–140.

BENTON, D. and ROBERTS, G. (1988) 'Effect of vitamin and mineral supplementation on intelligence of a sample of school children'. *Lancet*, pp. 140–143.

BERGA, P., BECKETT, P.R. and ROBERTS, D.J. (1986) 'Synergistic interactions between piracetam and dihydroergocristine in some animal models of cerebral hypoxia and ischaemia'. *Arzneimitteitors-chung*, 36, pp. 1314–1320.

BERGER, M.S., PITTS, L.H., LOVELY, M., EDWARDS, M.B.B. and BARTKOWSKI, H.M. (1985) 'Outcome from severe head injury in children and adolescents'. *Journal of Neurosurgery*, 62, pp. 194–199.

BERMAN, J.M. and FREDERICKSON, J.M. (1978) 'Vertigo after head injury — a five year follow-up' *Journal of Otolaryngology*, 7, pp. 237–245.

BHATARA, V.S., CLARK, D.L., ARNOLD, L.E., GUNSETT, R. and SMELTZER, D.J. (1981) 'Hyperkinesis treated by vestibular stimulation: an exploratory study', *Biological Psychiatry*, 16, pp. 269–279.

BICKNELL, J. (1983) 'The psychopathology of handicap'. *British Journal of Medical Psychology*, 56, pp. 167–178.

BISHOP, D. (1983) *Test for Reception of Grammar*, (published by the author).

BISHOP, D. and ROSENBLOOM, L. (1988) 'Childhood language disorders, classification and overview', in YULE, W. and RUTTER, M. (eds.) *Language Development and Disorders*, London, MacKeith Press.

BJORKLUND, A. and STENEVI, U. (1972) 'Nerve growth factor: stimulation of regenerative growth of central noradrenergic neurons' *Science*, 175, pp. 1251–1253.

BLACK, J.E. and GREENOUGH, W.T. (1986) 'Developmental approaches to the memory process', in MARTINEZ, J.L. and KESNER, R.P. (eds.) *Learning and Memory: a biological view*, Orlando, Academic Press.

BLACK, P., BLUMER, D., WELLNER, A.M. and WALKER, A.E. (1971) 'The head-injured child: time–course of recovery with implications for rehabilitation', in *Head-Injury: Proceedings of an International Symposium*, Edinburgh, Churchill Livingstone.

BLACK, P., JEFFRIES, J.J., BLUMER, D., WELLNER, A. and WALKER, A.E. (1969) 'The post-traumatic syndrome in children', in WALKER, A.E., CAVENESS, W.F. and CRITCHLEY, J.M. (eds.) *The Late Effects of Head Injury*, Edinburgh, Churchill Livingstone.

BLAND, B.H. and COOPER, R.M. (1970) 'Experience and vision of the posterior decorticate rat'. *Physiology and Behaviour*, 5, pp. 211–214.

BLAU, A. (1936) 'Mental changes following head trauma in children'. *Archives of Psychiatry and Neurology*, 35, pp. 723–728.

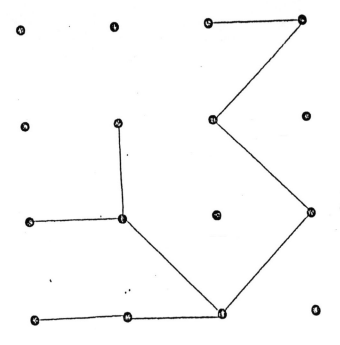

BLUSZTAJN, J.K. and WURTMAN, R.J. (1983) 'Choline and cholinergic neurons'. *Science*, 221, pp. 614–620.

BOGDANOVITCH, U.J.A., BAZAREVITCH, G.J.A. and KIRILLOV, A.L. (1975) 'The use of cholinesterase in severe head injury'. *Resuscitation*, 4, pp. 139–141.

BOLL, T.J. (1983) 'Minor head injury in children — out of sight but not out of mind'. *Journal of Clinical Child Psychology*, 12. pp. 74–80.

BONDY, S.C. and MORELO, B.S. (1971) 'Stimulus deprivation and cerebral blood flow'. *Experimental Neurology*, 31, pp. 200–206.

BOWE, J.L., CORNISH, E.J. and DAWSON, M. (1971) 'Evaluation of folic acid supplements in children taking phenytoin'. *Developmental Medicine and Child Neurology*, 13, pp. 343–354.

BOWMAN, K.M., BLOCH, A. and REICH, R. (1974) 'Psychiatric states following head injury in adults and children'. in FEIRING, E.H. (ed.) *Brock's Injuries of the Brain and Spinal Cord and their Coverings*, New York, Springer.

BRADSHAW, J.L. and NETTLETON, N.C. (1983) *Human Cerebral Asymmetry*, Englewood Cliffs, Prentice-Hall.

BRINK, J.D., GARRETT, A.L., HALE, W.R., WOO SAM, J. and NICKEL, V.L. (1970) 'Recovery of motor and intellectual function in children sustaining severe head injuries'. *Developmental Medicine and Child Neurology*, 12, pp. 565–571.

BRODAL, A. (1973) 'Self observations and neuroanatomical correlations after a stroke', *Brain*, 96, pp. 675–694.

BROMLEY, D.B. (1977) *Personality Description in Everyday Language*, Chichester, Wiley.

BROUWER, W.H. (1985) *Limitation of Attention After Closed Head Injury'*, Netherlands, Rijksuniversiteit, Groningen.

BROWN, G.W. and DAVIDSON, S. (1978) 'Social class, psychiatric disorder of mother and accidents to children', *Lancet*, 1, pp. 378–381.

BROWN, G., CHADWICK, O., SHAFFER, D., RUTTER, M. and TRAUB, M. (1981) 'A prospective study of children with head injuries. III Psychiatric sequelae'. *Psychological Medicine*, 11, pp. 63–78.

BRUCE, D.A. (1983) 'Outcome following head trauma in children', in SHAPIRO, K. (ed.) *Paediatric Head Trauma*, New York, Futura.

BRUCE, D.A., ALAVI, A., BILANIUK, L.T., DOLINSKAS, C., OBRIST, W.A., ZIMMERMAN, R.A. and UZZELL, B. (1981) 'Diffuse cerebral swelling following head injuries in children: the syndrome of "malignant oedema" '. *Journal of Neurosurgery*, 54, pp. 170–178.

BRUCE, D.A., RAPHAELY, R.C., GOLDBER, A.I., ZIMMERMAN, R.A., BILANIUK, L.T., SCHUT, L. and KHUL, D. (1978) 'Pathophysiology, treatment and outcome following severe head-injury in children', *Child's Brain*, 5, pp. 174–191.

BRUCE, D.A., SCHUT, L. and SUTTON, L.N. (1985) 'Pediatric Head Injury', in WILKINS, R.H. and RENGACHARY, S.S. (eds.) *Neurosurgery*, New York, McGraw-Hill.

BUCHANAN, A. and OLIVER, J.E. (1977) 'Abuse and neglect as a cause of mental retardation: A study of 140 children admitted to subnormality hospitals in Wiltshire'. *British Journal of Psychiatry*, 131, pp. 458–467.

BUCHTEL, H.A. (1987) 'Attention and vigilance after head trauma'. in LEVIN, H.S., GRAFMAN, J. and EISENBERG, H.M. (eds.) *Neurobehavioural Recovery from Head Injury*, New York, Oxford University Press.

BUCHWALD, J.S. (1975) 'Brain stem substrates of sensory information processing and adaptive behaviour'. *UCLA Forum in Medical Sciences*, 18, pp. 315–333.

BULL, J.P. and ROBERTS, B.J. (1973) 'Road accident statistics — a comparison of police and hospital information'. *Accident Analysis and Prevention*, 5, pp. 45–53.

BULL, N.L. (1985) 'Dietary habits of 15–25 year olds', *Human Nutrition*, 39A, Suppl. 1, pp. 1–68.

BUSCHKE, H. (1974) 'Components of verbal learning in children: analysis by selective reminding'. *Journal of Experimental Child Psychology*, 18, pp. 488–498.

BUSCHKE, H. and FULD, P.A. (1974) 'Evaluating storage, retention and retrieval in disordered memory and learning'. *Neurology*, 21, pp. 1019–1025.

BUTTNER, U., BUETTNER, U.W. and HENN, V. (1981) 'Vestibular nuclei activity and nystagmus in the alert monkey and their relation to optokinetic and vestibular stimulation', in GUALTIEROTTI, T. (ed.) *Vestibular System: function and morphology*, Berlin, Springer.

BUTTNER, U. and HENN, V. (1976) 'Thalamic unit activity in the alert monkey during natural vestibular stimulation', *Brain Research*, 103, pp. 127–132.

CAFFEY, J. (1972) 'On the theory and practice of shaking infants. Its potential residual effects of permanent brain damage and mental retardation', *American Journal of Diseases of Childhood*, 124, pp. 161–169.

CAFFEY, J. (1974) 'The whiplash shaken infant syndrome', *Paediatrics*, 54, pp. 306–403.

CAIRNS, E. and CANNOCK, T. (1978) 'Development of a more reliable version of the Matching Familiar Figures Test', *Developmental Psychology*, 14, pp. 555–560.

CALLAWAY, E. (1984) 'Human information processing: some effects of methylphenidate, age and scopolamine', *Biological Psychiatry*, 19, pp. 649–662.

CAMFIELD, C.S., CHAPLIN, S., DOYLE, A.B., SHAPIRO, S.H., CUMMINGS, C. and CAMFIELD, P.R. (1979) 'Side-effects of phenobarbitone in toddlers: behavioural and cognitive effects', *Journal of Paediatrics*, 95, pp. 361–365.

CAMPBELL, A.G.M. (1984) 'Children in a persistent vegetative state'. *British Medical Journal*, 289. pp. 1022–1023.

CARDENAS, D.D. (1987) 'Antipsychotics and their use after traumatic brain injury', *Journal of Head Trauma Rehabilitation*, 2, pp. 43–49.

CARTER, R.L., HOHENEGGER, M.K. and SATZ, P. (1982) 'Aphasia and speech organization in children', *Science*, 218, pp. 797–799.

CERMAK, L.S. (1982) *Human Memory and Amnesia*, New Jersey, Erlbaum.

CHADWICK, O. (1976) *Conference of the Meeting of the joint British–Dutch Head-Injury Workshop*, Oxford, UK (unpublished data).

CHADWICK, O. (1985) 'Psychological sequelae of head-injury in children', *Developmental Medicine and Child Neurology*, 27, pp. 72–75.

CHADWICK, O., RUTTER, M., BROWN, G., SHAFFER, D. and TRAUB, M. (1981) 'A prospective study of children with head injury II: cognitive sequelae', *Psychological Medicine*, 11, pp. 49–62.

CHADWICK, O., RUTTER, M., SHAFFER, D. and SHROUT, P. (1981) 'A prospective study of children with head injury IV: specific cognitive deficits', *Journal of Clinical and Experimental Neuropsychology*, 3, pp. 101–120.

CHADWICK, O., RUTTER, M., THOMPSON, J. and SHAFFER, D. (1981) 'Intellectual performance and reading skills after localized head-injury in children', *Journal of Child Psychology and Psychiatry*, 22, pp. 117–139.

CHADWICK, O. and RUTTER, M. (1984) 'Neuropsychological assessment'. in RUTTER, M. (ed.) *Developmental Neuropsychiatry*, Edinburgh, Churchill-Livingstone.

CHI, M.T.H. and GALLAGHER, J.D. (1982) 'Speed of processing: a developmental source of limitation', *Topics in Learning and Learning Disability*, 2, pp. 23–32.

CHILDS, A. (1987) 'Naltrexone in organic bulimia: a preliminary report', *Brain Injury*, 1, pp. 49–55.

CHOUX, M., GRISOLI, F. and PERGAUT, J.C. (1975) 'Extradural haematomas in children', *Child's Brain*, 1, pp. 337–347.

CHOW, K.L. and STEWART, D.L. (1972) 'Reversal of structural and functional effects of long term visual deprivation in cats', *Experimental Neurology*, 34, pp. 409–433.

CHUNG-A-ON, K.O., THOMAS, D.E., TIDMARSH, S.F., DICKERSON, J.W.T., SWEENEY, E.A. and SHAW, D.M. (1985) 'Vitamin deficiencies: a factor in senile dementia?, in SANDLER, M. and SILVERSTONE, T. (eds.) *Psychopharmacology and Food*, Oxford, Oxford University Press.

CLARK, C.R., GEFFEN, G.M. and GEFFEN, L.B. (1986) 'Role of monoamine pathways in attention and effort: effects of clonidine and methylphenidate in normal human adults'. *Psychopharmacology*, 90, pp. 35–39.

CLIFFORD, D.B., RUTHERFORD, J.L., HICKS, F.G. and ZORUMSKI, C.F. (1985) 'Acute effects of antidepressants on hippocampal seizures'. *Annals of Neurology*, 18, 692–697.

CLIFFORD ROSE, F., WHURR, R. and WYKE, M.A. (1988) *Aphasia*, London, Whurr Publishers.

CLIFTON, G.L. and ROBERTSON, C.S. (1986) 'Metabolic response to severe head injury', in MINER, M.E. and WAGNER, K.A. (eds.) *Neurotrauma: treatment, rehabilitation and related issues*, Boston, Butterworths.

CLIFTON, G.L., ROBERTSON, C.S. and CONTANT, C.F. (1985) 'Enteral hyperalimentation in head injury', *Journal of Neurosurgery*, 62, pp. 186–193.

CLIFTON, G.L., ROBERTSON, C.S., GROSSMAN, R.G., HODGE, S., FOLTZ, R. and GARZA, C. (1984) 'The metabolic response to severe head injury', *Journal of Neurosurgery*, 60, pp. 687–696.

CLIFTON, G.L., ZIEGLER, M.G. and GROSSMAN, R.G. (1981) 'Circulating catecholamines and sympathetic activity after head injury', *Neurosurgery*, 8, pp. 10–13.

COHEN, S.B. (1986) 'Educational reintegration and programming for children with head-injury', *Journal of Head Trauma Rehabilitation*, 1, pp. 22–29.

COHEN, S.B., JOYCE, C.M. and RHOADES, K.W. (1985) 'Educational programming for head-injured students'. in YLVISAKER, M. (ed.) *Head Injury Rehabilitation: children and adolescents*, London, Taylor and Francis.

COLLIGNON, R., HECAEN, H. and ANGELERGUES, G. (1968) 'A propos de 12 cas d'aphasie acquise de l'enfant'. *Acta Neurologica et Psychiatrica Belgica*, 68, pp. 245–277.

COMALI, P.E., WAPNER, S. and WERNER, H. (1962) 'Interference effects of Stroop colour–word test in childhood, adulthood, and ageing', *Journal of Genetic Psychology*, 100, pp. 47–53.

CONNERS, C.K. and BLOUIN, A.G. (1983) 'Nutritional effects on the behaviour of children', *Journal of Psychiatric Research*, 17, pp. 193–201.

CONNERS, C.K., CALDWELL, J., CALDWELL, L., SCHWAB, E., KRONSBERG, S., WELLS, K.C., LEONG, N., and BLOUIN, A.G. (1985) 'Experimental studies of sugar and aspartame on autonomic cortical and behavioural responses to sugar', cited by Spring (1986) op. cit.

COOPER, J.A. and FLOWERS, C.R. (1987) 'Children with a history of acquired aphasia: residual language and academic impairments', *Journal of Speech and Hearing Disorder* 52, pp. 251–262.

COOPER, J.R., BLOOM, F.E. and ROTH, R.H. (1986) *The Biochemical Basis of Neuropharmacology*, (5th Ed.), New York, Oxford University Press.

COPE, D.N. (1986) 'The pharmacology of attention and memory', *Journal of Head Trauma Rehabilitation*, 1, pp. 34–42.

CORBALLIS, M.C. (1983) *Human Laterality*, New York, Academic Press.

CORBETT, J.A. and TRIMBLE, M.R. (1984) 'Epilepsy and anticonvulsant medication', in RUTTER, M. (ed.) *Developmental Neuropsychiatry*, Edinburgh, Churchill Livingstone.

COUGHLAN, A.K. and HOLLOWS, S.E. (1985) *The Adult Memory and Information Processing Battery* (AMIPB) Leeds, Coughlan.

COWAN, W.M., FAWCETT, J.W., O'LEARY, D.D.M. and STANFIELD, B.B. (1984) 'Regressive events in neurogenesis', *Science*, 225, pp. 1258–1265.

CRAFT, A.W. (1975) 'Head injury in children', in VINKEN, P.J. and BRUYN, G.W. (eds.) *Handbook of Clinical Neurology*, Volume 23: *Injuries of the brain and skull*, New York, Elsevier.

CRAFT, A.W., SHAW, D.A. and CARTLIDGE, N.E.F. (1972) 'Head injuries in children', *British Medical Journal*, iv, pp. 200–203.

CRAVIOTO, J., DELICARDIE, E.R., and BIRCH, H.G. (1966) 'Nutrition, growth and neurointegrative development: an experimental ecological study'. *Pediatrics*, 38, pp. 319–372.

CRISOTOMO, E.A, DUNCAN, D.W., PROPST, M., DAWSON, D.V. and DAVIS, J.N. (1988) 'Evidence that amphetamine with physical therapy promotes recovery of motor function in stroke patients', *Annals of Neurology*, 23, pp. 94–97.

CROLL, P. and MOSES, D. (1985) *1 in 5: Assessment and Incidence of Special Educational Needs*, London, Routledge.

CROVITZ, H.F. (1987) 'Techniques to investigate post-traumatic and retrograde amnesia after head injury', in LEVIN, H.S., GRAFMAN, J. and EISENBERG, H.M. (eds.) *Neuropsychological Recovery from Head Injury*, New York, Oxford University Press.

CROVITZ, H.F. and DANIEL, W.F. (1987) 'Length of retrograde amnesia after head injury: a revised formula', *Cortex*, 23, pp. 695–698.

CULLUM, C.M. and BIGLER, E.D. (1985) 'Late effects of haematoma on brain morphology and memory in closed head injury', *International Journal of Neuroscience*, 28, pp. 279–283.

CUMMINS, B. (1987) 'A head injury polemic', *British Journal of Neurosurgery*, 1, pp. 6–8.

CURRY, S.H. (1981) 'Event related potentials as indicants of structural functional damage in closed head injury', *Progress in Brain Research*, 54, pp. 507–515.

CURZON, G., (1985) 'Effect of food intake on brain transmitter amine precursors and amine synthesis', in SANDLER, M. and SILVERSTONE, T. (eds.) *Psychopharmocology and Food*, Oxford, Oxford University Press.

DAS, J.P. and VARNHAGEN, C.K. (1986) 'Neuropsychological functioning and cognitive processing', in OBZRUT, J.E., and HYND, G.W. (eds.) *Child Neuropsychology Volume 1: Theory and Research*, New York, Academic Press.

DAVIDSON, L.L. and TAYLOR, E. (1987) 'Parental supervision does not explain the lack of association between overactivity and childhood injuries', *American Journal of Diseases in Children*, 141, 382.

DENNIS, M. and WHITAKER, H.A. (1977) 'Hemispheric equipotentiality and language acquisition', in SEGALOWITZ, S.J. and GRUBER, F.A. (eds.) *Language Development and Neurological Theory*, New York, Academic Press.

DEPARTMENT OF EDUCATION AND SCIENCE (1981) *Education Act*, London, HMSO.

DEPARTMENT OF HEALTH AND SOCIAL SECURITY (1987) *Hospital In-patient Enquiry*, London, HMSO.

DEPARTMENT OF TRANSPORT (1987) *Road Accidents in Great Britain*, 1986, London, HMSO.

De SALLES, A.A.F. and NEWLON, P.G. (1987) 'Electrophysiological assessment of mental function following head injury', *Surgical Neurology*, 27, 589.

DEUTSCH, J.A. (1971) 'The cholinergic synapse and the site of memory', *Science*, 174, pp. 788–794.

DEUTSCHMAN, C.S., KONSTANTINIDES, F.N., RAUP, S. THIENPRASIT, P., and CERRA, F.B. (1986) 'Physiological and metabolic responses to isolated closed head injury. I: Basal metabolic state: correlations of metabolic and physiological parameters with fasting and stressed controls', *Journal of Neurosurgery*, 64, pp. 89–98.

DEUTSCHMAN, C.S., KONSTANTINIDES, F.N., RAUP, S. and CERRA, F.B. (1987) 'Physiological and metabolic responses to isolated closed head injury. II: Effects of steroids on metabolism potentiation of protein wasting and abnormalities of substrate utilisation', *Journal of Neurosurgery*, 66, pp. 388–395.

De WIED, D., (1983) The importance of vasopressin in memory (letter). *Trends in Neuroscience*, 7, pp. 62–64.

DICKERSON, J.W.T. (1988a) 'The interrelationships of nutrition and drugs', in DICKERSON, J.W.T. and LEE, H.A. (eds.) *Nutrition in the Clinical Management of Disease*, (2nd. ed). London, Arnold.

DICKERSON, J.W.T. (1988b) 'Nutrition and disorders of the nervous system', in DICKERSON, J.W.T. and LEE, H.A. (eds.) *Nutrition in the Clinical Management of Disease*, (2nd. ed). London, Arnold.

DICKERSON, J.W.T., MERAT, A. and YUSUF, H.K.M. (1982) 'Effects of malnutrition on brain growth and development', in DICKERSON, J.W.T. and MCGURK, H. (eds.) *Brain and Behavioural Development*, Glasgow, Surrey University Press.

DICKERSON, J.W.T. and PAO, S-K. (1975) 'The effect of low protein diet and exogenous insulin on brain tryptophan and its metabolites in the weanling rat', *Journal of Neurochemistry*, 25, pp. 559–564.

DICKSTEIN, P.W. and TALLAL, P. (1987) 'Attentional capabilities of reading-impaired children during dichotic presentation of phonetic and complex non-phonetic sounds', *Cortex*, 23, pp. 237–249.

DILLON, H. and LEOPOLD, R.L. (1961) 'Children and the post-concussion syndrome', *Journal of American Medical Association*, 175, pp. 86–92.

DiROCCO, L., MAIRA, G., MEGLIO, M. and ROSSI, G.F. (1974) 'L-dopa treatment in comatose states due to cerebral lesions', *Journal of Neurological Sciences*, 18, pp. 169–176.

DOBBING, J. (1968) 'Vulnerable periods in the developing brain', in DAVISON, A.N. and DOBBING, J. (eds.) *Applied Neurochemistry*, Oxford, Blackwell.

DOUGLAS, V.I. (1984) 'Attentional and cognitive problems', in RUTTER, M. (ed.) *Developmental Neuropsychiatry*, Edinburgh, Churchill-Livingstone.

DRACHMAN, D.A. and SAHAKIAN, B.J. (1979) 'Effects of cholinergic agents on human learning and memory', in BARBEAU, A., GROWDON, H.H. and WURTMAN, R.J. (eds.) *Nutrition and the Brain* Volume 5: *Choline and Lecithin in Brain Disorders*, New York, Raven Press.

DUHAIME, A.C., GENNARELLI, T.A., THIBAULT, L.E., BRUCE, D.A., MARGULIES, S.S. and WISER, R. (1987) 'The shaken baby syndrome, a clinical, pathological and biomechanical study', *Journal of Neurosurgery*, 66, pp. 409–415.

EBELS, E.J. (1980) 'Maturation of the central nervous system', in RUTTER, M. (ed.) *Scientific Foundations of Developmental Psychiatry*, London, Heinemann.

EDVINSSON, L., OWMAN, C., ROSENGREN, E. and WEST, K.A. (1971) 'Brain concentrations of dopamine, noradrenaline, 5-hydroxytryptamine, and homovanillic acid during intracranial hypertension following traumatic brain injury in rabbits', *Acta Neurologica Scandinavica*, 47, pp. 458–463.

EGGER, J., CARTER, G.M., GRAHAM, T.J., GURNLEY, D. and SOOTHILL, J.F. (1985) 'Controlled trial of obligoantigenic treatment in the hyperkinetic syndrome', *Lancet*, I, pp. 540–545.

EIBEN, C.F., ANDERSON, T.P., LOCKMAN, L., MATTHEWS, D.J., DRYJA, R., MARTIN, J., BURRILL, C., GOTTESMAN, N., O'BRIAN, P. and WITTE, L. (1984) 'Functional outcome of closed head-injury in children and young adults', *Archives of Physical Medicine and Rehabilitation*, 65, pp. 168–170.

EMERY, P.W., GEISSLER, C.G., JUDD, P.A., THOMAS, J.E. and NAISMITH, D.J. (1988) 'Vitamin-mineral supplementation and non-verbal intelligence', *Lancet*, I, p. 407.

ENDERBY, P. (1983) *The Frenchay Dysarthria Test*, Windsor, NFER-Nelson.

ENGEL, G.L. (1977) 'The need for a new medical model: a challenge for biomedicine', *Science*, 196, pp. 129–136.

ENGEL, G.L. (1980) 'The clinical application of the biopsychosocial model', *American Journal of Psychiatry*, 137, pp. 535–544.

ESSER, G., SCHMIDT, M.H. and WITKOP, H.-J. '(1984) Wirksamkeit von carbamazepin bei hyperkinetischen kinderen,. *Zeitschrift fur Kinder und Jugendpsychiatrie*, 12, pp. 275–283.

ETIENNE, P., GAUGHIER, S., DASTOOR, D., COLLIER, B. and RATNER, J. (1979) 'Alzheimer's disease — clinical effect of lecithin treatment', in BARBEAU, A., GROWDON, J.H. and WURTMAN, R.J. (eds.) *Nutrition and the Brain* Volume 5: *Choline and Lecithin in Brain Disorders*, New York, Raven Press.

EVANS, B.M. (1978) 'Patterns of arousal in comatose patients', *Journal of Neurology, Neurosurgery and Psychiatry*, 39, pp. 392–402.

EVANS, B.M. (1979) 'Heart rate studies in association with electroencephalography as a means of assessing the progress of head injury', *Acta Neurochirurgica*, (Suppl.), 28, pp. 52–57.

EVANS, R.W., GUALTIERI, C.T. and PATTERSON, D.R. (1987) 'Treatment of chronic closed head injury with psychostimulant drugs: a controlled case study and appropriate evaluation procedure', *Journal of Nervous and Mental Diseases*, 175, pp. 106–110.

EWING-COBBS, L., FLETCHER, J.M., and LEVIN, H.S. (1985) 'Neuropsychological sequelae following paediatric head-injury'. in YLVISAKER, M. (ed.) *Head-injury Rehabilitation: children and adolescents*, London, Taylor and Francis.

EWING-COBBS, L., LEVIN, H.S., EISENBERG, H.M. and FLETCHER, J.M. (1987) 'Language functions following closed-head injury in children and adolescents', *Journal of Clinical and Experimental Neuropsychology*, 9, pp. 575–592.

FAY, G. and JANESHESKI, J. (1986) 'Neuropsychological assessment of head-injured children', *Journal of Head Trauma Rehabilitation*, 1, pp. 16–21.

FERCHMIN, P.A., BENNETT, E.L. and ROSENZWEIG, M.R. (1975) 'Direct contact with enriched environment is required to alter cerebral weights in rats', *Journal of Comparative and Physiological Psychology*, 88, pp. 360–367.

FERNSTROM, J.D. and WURTMAN, R.J. (1974) 'Nutrition and the brain', *Scientific American*, 230, pp. 84–91.

FERNSTROM, J.D., WURTMAN, R.J., HAMMARSTRAM-WIKLUND, B., RAND, W.M., MUNRO, H.N. and DAVIDSON, L.S. (1979) 'Diurnal variations in plasma concentrations of tryptophan, tyrosine, and other neutral amino acids: effect of dietary protein intake', *American Journal of Clinical Nutrition*, 32, pp. 1912–1922.

FERRIER, D. (1880) *Functions of the Brain*, New York, Putnam.

FERRY, P.C. (1986) 'Infant stimulation programs', *Archives of Neurology*, 43, pp. 281–282.

FIELD, J. H. (1976) *Epidemiology of head injuries in England and Wales*, London, HMSO.

FILLEY, C.M., CRANBERG, L.D., ALEXANDER, M.P. and HART, E.J. (1987) 'Neurobehavioural outcome after closed head-injury in childhood and adolescence', *Archives of Neurology*, 44, pp. 194–201.

FINGER, S. (1978) *Recovery from Brain Damage*, New York, Plenum Press.

FINGER, S. and STEIN, D.G. (1982) *Brain Damage and Recovery: research and clinical perspectives*, New York, Academic Press.

FINGER, S. and ALMLI, C.R. (1984) *Early Brain Damage*, Volume 2: *Neurobiology and Behaviour*, New York, Academic Press.

FINGER, S., LeVERE, T.E., ALMLI, C.R. and STEIN, D.G. (1988) *Brain Injury and Recovery: theoretical and controversial issues*, New York, Plenum Press.

FISHER, C.M. (1983) 'Abulia minor versus agitated behaviour', *Clinical Neurosurgery*, 31, pp. 9–31.

FISHER-THOMPSON, D. and THELEN, E. (1986) 'The effects of supplemented vestibular stimulation on stereotyped behaviour and development in normal infants', *Physical and Occupational Therapy in Paediatrics*, 6, pp. 57–67.

FLACH, J. and MALMROS, R. (1972) 'A longterm follow-up of children with severe head-injury', *Scandinavian Journal of Rehabilitation Medicine*, 4, pp. 9–15.

FLETCHER, C.M. (1973) *Communication in Medicine*, London, Nuffield Provincial Hospitals Trust.

FLETCHER, J.M. and LEVIN, H.S. (1987) 'Neurobehavioural effects of brain injury in children', in ROUTH, D.K. (ed.) *Handbook of Paediatric Psychology*, New York, Guilford Press.

FLETCHER, J.M., MINER, M. and EWING-COBBS, L. (1987) 'Age and recovery from head injury in children: developmental issues', in LEVIN, H.S., GRAFMAN, J. and EISENBERG, H.M. (eds.) *Neurobehavioural Recovery from Head Injury*, New York, Oxford University Press.

FLETCHER, J.M. and TAYLOR, H.G. (1984) 'Neuropsychological approaches to children: towards a developmental neuropsychology', *Journal of Clinical and Experimental Neuropsychology*, 6, pp. 34–56.

FORD, F.R. (1937) Cited by Guttman (1942).

FRANKLIN, M.B. and BARTEN, S.S. (1988) *Child Language: A Reader*, Oxford, Oxford University Press.

FREEDMAN, L.S., SAUNDERS, M.P. and BRIGGS, M. (1986) 'Analysis of head injuries admitted to the Oxford Regional Neurosurgical Unit 1980–1982', *Injury*, 17, pp. 113–116.

FREEMAN, E.A. (1987) *The Catastrophe of Coma*, Queensland, Bateman.

FREY, A. (1976) cited by Pardridge, W.M. (1986) 'Potential effects of the dipeptide sweetener Aspartame on the brain', in WURTMAN, R.J. and WURTMAN, J.J. (eds.) *Nutrition and the Brain*, Volume 7, New York, Raven Press.

FRIBERG, L., OLSEN, T.S., ROLAND, P.E., PAULSON, O.B. and LASSEN, N.A. (1985) 'Focal increase of bloodflow in the cerebral cortex of man during vestibular stimulation', *Brain*, 108, pp. 609–623.

FRIEDMAN, S.L., KLIVINGTON, K.A. and PETERSON, R.W. (1986) *The Brain, Cognition and Education*, New York, Academic Press.

FRUIN, A.H., TAYLOR, C. and PETTIS, M.S. (1986) 'Caloric requirements in patients with severe head injuries', *Surgical Neurology*, 25, pp. 25–28.

FULD, P.A. and FISHER, P. (1977) 'Recovery of intellectual ability after closed head-injury', *Developmental Medicine and Child Neurology*, 19, pp. 495–502.

FULLER, J.L. (1967) 'Experimental deprivation and later behaviour', *Science*, 158, pp. 1645–1652.

FURNHAM, A. and GIBBS, M. (1984) 'School children's attitudes towards the handicapped', *Journal of Adolescence*, 7, pp. 99–117.

GADDES, W.H. (1986) 'Brain function and classroom learning, in FLEHMIG, I. and STERN, L. (eds.) *Child Development and Learning Behaviour*, Stuttgart, Fischer.

GADDES, W.H. and CROCKETT, D.J. (1975) 'The Spreen-Benton aphasia tests; normative data as a measure of language development', *Brain and Language*, 2, pp. 257–280.

GADISSEAUX, P., WARD, J.D., YOUNG, H.F. and BECKER, D.P. (1984) 'Nutrition and the neurosurgical patient', *Journal of Neurosurgery*, 60, pp. 219–232.

GADISSEAUX, P. (1985) 'Nutrition and CNS trauma', in BECKER, D.M. and POVLISHOCK, J.T., (eds.) *Central Nervous System Trauma Status Report*, Maryland, NIH.

GAGE, F.H. and VARON, S. (1988) 'Trophic hypothesis of neuronal cell death and survival', in FINGER, S., LeVERE, T.E., ALMLI, C.R. and STEIN, D.G. (eds.) *Brain Injury and Recovery: Theoretical and Controversial Issues*, New York, Plenum Press.

GAIDOLFI, E. and VIGNOLO, L.A. (1980) 'Closed head injury of school-aged children: Neuropsychological sequelae in early adulthood', *Italian Journal of Neuroscience*, 1, pp. 65–73.

GALLIARD, L. (1961) *Les Sequelles Cochleo-Vestibulaires des Traumatismes Craniens Fermes: étude clinique et medico-legale*, Paris, Masson and Cie.

GALABURDA, A.M. and KEMPER, T.L. (1979) 'Cytoarchitectonic abnormalities in developmental dyslexia: a case study', *Annals of Neurology*, 6, pp. 94–100.

GANNON, R.P., WILLSON, G.N., ROBERTS, M.E. and PEARSE, H.J. (1978) 'Auditory and vestibular damage in head injuries at work', *Archives of Otolaryngology*, 104, pp. 404–408.

GASH, D.M. and THOMAS, G.J. (1983) 'What is the importance of vasopressin in memory processes?', *Trends in Neuroscience*, 6, pp. 197–198.

GENNARELLI, T.A. and THIBAULT, L.E. (1985) 'Biological models of head injuries', in BECKER, D.P. and POVLISHOCK, J.T. (eds.) *Central Nervous System Trauma Status Report*, Maryland, NIH.

GENNARELLI, T.A., ADAMS, J.H. and GRAHAM, D.I. (1986) 'Diffuse axonal injury — a new conceptual approach to an old problem', in BAETHMANN, A., GO, K.G. and UNTERBERG, A. (eds.) *Mechanisms of Secondary Brain Damage*, New York, Plenum Press.

GESCHWIND, N. (1982) 'Disorders of attention: a frontier in neuropsychology', *Philosophical Transcripts of the Royal Society*, London, B298, pp. 173–185.

GESCHWIND, N. and GALABURDA, A.M. (1985) 'Cerebral lateralization: Biological mechanisms, associations, and pathology: A hypothesis and a program for research', *Archives of Neurology*, 42, pp. 428–459.

GIBSON, E. and RADER, N. (1979) 'Attention: perceiver as performer', in HALE, G.A. and LEWIS, M. (eds.) *Attention and Cognitive Development*, New York, Plenum Press.

GIURGEA, C. (1973) 'The "nootropic" approach to the pharmacology of the integrative activity of the brain', *Conditional Reflex*, 8, pp. 108–115.

GLENN, M.B. (1986) 'CNS stimulants: applications for traumatic brain-injury', *Journal of Head Trauma Rehabilitation*, 1, pp. 74–76.

GLUCKSMAN, A. (1951) 'Cell death in normal vertebrate ontogeny', *Biological Reviews*, 26, pp. 59–86.

GOFFINET, M. and EVERARD, P.H. (1986) 'Neurotransmitters, receptors and embryonic brain development', in FLEHMIG, I. and STERN, L. (eds.) *Child Development and Learning Behaviour*, Stuttgart: Fischer.

GOLDBERG, E. and COSTA, L.D. (1981) 'Hemisphere differences in the acquisition and use of descriptive systems', *Brain and Language*, 14, pp. 144–173.

GOLDBERG, E., GERSTMAN, L.J., MATTIS, S., HUGHES, J.E.O., SIRIO, C.A. and BILDER, R.M. (1982) 'Selective effects of cholinergic treatment on verbal memory in post-traumatic amnesia', *Journal of Clinical and Experimental Neuropsychology*, 4, pp. 219–234.

GOLDMAN-RAKIC, P.S., ISSEROFF, A., SCHWARTZ, M.L. and BUGBEE, N.M. (1983) 'The neurobiology of cognitive development', in HAITH, M.M. and CAMPOS, J.J. (eds.) *Mussen's Handbook of Child Psychology* (4th ed), vol. II: *Infancy and Developmental Psychology*, New York, Wiley.

GOLDSTEIN, F.C. and LEVIN, H.S. (1985) 'Intellectual and academic outcome following closed head injury in children and adolescents: research strategies and empirical findings', *Developmental Neuropsychology*, 1, pp. 195–214.

GOLDSTEIN, L.H. and OAKLEY, D.A. (1985) 'Expected and actual behavioural capacity after diffuse reduction in cerebral cortex: a review and suggestions for rehabilitative techniques with the mentally handicapped and head injured', *British Journal of Clinical Psychology*, 24, pp. 13–14.

GOODGLASS, H. and KAPLAN, E. (1972) *The Assessment of Aphasia and Related Disorders*, Philadelphia, Lea and Febiger.

GOODMAN, C.S. (1984) 'Serotonergic recognition during neuronal development', *Science*, 225, pp. 1271–1279.

GOODMAN, R. (1986) 'Hemispherectomy and its alternatives in the treatment of intractable epilepsy in patients with infantile hemiplegia', *Developmental Medicine and Child Neurology*, 28, pp. 251–258.

GOODMAN, R. (1987) 'The developmental neurobiology of language', in YULE, W. and RUTTER, M. (eds.) *Language Development and Disorders. Clinics in Developmental Medicine* Nos. 101/102, London, MacKeith Press/Blackwell.

GORDON, H.W. (1983) 'Music and the right hemisphere', in YOUNG, A.W. (ed.) *Functions of the Right Cerebral Hemisphere*, London, Academic Press.

GREEN, D. (1985) *Head Injury in Adolescence: the Impact of Self.* Paper presented at the Sixth International Congress on Personal Construct Psychology, Cambridge University, August.

GREENBERG, D.A. (1986) 'Calcium channel antagonists and the treatment of migraine'. *Clinical Neuropharmacology*, 9, pp. 311–328.

GREENOUGH, W.T. (1975) 'Experiential modification of the developing brain', *American Scientist*, 63, pp. 37–46.

GREENOUGH, W.T., FASS, B. De VOOGD, T.J. (1976) 'The influence of experience on recovery from brain damage in rodents', in WALSH, R.N. and GREENOUGH, W.T. (eds.) *Environments as Therapy for Brain Dysfunction*. London, Plenum Press.

GREENWOOD, C.T. and RICHARDSON, D.P. (1979) 'Nutrition during adolescence', *World Review of Nutrition and Diet*, 33, pp. 1–41.

GRIFFITHS, M.V. (1979) 'The incidence of auditory and vestibular concussion following minor head injury', *Journal of Laryngology and Otology*, 93, pp. 253–265.

GRONWALL, D. (1987) 'Advances in the assessment of attention and information processing after head injury', in LEVIN, H.S., GRAFMAN, J. and EISENBERG, H.M. (eds.) *Neurobehavioural Recovery from Head Injury*, New York, Oxford University Press.

GROSSMAN, R.G. and GILDENBERG, P.L. (1982) *Head Injury: Basic and Clinical Aspects*, New York, Raven Press.

GROTE, E.H. (1981) 'CNS control of glucose metabolism', *Acta Neurologica Chirurgica* (Suppl.) 31, pp. 1–16.

GROWDON, J.H. (1979) 'Ways to predict clinical responses to lecithin administration,' in BARBEAU, A., GROWDON, J.H. and WURTMAN, R.J. (eds.) *Nutrition and the Brain* Volume 5: *Choline and Lecithin in Brain Disorders*, New York, Raven Press.

GUALTIERI, C.T. (1987) *Pharmacotherapy and the neurobehavioural sequelae of traumatic brain-injury*, Unpublished manuscript.

GUALTIERI, C.T. (1988) 'Pharmacotherapy and the neurobehavioural sequelae of traumatic brain-injury', *Brain Injury*, 2, pp. 101–129.

GULBRANDSEN, G.B. (1984) 'Neuropsychological sequelae of light head injuries in older children six months after trauma', *Journal of Clinical Neuropsychology*, 6, pp. 257–268.

GUTTMAN, E. (1942) 'Aphasia in children', *Brain*, 65, pp. 205–219.

HAAS, J.F., COPE, D.N. and HALL, K. (1987) 'Premorbid prevalence of poor academic performance in severe head injury', *Journal of Neurology, Neurosurgery and Psychiatry*, 50, pp. 52–56.

HATCHINSKI, V. (1986) 'Infant stimulation programs', *Archives of Neurology*, 43, pp. 283–286.

HADLEY, M.N., GRAHAM, T.W., HARRINGTON, T., SCHILLER, W.R., McDERMOTT, N.K. and POSILLICO, D.B. (1986) 'Nutritional support and neurotrauma: a critical review of early nutrition in 45 acute head-injury patient', *Neurosurgery*, 19, pp. 367–373.

HAIDER, W., BENZER, H., KRYSTOF, G., LACKNER, F., MAYRHOFER, O., STEINBEREITHNER, K., IRSIGLER, K., KORN, A., SCHLICK, W., BINDER, H. and GERSTENBRAND, F. (1975) 'Urinary catecholamines in excretion and thyroid hormone blood level in the course of severe acute brain damage', *European Journal of Intensive Care Medicine*, 1, pp. 115–123.

HALL, J.W., MUSAN, H.F. and GENNARELLI, T.A. (1982) 'Auditory function in acute severe head injury', *Laryngoscope*, 92, pp. 883–890.

HAMILL, R.W., WOOLF, P.D., McDONALD, J.V., LEE, L.A. and KELLY, M. (1987) 'Catecholamines predict outcome in traumatic brain injury', *Annals of Neurology*, 21, pp. 438–443.

HANDEL, S.F. and PERALES, D.P. (1986) 'Injury prevention', in MINER, M.E. and WAGNER, K.A. (eds.) *Neurotrauma: treatment, rehabilitation and related issues*, Boston, Butterworths.

HANNAY, H.J., LEVIN, H.S. and GROSSMAN, R.G. (1979) 'Impaired recognition memory after head injury', *Cortex*, 15, pp. 269–283.

HARRELL, L.E., RAWBSON, R. and BALAGURA, S. (1974) 'Acceleration of functional recovery following lateral hypothalamic damage by means of electrical stimulation in the lesioned areas', *Physiology and Behaviour*, 12, pp. 897–899.

HART, T., HAYDEN, M.E. and McDOWELL, J. (1986) 'Rehabilitation of severe brain injury: when you stick to the facts, you cut the losses', in MINER, M.E. and WAGNER, K.A. (eds.) *Neural Trauma II*, Boston, Butterworths.

HASTINGS, J.E. and BARKLEY, R.A. (1978) 'A review of psychophysiological research with hyperkinetic children', *Journal of Abnormal Child Psychology*, 6, pp. 413–447.

HAYES, P.E. and KRISTOFF, C.A. (1986) 'Adverse reactions to five new antidepressants', *Clinical Pharmacology*, 5, pp. 471–480.

HAYES, R.L., PECHURA, C.M., KATAYAMA, Y., POVLISHOCK, J.T., GIEBEL, M.L. and BECKER, D.P. (1984) 'Activation of pontine cholinergic sites implicated in unconsciousness following cerebral concussion in the cat', *Science*, 223, pp. 301–303.

HAYES, R.L., LYETH, B.G., DIXON, C.E., STONNINGTON, H.H. and BECKER, D.P. (1985) 'Cholinergic antagonist reduces neurological deficits following cerebral concussion in the rat', *Journal of Cerebral Blood Flow and Metabolism*, 5 (Suppl. 1), pp. 395–396.

HEARD, C.W., GRIFFITH, R.B., SMITH, T.K., DALY, J.M. and DUDRICK, S.J. (1983) cited by GADISSEAUX, P. (1985) 'Nutrition and CNS trauma', in BECKER, D.M. and POVLISHOCK, J.T. (eds.) *Central Nervous System Trauma Status Report*, Maryland, NIH.

HEBB, D.O. (1942) 'The effect of early and late brain injury upon test scores, and the nature of normal adult intelligence', *Proceedings of the American Philosophical Society*, 85, pp. 275–292.

HEBB, D.O. (1949) *The Organisation of Behaviour*, New York, Wiley.

HECAEN, H. (1976) 'Acquired aphasia in children and the ontogenesis of hemispheric specialization', *Brain and Language*, 3, pp. 114–134.

HECAEN, H. (1983) 'Acquired aphasia in children: revisited', *Neuropsychologia*, 21, pp. 581–587.

HEILMAN, K., and van den ABEL, T. (1980) 'Right hemisphere dominance for attention', *Neurology*, 30, pp. 327–330.

HEIRD, W.C., Driscoll, J.M., Schullinger, J.N., Grebin, B., Winters, R.W. (1972) 'Intravenous alimentation in paediatric patients. *Journal of Paediatrics*, 8, pp. 351–372.

HEISKANEN, O. and KASTE, M. (1974) 'Late prognosis of severe brain injury in children', *Developmental Medicine and Child Neurology*, 16, pp. 11–14.

HELD, R. and HEIN, A. (1963) 'Movement produced stimulation in the development of visually-guided behaviour', *Journal of Comparative and Physiological Psychology*, 56, pp. 872–876.

HENDRICK, E.B., HARWOOD-NASH, D.C.F. and HUDSON, A.R. (1964) Head injuries in children: a survey of 4465 consecutive cases at the Hospital for Sick Children, Toronto', *Clinical Neurosurgery*, 11, pp. 46–65.

HILL, A.E. and ROSENBLOOM, L. (1986) 'Disintegrative psychosis of childhood: teenage follow-up', *Developmental Medicine and Child Neurology*, 28, pp. 34–40.

HILL, P. (1985) 'The diagnostic interview with the individual child', in RUTTER, M. and HERSOV, L. (eds.) *Child and Adolescent Psychiatry: modern approaches* (2nd ed). Oxford, Blackwell Scientific.

HISCOCK, M. and KINSBOURNE, M. (1987) 'Specialisation of the cerebral hemispheres: indications for learning', *Journal of Learning Disabilities*, 27, pp. 130–143.

HOBBS, C.A., GRATTAN, E. and HOBBS, J.A. (1979) 'Classification of injury severity by length of stay in hospital', *TRRL Laboratory Report 871*, Crowthorne, Transport and Road Research Laboratory.

HOCK, R.A. (1984) *The Rehabilitation of a Child with a Traumatic Brain Injury*, Springfield, Charles C. Thomas.

HORTNAGEL, H., HAMMERLE, A.F., HACKL, J.M., BRUCKE, T., and RUMPL, E. (1980) 'The activity of the sympathetic nervous system following severe head injury', *Intensive Care Medicine*, 6, pp. 169–177.

HOWARD, D., PATTERSON, K., FRANKLIN, V.O. and MORTON, J. (1985) 'Treatment of word retrieval deficits in aphasia', *Brain*, 108, pp. 817–829.

HUNT, E. (1980) 'Intelligence as an information processing concept', *British Journal of Psychology*, 71, pp. 449–474.

HUTTENLOCHER, P.R. (1979) 'Synaptic density in human frontal cortex — developmental changes and effects of aging', *Brain Research*, 163, pp. 195–205.

IKEDA, Y. and NAKAZAWA, S. (1984) 'Plasma norepinephrine levels among patients with acute head injury', *Journal of the Nippon Medical School*, 51, pp. 643–644.

IRLE, E. and MARKOWITSCH, H.J. (1987) 'Basal forebrain lesioned monkeys are severely impaired in tasks of associative and recognition memory', *Annals of Neurology*, 22, pp. 735–743.

ISAACSON, R.L. (1975) 'The myth of recovery from early brain damage', in ELLIS, N.R. (ed.) *Aberrant Development in Infancy*, Potomac, Erlbaum.

ITO, H., MIWA, E. and ONODRA, Y. (1977) 'Growing skull fracture of childhood: with reference to the importance of the brain injury and its pathogenetic consideration', *Child's Brain*, 3, pp. 116–126.

IVERSEN, S.D. and IVERSEN, L.L. (1981) *Behavioural Pharmacology*, 2nd ed. Oxford, Oxford University Press.

JACKSON, R.D., CORRIGAN, J.D. and ARNETT, J.A. (1985) 'Amitriptyline for agitation in head injury', *Archives of Physical Medicine and Rehabilitation*, 66, pp. 180–181.

JAFFE, K.M. (1986) 'Paediatric head injury', *Journal of Head Trauma Rehabilitation*, 1, pp. 1–73.

JAMES, W. (1899) *Talks to Teachers*, London, Longman.

JANOWSKY, J.S. and FINLAY, B.L. (1986) 'The outcome of perinatal brain damage: the role of normal neuronal loss and axonal retraction', *Developmental Medicine and Child Neurology*, 28, pp. 375–389.

JEFFERY, R. (1980) 'The developing brain and child development', in WITTROCK, M.C. (ed.) *The Brain and Psychology*, New York, Academic Press.

JELLINGER, K. (1983) 'The neuropathology of paediatric head injury', in SHAPIRO, K. (ed.) *Paediatric Head Trauma*, New York, Futura.

JENNETT, B. and TEASDALE, G. (1977) 'Aspects of coma after severe head injury', *Lancet*, 1, pp. 734–737.

JENNETT, B. and TEASDALE, G. (1981) *Management of Head Injuries*, 1st ed., Philadelphia, Davis.

JOHNSON, D.A. (1989) 'Attention, children and head injury' in CRAWFORD, J. and PARKER, D.M. (eds.) *Advances in Clinical and Experimental Neuropsychology*, London, Plenum Press.

JOHNSON, D.A. and ALMLI, C.R. (1978) 'Age, brain damage and performance', in FINGER, S. (ed.) *Recovery from Brain Damage*, New York, Plenum Press.

JOHNSON, D.A., RICHARDS, D. and ROETHIG-JOHNSTON, K. (1988) *Biochemical and physiological indices of arousal in acute severe head trauma* (in preparation).

JOHNSON, D.A. and ROETHIG-JOHNSTON, K. (1988) 'Stopping the slide of head-injured children', *Special Children*, 15, pp. 18–20.

JOHNSON, D.A. and ROETHIG-JOHNSTON, K. (1988) 'Coma stimulation: a challenge for occupational therapists', *British Journal of Occupational Therapy*, 51, pp. 88–90.

JOHNSON, D.A., ROETHIG-JOHNSTON, K. and MIDDLETON, J. (1988) 'CHIPASAT: the development of an attentional test for head-injured children: Information processing in a normal sample', *Journal of Child Psychology and Psychiatry*, 29, pp. 199–208.

JOHNSON, L.C. and LUBIN, A. (1967) 'The orienting reflex during waking and sleeping', *Electroencephalography and Clinical Neurophysiology*, 22, pp. 11–21.

JOHNSON, L.C. and LUBIN, A. (1972) 'On planning psychophysiological experiments', in GREENFIELD, N.S. and STERNBACH, R.A. (eds.) *Handbook of Psychophysiology*, New York, Holt Rinehart Winston.

JORDAN, F.M., OZANNE, A.E. and MURDOCH, B.E. (1988), 'Longterm speech and language disorders subsequent to closed head injury in children', *Brain Injury*, 2, pp. 179–185.

JOURNAL OF HEAD TRAUMA REHABILITATION (1987) *Psychopharmacology*, 2, pp. 1–76.

JUNCOS, J.L., FABRINI, G., MOURADIAN, N.M., SERATI, C. and CHASE, N. (1987) 'Dietary influences on the anti-Parkinsonian response to levadopa', *Archives of Neurology*, 44, pp. 1003–1005.

KAHNEMANN, D. (1973) *Attention and Effort*, New Jersey, Prentice Hall.

KAIL, R. (1979) *The Development of Memory in Children*, San Francisco, Freeman.

KAIL, R. (1986) 'Sources of age differences in speed of processing', *Child Development*, 57, pp. 969–987.

KAIL, R. and BISANZ, J. (1982) 'Information processing and cognitive development', *Advances in Child Development and Behaviour*, 17, pp. 45–81.

KAISER, G., RUDEBERG, I., FANKHAUSER, I. and ZUMBUHL, C. (1986) 'Rehabilitation medicine following severe head injury in infants and children', in RAIMONDI, A.J., CHOUX, M. and DiROCCO, C. (eds.) *Head Injury in the Newborn and Infant*, New York, Springer.

KANDEL, E. (1982) 'The origins of modern neuroscience', *Annual Review of Neuroscience*, 5, pp. 299–304.

KANTNER, R.M., CLARK, D.L., ATKINSON, J. and PAULSON, G. (1982) 'Effects of vestibular stimulation in seizure-prone children, an EEG Study', *Physical Therapy*, 62, pp. 16–21.

KARCZMAR, A.G. (1979) 'Overview: cholinergic drugs and behaviour; what effects may be expected from a cholinergic diet', in BARBEAU, A., GROWDON, J.H. and WURTMAN, R.J. (eds.) *Nutrition and the Brain*, Volume 5: *Choline and Lecithin in Brain Disorders*, New York, Raven Press.

KARPIAK, S.E., LI, Y.S. and MAHADIK, S.P. (1987) 'Ganglioside treatment: reduction of CNS injury and facilitation of functional recovery', *Brain Injury*, 1, pp. 161–170.

KASAMATSU, T., PETTIGREW, J.D. and ARY, M. (1979) 'Restoration of visual cortical plasticity by local microperfusion of norepinephrine', *Journal of Comparative Neurology*, 185, pp. 163–182.

KATZ, J. (1985) *Handbook of Clinical Audiology* (3rd. ed.), Baltimore, Williams and Wilkins.

KAY, D., KERR, T.A. and LASSMAN, L.P. (1971) 'Brain trauma and the post-concussional syndrome', *Lancet*, II, pp. 1052–1055.

KELLY, G.A. (1955) *The Psychology of Personal Constructs*, Vols 1 and 2, New York, Norton.

KEWMAN, D.E., YANUS, B. and KIRSCH, N. (1988) 'Assessment of distractability in auditory comprehension after traumatic brain Injury', *Brain injury*, 2, pp. 131–138.

KINSBOURNE, M. (1971) 'The minor cerebral hemisphere as a source of aphasic speech', *Archives of Neurology*, 25, pp. 302–306.

KITAMURA, K. (1981) 'Therapeutic effects of pyritinol on sequelae of head injuries', *Journal of International Medical Research*, 9, pp. 215–221.

KLAUBER, M.R., BARRETT-CONNOR, E., MARSHALL, L.F. and BOWERS, S.A. (1981) 'The epidemiology of head injury', *American Journal of Epidemiology*, 113, pp. 505–509.

KLIVINGTON, K.A. (1986) 'Building bridges among neuroscience, cognitive psychology and education', in FRIEDMAN, S.L., KLIVINGTON, K.A. and PETERSON, R.W. (eds.) *The Brain, Cognition and Education*, New York, Academic Press.

KLONOFF, H. (1971) 'Head injuries in children: predisposing factors, accident conditions, accident proneness and sequelae', *American Journal of Public Health*, 61, pp. 2405–2417.

KLONOFF, H. and LOW, M. (1974) 'Disordered brain function in young children and early adolescents: neuropsychological and electroencephalographic correlates', in REITAN, R.M. and DAVIDSON, L.A. (eds.) *Clinical Neuropsychology: Current Status and Applications*, New York, Wiley.

KLONOFF, H., LOW, M.D. and CLARK, C. (1977) 'Head injuries in children: a prospective five year follow-up', *Journal of Neurology, Neurosurgery and Psychiatry*, 40, pp. 1211–1219.

KLOVE, H. (1987) 'Activation, arousal and neuropsychological rehabilitation', *Journal of Clinical and Experimental Neuropsychology*, 9, pp. 297–309.

KNOWLES, W., MASIDLOVER, M. and SMITH, D. (1982) *The Derbyshire Language Scheme* (published by the authors).

KOCHHAR, A., ZIVIN, J.A., LYDEN, P.D. and MAZZARELLA, V. (1988) 'Glutamate antagonist therapy reduces neurologic deficits produced by focal central nervous system ischaemia', *Archives of Neurology*, 45, pp. 148–153.

KORSCHING, S., (1986) 'The role of nerve growth factor in the central nervous system', *Trends in Neuroscience*, 9, pp. 570–573.

KRAEMER, G.W. (1985) 'The primate social environment, brain neurochemical changes and psychopathology', *Trends in Neuroscience*, 8, pp. 339–340.

KROMER, L.F., BJORKLUND, A. and STENEVI, U. (1981) 'Innervation of embryonic implants by regenerating axons of cholinergic septal neurones in the adult rat', *Brain Research*, 210, pp. 153–171.

LABADARIOS, D., OBUWA, G., LUCAS, E.G., DICKERSON, J.W.T. and PARKE, D.V. (1978) 'The effects of chronic drug administration on hepatic enzyme induction and folate metabolism' *British Journal of Clinical Pharmacology*, 5, pp. 167–173.

LANDAU, W. M. and KLEFFNER, F. (1957) 'Syndrome of acquired aphasia with convulsive disorder in children', *Neurology*, 7, pp. 523–530.

LANGE-COSACK, H., WIDER, B., SCHLESNER, H.J., FRUMME, T. and KUBICKI, S. (1979) 'Prognosis of brain injuries in young children (1 until 5 years of age)', *Neuropaediatrie*, 10, pp. 105–127.

LANGFITT, T.W. and GENNARELLI, T.A. (1982) 'Can the outcome of head injury be improved?' *Journal of Neurosurgery*, 56, pp. 19–25.

LANGFITT, T.W., OBRIST, W.D., ALAVI, A., GROSSMAN, R., ZIMMERMAN, J., JAGGI, B., UZZELL, B., REIVICH, M. and PATTON, D. (1987) 'Regional structure and function in head-injured patients: correlation of CT, MRI, PET, CBF and neuropsychological assessment', in LEVIN, H.S., GRAFMAN, J. and EISENBERG, H.M. (eds.) *Neurobehavioural Recovery from Head Injury*, New York, Oxford University Press.

LANGLEY, J. (1984) 'Injury control psychosocial considerations', *Journal of Child Psychology and Psychiatry*, 25, pp. 349–356.

LAUDER, J. and KREBS, H. (1978) 'Serotonin as a differentiation signal in early neurogenesis', *Developmental Neuroscience*, 1, pp. 15–30.

LAURENCE, S. and STEIN, D.G. (1978) 'Recovery after brain damage and the concept of localisation of function', in FINGER, S., (ed.) *Recovery from Brain Damage*. London, Plenum Press.

LAYTON, B.S., CORRICK, G.E. and TOGA, A.W. (1978) 'Sensory restriction and recovery of function', in FINGER, S. (ed.) *Recovery from Brain Damage*. New York, Plenum Press.

LEA, J. (1970) *The colour pattern scheme: A method of remedial language teaching*, Oxted, Surrey, Moorhouse School.

LEAHY, L.F., HOLLAND, A.C. and FRATTALLI, C.M. (1987) 'Persistent deficits following children's head-injury ', *Paper presented to International Neuropsychology Society*, Washington, USA.

LEE, H.A. (1988) 'Parenteral nutrition', in DICKERSON, J.W.T. and LEE, H.A. (eds.) *Nutrition in the Clinical Management of Disease* (2nd. ed), London, Arnold.

LEES, J. (1989) *A Linguistic Investigation of Acquired Childhood Aphasia*, Unpublished MPhil Thesis, London, City University.

Le FEVER, F.F. (1986) 'What can the coma patient hear?: exploratory evaluations using the cardiac deceleration response (abstract)', *Journal of Clinical and Experimental Neuropsychology*, 8, p. 141.

LENNEBERG, E. (1967) *Biological Foundations of Language*, New York, Wiley.

LeVERE, T.E. (1988) 'Neural system imbalances and the consequences of large brain injuries', in FINGER, S., LeVERE, T.E., ALMLI, C.R. and STEIN, D.G., (eds.) *Brain Injury and Recovery: Theoretical and Controversial Issues*, London, Plenum Press.

LEVIN, H.S. (1985) 'Neurobehavioural outcome', in BECKER, D.B. and POVLISHOCK, J.T. (eds.) *Central Nervous System Trauma Status Report*, Maryland, NIH.

LEVIN, H.S. (1986) 'Learning and memory', in HANNAY, J. (ed.) *Experimental Techniques in Human Neuropsychology*, New York, Oxford University Press.

LEVIN, H.S., AMPARO, E., EISENBERG, H.M., WILLIAMS, D.H., HIGH, W.M., McCARDLE, C.B. and WEINER, R.L. (1987) 'Magnetic resonance imaging and computerized tomography in relation to the neurobehavioural sequelae of mild and moderate head injuries', *Journal of Neurosurgery*, 66, pp. 706–713.

LEVIN, H.S. and EISENBERG, H.M. (1979) 'Neuropsychological outcome of closed head injury', *Childs Brain*, 5, pp. 281–292.

LEVIN, H.S., BENTON, A. and GROSSMAN, R. (1982) *Neurobehavioural Consequences of Head-Injury*, Oxford, Oxford University Press.

LEVIN, H.S., EISENBERG, H.M. and MINER, M.E. (1983) 'Neuropsychological findings in head-injured children', in SHAPIRO, K. (ed.) *Paediatric Head Injury*, New York, Futura.

LEVIN, H.S., EWING-COBBS, L. and BENTON, A.L. (1984) 'Age and recovery from brain damage', in SCHEFF, S.W., (ed.) *Aging and Recovery of Function in the Central Nervous System*, New York, Plenum Press.

LEVIN, H.S., GRAFMAN, J. and EISENBERG, H.M. (1987) *Neurobehavioural Recovery from Head Injury*, Oxford, Oxford University Press.

LEVIN, H.S., EISENBERG, H.M., WIGG, N.R. and KOBAYASHI, K. (1982) 'Memory and intellectual ability after head-injury in children and adolescents', *Neurosurgery*, 11, pp. 668–673.

LEVIN, H.S., GOLDSTEIN, F.C., HIGH, W.M. and EISENBERG, H.M. (1988) 'Disproportionately severe memory deficit in relation to normal intellectual function after closed head-injury', *Journal of Neurology, Neurosurgery and Psychiatry*, 51, pp. 1294–1301.

LEVIN, H.S., GROSSMAN, R.G., ROSE, J.E. and TEASDALE, G. (1979) 'Long term neuropsychological outcome of closed head injury', *Journal of Neurosurgery*, 50, pp. 412–422.

LEVIN, H.S., MADISON, C.F., BAILEY, C.B., MEYERS, C.A., EISENBERG, H.M. and GUINTO, F.C. (1983) 'Mutism after closed head injury', *Archives of Neurology*, 40, pp. 601–606.

LEVIN, H.S., PETERS, B.H. and KALISKY, Z. (1986) 'Effects of oral physostigmine and lecithin on memory and attention in closed head-injured patients', *Central Nervous System Trauma*, 3, pp. 333–342.

LEVIN, H.S., WILLIAMS, D., CROFFORD, M.J., HIGH, W.M., EISENBERG, H.M., AMPARO, E.G., GUINTO, F.C., KALISKY, Z., HANDEL, S.F. and GOLDMAN, A.M. (1988) 'Relationship of depth of brain lesions to consciousness and outcome after closed head injury', *Journal of Neurosurgery*, 69, pp. 861–866.

LEVINE, M.J. (1976) 'Physiological responses in intrasensory and intersensory integration of auditory and visual signals by normal and deficit readers', in BAKKER, O. and KNIGHT, R. (eds.) *The Neuropsychology of Learning Disorders: Theoretical Approaches*, Baltimore, University Park Press.

LEVINE, M.J. (1984) 'Physiological responses in the cognitive processing of bisensory tasks in closed head injury', *Paper presented at the International Neuropsychology Society*, Houston, Texas.

LEVINE, M.J., GUERMAY, M. and FRIEDRICH, D. (1987) 'Psychophysiological responses in closed head injury', *Brain Injury*, 1, pp. 171–181.

Le WINN, E.B. (1980) 'The coma arousal team', *Royal Society of Health Journal*, 100, pp. 19–20.

Le WINN, E.B. and DIMANCESCU, M. (1978) 'Environmental deprivation and enrichment in coma', *Lancet*, II, pp. 156–157.

LEZAK, M.D. (1983) *Neuropsychological Assessment* (2nd. ed). New York, Oxford University Press.

LEZAK, M.D. (1988a) 'IQ:RIP', *Journal of Clinical and Experimental Neuropsychology*, 10, pp. 351–361.

LEZAK, M.D. (1988b) 'Brain damage is a family affair', *Journal of Clinical and Experimental Neuropsychology*, 10, pp. 111–123.

LINDENBERG, R., RISCHER, R.S. and DURLACHER, S. (1955) 'The pathology of the brain in blunt head injuries of infants and children', in *Proceedings of the Second International Congress of Neuropathology*, Amsterdam, Excerpta Medica.

LINDSLEY, D.B. (1960) 'Attention, consciousness, sleep and wakefulness', in FIELD, J., MAGOUN, W. and HALL, V.E. (eds.) *Handbook of Physiology 3: Neurophysiology*, Washington: American Physiological Society.

LIPPER, S. and TUCHMAN, M.M. (1976) 'Treatment of chronic post-traumatic organic brain syndrome with dextroamphetamine: first reported case', *Journal of Nervous and Mental Disease*, 162, pp. 366–371.

LOISELLE, D.L., STAMM, J.S., MAITINSKY, C. and WHIPPLE, S.C. (1980) 'Evoked potential and behavioural signs of attentive dysfunction in hyperactive boys', *Psychophysiology*, 17, pp. 193–201.

LUERSSEN, T.G., KLAUBER, M.R. and MARSHALL, L.F. (1988) 'Outcome from head injury related to patient's age', *Journal of Neurosurgery*, 68, pp. 409–416.

LUK, S.-L., THORLEY, G. and TAYLOR, E. (1987) 'Gross overactivity: a study of direct observation', *Journal of Psychopathology and Behavioural Assessment*, 9, pp. 173–182.

LUND, R.D. (1978) *Development and Plasticity of the Brain*, New York, Oxford University Press.

LURIA, A.R. (1963) *Restoration of Function after Brain-injury*, Oxford, Pergamon Press.

LURIA, A.R. (1972) *The Man with a Shattered World*, Harmondsworth, Penguin Books.

LURIA, A.R. (1973) *The Working Brain*, Harmondsworth, Penguin Books.

LURIA, A.R., NAYDIN, V. and TSVETKOVA, L. (1969) 'Restoration of higher cortical function following local brain damage', in VINKEN, G.W. and BRUYN, P.J. (eds.) *Handbook of Clinical Neurology*, Volume 3. Amsterdam, North Holland.

LUTSCHG, J., PFENNINGER, J. and LUDIN, H.P. (1983) 'Brain stem auditory evoked potentials and early smatosensory evoked potentials in neuro-intensively treated comatose children'. *American Journal of Diseases of Childhood*, 137, pp. 41–46.

LUXON, L.M. (1988) 'Methods of examination — audiological and vestibular', in LUDMAN, H. (ed.) *Mawson's Diseases of the Ear* (5th edition) London, Arnold.

LYNN, R. (1966) *Attention, Arousal and the Orienting Reaction*, Oxford, Pergamon Press.

McCABE, R.J.R. and GREEN, D. (1987) 'Rehabilitating severely head-injured adolescents: three case reports', *Journal of Child Psychology and Psychiatry*, 28, pp. 111–126.

McCLAIN, C.J., TWYMAN, D.L., OTT, L.G., RAPP, R.P., TIBBS, P.A., NORTON, J.A., KASARSKIS, E.J., DEMPSEY, R.J. and YOUNG, B. (1986) 'Serum and urine zinc response in head injury patients', *Journal of Neurosurgery*, 64, pp. 224–230.

McCLELLAND, C.Q., REKATE, H., KAUFMAN, B. and BERSSE, L. (1980) 'Cerebral injury in child abuse: a changing profile', *Child's Brain*, 7, pp. 225–235.

McGEAR, P.L. and McGEAR, E.G. (1979) 'Essential cholinergic pathways', in BARBEAU, A., GROWDON, J.H. and WURTMAN, R.J. (eds.) *Nutrition and the Brain* Volume 5: *Choline and Lecithin in Brain Disorders*, New York, Raven Press.

McGUINNESS, D. and PRIBRAM, K. (1980) 'The neuropsychology of attention: emotional and motivational controls', in WITTROCK, M.C. (ed.) *The Brain and Psychology*, New York, Academic Press.

McKENNA, P. and WARRINGTON, E. (1983) *The Graded Naming Test*, Windsor, NFER-Nelson.

McLAURIN, R.L. and KING, L.R. (1975) 'Metabolic effects of head injury', in VINKEN, P.J. and BRUYN, G.W. (eds.) *Handbook of Clinical Neurology*, Volume 23: *Injuries of the Brain and Skull*, Amsterdam, Elsevier.

McLEAN, A., STANTON, K.M., CARDENAS, D.D. and BERGERUD, D.B. (1987) 'Memory retraining combined with the use of oral physostigmine', *Brain Injury*, 1, pp. 145–159.

McMILLAN, T.M. (1984) 'Investigation of everyday memory in normal subjects using the subjective memory questionnaire', *Cortex*, 20, pp. 333–347.

McMILLEN, M.E., MULE, L.N. and LEES, J.A. (1987) 'Acquired neurological insult in children; current management issues — USA/UK', *Presented at the 8th Annual Traumatic Head Injury Programme*, Braintree, Mass.

MACCARIO, M., BACKMAN, J.R. and KOREIN, J. (1972) 'Paradoxical caloric response in altered states of consciousness', *Neurology*, 22, pp. 781–8.

MACKLER, B., PERSON, R., MILLER, L.R., INAMDAR, A.R. and FINCH, C.A. (1978) 'Iron deficiency in the rat: biochemical studies of brain metabolism', *Paediatric Research*, 12, pp. 217–220.

MAKINO, H. and MATSUSHITA, T. (1981) 'Prognosis of vertigo following cranio-cervical injury', *Auris Nasus Larynx (Tokyo)*, 8, pp. 1–10.

MAKISHIMA, K. and SNOW, J.B. (1975) 'Pathogenesis of hearing loss: head injury', *Archives of Otolaryngology*, 101, pp. 426–436.

MAKISHIMA, K. and SNOW, J.B. (1976) 'Histopathological correlates of otoneurological manifestations following head trauma', *The Laryngoscope*, February, pp. 1303–1314.

MANHEIMER, D.I. and MELLINGER, G.D. (1967) 'Personality characteristics of the child accident repeater, *Child Development*, 38, pp. 491–513.

MARKOWITZ, J.C. and BROWN, R.P. (1987) 'Seizures with neuroleptics and antidepressants', *General Hospital Psychiatry*, 9, pp. 135–141.

MARSDEN, C.D. (1987) 'Movement disorders', in WEATHERALL, D.J., LEDINGHAM, J.G.G. and WARRELL, D.A. (eds.) *Oxford Textbook of Medicine*, (2nd ed.) Volume II. Oxford, Oxford University Press.

MARSHALL, J.F. (1984) 'Brain function, neural adaptations and recovery from injury', *Annual Review of Psychology*, 35, pp. 277–308.

MARTIN, H.P. (1980) 'The consequences of being abused and neglected', in KEMPE, C.H. and HELFER, R.E. (eds.) *The Battered Child* (3rd ed.) Chicago, University of Chicago Press.

MARTI-NICOLOVIUS, M., PORTELL-CORTES, I. and MORGADO-BERNAL, I. (1984) 'Intracranial self stimulation after paradoxical sleep deprivation induced by platform methods in rats', *Physiology and Behaviour*, 33, pp. 165–167.

MASSARO, T.F. and WIDMAYER, P. (1981) 'The effect of iron deficiency on cognitive performance in the rat', *Medical and General Clinical Nutrition*, 34, pp. 864–870.

MECK, W.H. and CHURCH, R.M. (1987) 'Nutrients that modify the speed of internal clock and memory storage processes', *Behavioural Neuroscience*, 101, pp. 465–475.

MEPSTEAD, J. (1988) 'Teachers attitudes'. *Special Children*, 17, pp. 14–15.

MESULAM, M.M. (1981) 'A cortical network for directed attention and unilateral neglect', *Annals of Neurology*, 10, pp. 309–325.

MEUDELL, P., MAYES, A. and NEARY, D. (1980) 'Amnesia is not caused by cognitive slowness', *Cortex*, 16, pp. 413–420.

MIDDLETON, J. (1989) 'Thinking about head injury in childhood', *Journal of Child Psychology and Psychiatry*, (in press).

MILLER, C. (1985) 'Hope for coma patients?' *Medical World News*, February, pp. 69–70.

MINDE, K. (1986) 'Hyperactive syndrome', in REMSCHMIDT, H. and SCHMIDT, M. (eds.) *Child and Adolescent Psychiatry in Clinical Practice*, Stuttgart, Thieme.

MINDERHOUD, J.M., HUIZENGA, J. and VAN WOERKOM, T.C.A.M. (1982) 'Patterns of recovery after severe head injury', *Clinical Neurology and Neurosurgery*, 84, pp. 15–28.

MINDERHOUD, J.M., VAN WOERKOM, T.C.A.M. and VAN WEERDEN, T.W. (1976) 'On the nature of brain stem disorders in severely head-injured patients. II: A study in caloric vestibular reactions with neurotransmitter treatment', *Acta Neurochirurgica*, 32, pp. 23–35.

MINDUS, P., CRONHOLM, B., LEVANDER, S.E. and CHALLYNG, D. (1976) 'Piracetam-induced improvement of mental performance: controlled study on normal ageing individuals', *Acta Psychiatrica Scandinavica*, 54, pp. 150–160.

MINER, M.E., FLETCHER, J.M. and EWING-COBBS, L. (1986) 'Recovery versus outcome after head injury in children', in MINER, M.E. and WAGNER, K.A. (eds.) *Neurotrauma: Treatment, Rehabilitation and Related Issues*, Boston, Butterworths.

MINER, M.E. and KOPANIKY, D.R. (1986) 'Cardiopulmonary changes after head-injury', in MINER, M.E. and WAGNER, K.A. (eds.) *Neurotrauma: Treatment, Rehabilitation and Related Issues*, Boston, Butterworths.

MINER, M.E. and WAGNER, K.A. (1986) *Neurotrauma: Treatment, Rehabilitation and Related Issues*, Boston, Butterworths.

MISHKIN, M. and APPENZELLER, T. (1987) 'The anatomy of memory', *Scientific American*, 256, pp. 62–71.

MITCHELL, D.P. and STONE, P. (1973) 'Temporal bone fractures in children', *Canadian Journal of Otolaryngology*, 2, pp. 156–162.

MOLNAR, G.E. and PERRIN, J.C.S. (1983) 'Rehabilitation of children with head injury', in SHAPIRO, K. (ed.) *Paediatric Head Trauma*, New York, Futura.

MORGAN, B.L.G. (1978) 'Effects of hormonal and other factors on growth and development', in DICKERSON, J.W.T. and McGURK, H. (eds.) *Brain and Behavioural Development*, Glasgow, Surrey University Press.

MORGAN, B.L.G. and WINICK, M. (1980) 'Effects of environmental stimulation on brain N-acetyl-neuraminic acid content and behaviour', *Journal of Nutrition*, 110, pp. 425–432.

MORGAN, S.F. (1982) 'Measuring long term memory storage and retrieval in children', *Journal of Clinical and Experimental Neuropsychology*, 4, pp. 77–85.

MOORE, J. (1980) 'Neuroanatomical considerations relating to recovery of function following brain injury', in BACH-Y-RITA, P. (ed.) *Recovery of Function: theoretical considerations for brain injury rehabilitation*, Bern, Huber.

MOORE, R.Y. (1980) 'The reticular formation: monoamine systems', in HOBSON, J.A. and BRAZIER, M.A.B. (eds.) *The Reticular Formation Revisited: specifying function for a non-specific system*, New York, Raven Press.

MORRIS, R.G., KANDEL, E.R. and SQUIRE, L.R. (1988) 'The neuroscience of learning and memory: cells, neural circuits and behaviour', *Trends in Neuroscience*, 11, pp. 125–127.

MORTIMER, J.A. and PIROZZOLO, F.J. (1985) Remote effects of head trauma, *Developmental Neuropsychology*, 1, pp. 215–229.

219

MOSKOVITCH, M. (1979) 'Information processing and the cerebral hemispheres', in GAZZANIGA, M.S. (ed.) *Handbook of Behavioural Neurology* Volume 2: *Neuropsychology*, New York, Plenum Press.

MUSSEN, P. and EISENBERG-BERG, N. (1977) *Roots of Caring, Sharing and Helping: the development of pro-social behaviour in children*, San Francisco, Freeman.

MYSIW, W.J. and JACKSON, R.D. (1987) 'Tricyclic antidepressant therapy after traumatic brain injury', *Journal of Head Trauma Rehabilitation*, 2, pp. 34–42.

MYSIW, W.J., JACKSON, R.D. and CORRIGAN, J.D. (1988) 'Amitriptyline for post-traumatic agitation', *American Journal of Physical Medicine Rehabilitation*, 67, pp. 29–33.

NAISMITH, D.J., NELSON, M., BURLEY, V.J. and GATENBY, S.J. (1988) 'Can children's intelligence be increased by vitamin and mineral supplements?' *Lancet*, II, pp. 335.

NAUGHTON, J.A.L. (1971) 'The effects of severe head injuries in children — psychological aspects', in *Head Injuries: Proceedings of an International Symposium*, Edinburgh, Churchill Livingstone.

NAYAK, A. (1980) 'Plasma biogenic amines in head injury', *Journal of Neurological Sciences*, 47, pp. 211–219.

NELSON, M. and NAISMITH, D.J. (1979) 'The nutritional status of poor children in London'. *Journal of Human Nutrition*, 33, pp. 33–45.

NEWTON, A. and JOHNSON, D.A. (1986) 'Social adjustment after severe head injury I: performance, anxiety or esteem?', *British Journal of Clinical Psychology*, 24, pp. 225–234.

NIMH (1984) *The Neuroscience of Mental Health*, Maryland, National Institute of Mental Health.

NISSEN, M.J. (1986) 'Neuropsychology of attention and memory', *Journal of Head Trauma Rehabilitation*, 1, pp. 13–21.

NIXON, J., JACKSON, R.H. and HAYES, H.R.M. (1987) *Childhood falls involving stairs and bannisters*, London, Department of Trade and Industry.

NONNEMAN, A.J., CORWIN, J.V., SAHLEY, C.L. and VICEDOMINI, J.P. (1984) 'Functional development of the prefrontal system', in FINGER, S. and ALMLI, C.R. (eds.) *Early Brain Damage*, Volume 2. New York, Academic Press.

ODDY, M. (1984a) 'Head injury during childhood: psychological implications', in BROOKS, D.N. (ed.) *Closed Head Injury: psychological, social and family consequences*, Oxford, Oxford University Press.

ODDY, M. (1984b) 'Head injury and social adjustment', in BROOKS, D.N. (ed.) *Closed Head Injury: psychological, social and family consequences*, Oxford, Oxford University Press.

OFFICE OF POPULATION CENSUSES AND SURVEYS (1985) *Mortality Statistics, Cause*, 1984. Series DH2, No 11, London, HMSO.

OKEN, B.S. and CHIAPPA, K.H. (1985) 'Electroencephalography and evoked potentials in head trauma', in BECKER, D.B. and POVLISHOCK, J.T. (eds.) *Central Nervous System Trauma Status Report*, Maryland, NIH.

OLBRICH, H.M., NAU, H.E., LODERMANN, E., ZERBIN, D. and SCHMIT-NEURERBURG, K.P. (1986) 'Evoked potential assessment of mental function during recovery from severe head injury', *Surgical Neurology*, 26, pp. 112–118.

OLDER, M.W.J., EDWARDS, D. and DICKERSON, J.W.T. (1980) 'A nutrient survey in elderly women with femoral neck fractures', *British Journal of Surgery*, 67, pp. 884–886.

OLIVER, J.E. (1975) 'Microcephaly following baby battering and shaking', *British Medical Journal*, ii, pp. 262–264.

OMMAYA, A.C. (1979) 'Indices of neural trauma', in POPP, A.J. (ed.) *Neural Trauma*, New York, Raven Press.

OMMAYA, A.K. and GENNARELLI, T.A. (1974) 'Cerebral concussion and traumatic unconsciousness: correlation of experimental and clinical observations on blunt head injuries', *Brain*, 97, pp. 633–654.

ORNITZ, E.M. (1983) 'Normal and pathological maturation of vestibular function in the human child', in ROMAND, R. (ed.) *Development of Auditory and Vestibular Systems*, New York, Academic Press.

PANKSEPP, J. (1986) 'The neurochemistry of behaviour', *Annual Review of Psychology*, 37, pp. 77–107.

PAPAKOSTOPOULOS, D. (1985) *Clinical and Experimental Neuropsychophysiology*, London, Croom Helm.

PAPANICOLAOU, A. C. (1987) 'Electrophysiological methods for the study of attentional deficits in head injury', in LEVIN, H. S., GRAFMAN, J. and EINSENBERG, H. M. (eds.) *Neurobehavioural Recovery from Severe Head Injury*, New York, Oxford University Press.

PAPANICOLAOU, A.C., LEVIN, H.S., EISENBERG, H.M., MOORE, B.D., GOETHE, K.E. and HIGH,

W.M., Jnr. (1984) 'Evoked potential correlates of post-traumatic amnesia after closed head injury', *Neurosurgery*, 14, pp. 676–678.

PAPUROV, G. and CHOLAKOV, D. (1970) 'Change in hearing in patients with acute craniocerebral injury', *Zhushn Nos Gorlov Boleznei*, 30, pp. 47–49.

PARDRIDGE, W.M. (1986) 'Potential effects of the dipeptide sweetener Aspartame on the brain, in WURTMAN, R.J. and WURTMAN, J.J. (eds.) *Nutrition and the Brain*, Volume 7. New York, Raven Press.

PARKES, J.D. (1985) *Sleep and its Disorders*, New York, Saunders.

PARMELEE, D.X. and O'SHANICK, G.J. (1987) 'Neuropsychological intervention with head-injured children and adolescents', *Brain Injury*, 1, pp. 41–48.

PATTERSON, K. VARGHA-KHADEM, F. and POLKEY, C.E. (1988) 'Reading with one hemisphere', *Brain* 112, p. 39–63.

PAVLOV, I.P. (1960) *Conditioned Reflexes*, New York, Dover Publications.

PEARSON, B.W. and BARBER, H. (1973) 'Head injury: some otoneurological sequelae', *Archives of Otolaryngology*, 97, pp. 81–84.

PEDDER, J.B., HAGUES, S.B., MACKAY, G.M. and ROBERTS, B.J. (1981) 'A study of two-wheeled vehicle casualties at a city hospital', *Proceedings of the 6th International IRCOBI Conference*, Bron, IRCOBI.

PEERLESS, S.J. and GRIFFITHS, J.C. (1975) 'Plasma catecholamines following subarachnoid haemorrhage', in SMITH, R.R. and ROBERTSON, J.T. (eds.) *Subarachnoid Haemorrhage and Cerebrovascular Spasm*, Illinois, C.C. Thomas.

PERECMAN, E. (1987) *The Frontal Lobes Revisited*, New York, IRBN Press.

PFURTSCHELLER, G., SCHWARZ, G. and LIST, W. (1986) 'Long lasting EEG reactions in comatose patients after repetitive stimulation', *Electroencephalography and Clinical Neurophysiology*, 64, pp. 402–410.

PIAGET, J. (1954) *The Construction of Reality in the Child*, New York, Basic Books.

PINCUS, J.H. and BARRY, K.M. (1987) 'Plasma levels of amino acids correlate with motor fluctuations in Parkinsonism', *Archives of Neurology*, 44, pp. 1006–1009.

PINCUS, J.H. and BARRY, K.M. (1988) 'Protein redistribution diet restores motor function in patients with dopa-resistant "off" periods', *Neurology*, 38, pp. 481–483.

PIONTKOWSKI, D. and CALFEE, R. (1979) 'Attention in the classroom', in HALE, G.A. and LEWIS, M. (eds.) *Attention and Cognitive Development*, New York, Academic Press.

PIPER, M. and PLESS, L. (1980) 'Early intervention for infants with Down's Syndrome: A controlled trial', *Paediatrics*, 65, pp. 463–467.

PLUM, F. and POSNER, J.B. (1982) *The Diagnosis of Stupor and Coma*, (3rd ed.) Philadelphia, Davis.

POLLITT, E., LEWIS, N.L., GARZA, C. and SHULMAN, R.J. (1983) 'Fasting and cognitive function', *Journal of Psychiatric Research*, 17, pp. 169–174.

PORCH, B. (1972) *The Porch Index of Communicative Ability in Children*, California Consulting Psychologist Press.

PORTA, M., BAREGGI, S.R. and COLLICE, M. (1975) 'Homovanillic acid and 5-hydroxyindole-acetic acid in the CSF of patients after a severe head injury. II. Ventricular CSF concentration in acute brain post-traumatic syndromes', *European Neurology*, 13, pp. 545–554.

POSNER, M.I. (1987) 'Selective attention in head injury,' in LEVIN, H.S., GRAFMAN, J. and EISENBERG, H.M. (eds.) *Neurobehavioural Recovery from Head Injury*, New York, Oxford University Press.

POSNER, M.I. and PRESTI, D.E. (1987) 'Selective attention and cognitive control', *Trends in Neuroscience*, 10, pp. 13–16.

POULSON, J. and ZILSTROFF, K. (1972) 'Prognostic value of the caloric vestibular test in the unconscious patient with cranial trauma', *Acta Neurologica Scandinavica*, 48, pp. 282–292.

PRATAP-CHAND, R., SINNIAH, M. and SALEM, F.A. (1988) 'Cognitive evoked potential (P300): a metric for cerebral concussion', *Acta Neurologica Scandinavica*, 78, pp. 185–189.

PRIBRAM, K. and McGUINNESS, D. (1975) 'Arousal, activation and effort in the control of attention', *Psychological Review*, 82, pp. 116–149.

PRIOR, M. and SANSON, A. (1986) 'Attention deficit disorder with hyperactivity: A critique', *Journal of Child Psychology and Psychiatry*, 27, pp. 307–320.

PROCTOR, B., GURDJIAN, E.S. and WEBSTER, J.E. (1956) 'The ear in head trauma', *Laryngoscope*, 66, pp. 16–61.

PRUGH, D. and ECKHARDT, L.O. (1980) 'Stages and phases in the response of children and adolescents to illness or injury', *Advances in Behavioural Paediatrics*, 1, pp. 181–194.

PRUGH, D. and TAGIURI, C.K. (1954) 'Emotional aspects of the respirator care of patients with polio-myelitis', *Psychosomatic Medicine*, 16, p. 104.

PUDENZ, R.H. and SHELDON, C.H. (1946) 'The lucite calvarium: a method for direct observation of the brain', *Journal of Neurosurgery*, 3, pp. 487–505.

QUERA-SELVA, M.A. and GUILLEMINAULT, C. (1987) 'Post traumatic central sleep apnoea in the child', *Journal of Paediatrics*, 110, pp. 906–909.

QUINE, L. and PAHL, J. (1987) 'First diagnosis of severe handicap: a study of parental reactions', *Developmental Medicine and Child Neurology*, 29, pp. 232–242.

QUINE, S., PIERCE, J.P. and LYLE, D.M. (1988) 'Relatives as lay-therapists for the severely head-injured', *Brain Injury*, 2, pp. 139–150.

RAIMONDI, A.J., CHOUX, M. and DI ROCCO, C. (1986) *Head Injuries in the Newborn and Infant*, New York, Springer Verlag.

RAPIN, I. (1982) *Children with Brain Dysfunction*, New York, Raven Press.

RAPIN, I. (1986) 'Cerebral dysfunction in children: A need for more specificity', in FLEHMIG, I. and STERN, L. (eds.) *Child Development and Learning Behaviour*, Stuttgart, Fischer.

RAPOPORT, J.L. (1984) 'The use of drugs: trends in research', in RUTTER, M. (ed.) *Developmental Neuro-psychiatry*, Edinburgh, Churchill-Livingstone.

RAPP, R.P., YOUNG, B., TWYMAN, D., BIVINS, B.A., HAACK, D., TIBBS, P.A. and BEAN, J.R. (1983) 'The favourable effect of early parenteral feeding on survival in head-injured patients', *Journal of Neurosurgery*, 58, pp. 906–912.

RASKIN, L.A., SHAYWITZ, B.A., SHAYWITZ, S.E., COHEN, D.J. and ANDERSON, G.M. (1984) 'Early brain damage and attentional deficit disorder: an animal model', in ALMLI, C.R. and FINGER, S. (eds.) *Early Brain Damage* Volume 1: *Research Orientations and Clinical Perspectives*, New York, Academic Press.

REIVICH, M., GUR, R. and ALAVI, A. (1983) 'Positron emission tomographic studies of sensory stimuli, cognitive processes and anxiety', *Human Neurobiology*, 2, pp. 25–33.

RENFREW, C. (1972) *The Word Finding Vocabulary Test* (published by author).

RENNER, M.J. and ROSENZWEIG, M.R. (1987) *Enriched and Impoverished Environments: effects on brain and behaviour*, New York, Springer.

REYNELL, J. (1977) *The Reynell Developmental Language Scales* (revised), Windsor, NFER-Nelson.

REYNOLDS, C.R. and GUTKIN, T.B. (1979) 'Predicting the pre-morbid intellectual status of children using demographic data', *Clinical Neuropsychology*, 1, pp. 36–38.

RICCIUTI, H.N. (1981) 'Adverse environmental and nutritional influences on mental development: a perspective', *Journal of the American Dietetic Association*, 79, pp. 115–120.

RICHARDSON, F. (1963) 'Some effects of severe head injury: a follow-up study of children and adolescents after protracted coma', *Developmental Medicine and Child Neurology*, 5, pp. 471–482.

RIESEN, A.H. (1975) *The Developmental Neuropsychology of Sensory Deprivation*, New York, Academic Press.

RIPPERE, V. (1983) 'Food additives and hyperactive children: a critique of Conners', *British Journal of Clinical Psychology*, 22, pp. 19–32.

RISBERG, J. (1986) 'Regional cerebral blood flow', in HANNAY, H.J. (ed.) *Experimental Techniques in Human Neuropsychology*, New York, Oxford University Press.

RIVERA, F., TANAGUCHI, T., PARISH, R.A., STIMAC, G.K. and MUELLER, B., (1987) 'Poor prediction of positive computed tomographic scans by clinical criteria in symptomatic paediatric head trauma', *Paediatrics*, 80, pp. 579–584.

ROBINSON, R.J.R. (1987) 'The causes of language disorder: introduction and overview', *Proceedings of the First International Symposium of Specific Speech and Language Disorders in Children*, Reading, AFASIC.

ROLAND, P. and FRIBERG, L. (1983) 'Are cortical cerebral blood flow increases during brain work in man due to synaptic excitation or inhibition?' *Journal of Cerebral Blood Flow and Metabolism*, 3, pp. 244–245.

ROLLS, E.T. (1985) 'The neurophysiology of feeding', in SANDLER, M. and SILVERSTONE, T. (eds.) *Psychopharmacology and Food*, Oxford, Oxford University Press.

ROSE, F.D. (1988) 'Environmental enrichment and recovery of function following brain damage', *Medical Science Research*, 16, pp. 257–263.

ROSENZWEIG, M.R., BENNETT, E.L. and DIAMOND, M.C. (1972) 'Brain changes in response to experience', *Scientific American*, 226, pp. 22–29.

ROSENZWEIG, M.R., BENNETT, E.L., DIAMOND, M.C., WU, S-Y, SLAGLE, R.W. and SAFFRAN, E. (1969) 'Influences of environmental complexity and visual stimulation on development of occipital cortex in the rat', *Brain Research*, 14, pp. 427–445.

ROSENZWEIG, M.R. (1980) 'Animal models for effects of brain lesions and for rehabilitation', in BACH Y RITA, R. (ed.) *Recovery of Function: theoretical considerations for brain injury rehabilitation*, Stuttgart, Huber.

ROSNER, M.J. (1987) 'Cerebral perfusion: link between ICP and systemic circulation', in WOOD, J.H. (ed.) *Cerebral Blood Flow: physiologic and clinical aspects*, New York, McGraw-Hill.

ROSS, E.D. and STEWART, R.M. (1981) 'Akinetic mutism from hypothalamic damage: successful treatment with dopamine agonists', *Neurology*, 31, pp. 1435–1439.

ROTH, C. (1983) 'Factors affecting developmental change in speed of processing', *Journal of Experimental Child Psychology*, 35, pp. 509–528.

ROURKE, B.P., BAKKER, D.A., FISK, J.L. and STRANG, J.D. (1983) *Child Neuropsychology: an introduction to theory, research and clinical practice*, New York, Guildford Press.

ROWBOTHAM, G.F., MACIVER, I.N., DICKSON, J. and BOUSFIELD, M.E. (1954) 'Analysis of 1400 cases of acute injury to the head', *British Medical Journal*, March 27th, pp. 726–730.

ROWE, M.J. and CARLSON, C. (1980) 'Brainstem auditory evoked potentials in post-concussion dizziness', *Archives of Neurology*, 37, pp. 679–683.

ROY, C.S. and SHERRINGTON, M.B. (1890) 'On the regulation of the blood supply to the brain', *Journal of Physiology*, 11, p. 85.

RUNE, V. (1970) 'Acute head injuries in children', *Acta Paediatrica Scandinavica*, Supplement 209.

RUSSELL, J. (1978) *The Acquisition of Knowledge*, London, MacMillan.

RUSSELL, W.R. (1959) *Brain, Learning and Memory*, Oxford, Oxford University Press.

RUSSELL, W.R. (1971) *The Traumatic Amnesias*, Oxford, Oxford University Press.

RUTHERFORD, W.H., GREENFIELD, T., HAYES, H.R.M. and NELSON, J.K. (1985) *The medical effects of seat belt legislation in the United Kingdom*, London, HMSO.

RUTTER, M. (1968) *Scale B (2)*, London, Institute of Psychiatry.

RUTTER, M. (1981) 'Psychological sequelae of brain damage in children', *American Journal of Psychiatry*, 138, pp. 1533–1544.

RUTTER, M. (1984) 'Issues and prospects in developmental neuropsychiatry, in RUTTER, M. (ed.) *Developmental Neuropsychiatry*, Edinburgh, Churchill Livingstone.

RUTTER, M., CHADWICK, O. and SHAFFER, D. (1984) 'Head Injury', in RUTTER, M. (ed.) *Developmental Neuropsychiatry*, Edinburgh, Churchill Livingstone.

RUTTER, M., CHADWICK, O., SHAFFER, D. and BROWN, G. (1980) 'A prospective study of children with head injuries I: design and methods', *Psychological Medicine*, 10, pp. 633–645.

RUTTER, M., GRAHAM, P. and YULE, W. (1970) 'A Neuropsychiatric Study in Childhood', *Clinics in Developmental Medicine*, Nos. 35–36. London, SIMP-Heinemann.

ST. JAMES-ROBERTS, I. (1979) 'Neurological plasticity, recovery from brain insult, and child development', in REESE, H.W. and LIPSITT, L.P. (eds.) *Advances in Child Behaviour and Development*, Volume 14, New York, Academic Press.

SACHS, E.J.R. (1957) 'Acetylcholine and serotonin in the spinal fluid', *Journal of Neurosurgery*, 14, pp. 22–27.

SAMPSON, H. (1956) 'Pacing and performance in a serial addition task', *Canadian Journal of Psychology*, 10, pp. 219–225.

SANDLER, A.G. and McLAIN, S.C. (1987) 'Sensory reinforcement: effects of response contingent vestibular stimulation on multiply handicapped children'. *American Journal of Mental Deficiency*, 91, pp. 373–378.

SAPOLSKY, R.M. (1987) 'Glucocorticoids and hippocampal damage', *Trends in Neuroscience*, 10, pp. 346–349.

SATTERFIELD, J.D.M. (1976) 'Neurophysiological studies with hyperkinetic children', in CANTWELL, P. (ed.) *The Hyperkinetic Child*, New York, Spectrum.

SAVAGE, R. (1987) Educational issues for the head-injured adolescent and young adult; *Journal of Head Trauma Rehabilitation*, 2, pp. 1–10.

SAVAKI, H.E. LEVIS, G.M. (1977) 'Changes in rat brain gangliosides following active avoidance conditioning', *Pharmacology, Biochemistry and Behaviour*, 7, pp. 7–12.

SCHADE, J.P. and VAN GROENIGEN, W.B. (1961) 'Structural organization of the human cerebral cortex. I. Maturation of the middle frontal gyrus', *Acta Anatomica*, 47, pp. 74–111.

SCHNEIDER, G.E. (1979) 'Is it really better to have your brain lesion early? A revision of the Kennard principle', *Neuropsychologica*, 17, pp. 557–583.

SCHNEIDER, W. and SHIFFRIN, R.M. (1977) 'Controlled and automatic human information processing: 1 — detection, search and attention', *Psychological Review*, 84, pp. 1–66.

SCHUKNECHT, H.F., NEFF, W.D. and PERLMANN, H.B. (1951) 'An experimental study of auditory damage following blows to the head', *Annals of Otology, Rhinology and Laryngology*, 60, pp. 273–290.

SCHUKNECHT, H.F. (1969) 'Cupulolithiasis', *Archives of Otolaryngology*, 90, pp. 765–778.

SCHWARZ, S. (1964) 'Effects of neocortical lesions and early environmental factors on adult rat behaviour', *Journal of Comparative and Physiological Psychology*, 57, pp. 72–77.

SHAFFER, D., CHADWICK, O. and RUTTER, M. (1975) 'Psychiatric outcome of localized head injury in children', in PORTER, R. and FITZSIMONS, D. (eds.) *Outcome of Severe Damage to the Nervous System*, Ciba Foundation Symposium No 34. Amsterdam, Elsevier.

SHAPIRO, K. (1985) 'Head injury in children', in BECKER, D.P. and POVLISHOCK, J.T. (eds.) *Central Nervous System Trauma Status Report*, Maryland, NIH.

SHAPIRO, R. (1979) 'Temporal bone fractures in children', *Otolaryngology, Head and Neck Surgery*, 87, pp. 323–329.

SHAROV, T., and SHLOMO, L. (1986) 'Stimulation of infants with Down's Syndrome: Long term effects', *Mental Retardation*, 24, pp. 81–86.

SHEER, D.E. and SCHROCK, B. (1986) 'Attention', in HANNAY, H.J. (ed.) *Experimental Techniques in Human Neuropsychology*, New York, Oxford University Press.

SHIROMANI, P.J., GILLIN, J.C. and HENRIKSEN, S.J. (1987) 'Acetylcholine and the regulation of REM sleep: basic mechanisms and clinical implications for affective illness and narcolepsy', *Annual Review of Pharmacology and Toxicology*, 27, pp. 137–156.

SIMEON, J., WATERS, B. and RESNICK, M. (1980) 'Effects of piracetam in children with learning disorders', *Psychopharmacology Bulletin*, 16, pp. 65–66.

SIMPSON, D. and REILLY, P. (1982) 'Paediatric coma scale', *Lancet* II, p. 450.

SINCLAIR, D. (1978) *Human Growth after Birth*, (3rd. ed.) London, Oxford University Press.

SKINNER, B.F. (1953) *Science and Human Behaviour*, New York, Macmillan.

SMITH, A. (1972) 'Dominant and nondominant hemispherectomy', in SMITH, W.L. (ed.) *Drugs, Development and Cerebral Function*, Springfield, Charles C. Thomas.

SMITH, A. and SUGAR, O. (1975) 'Development of above normal language and intelligence 21 years after left hemispherectomy', *Neurology*, 25, p. 813–818.

SPEAR, L.P. and SCALZO, F.M. (1985) 'Ontogenetic alterations in effects of food and or maternal deprivation on 5-HT, 5-HIAA, and 5-HIAA:5-HT ratios', *Developmental Brain Research*, 18, pp. 143–157.

SPEAR, P.D. (1979) 'Behavioural and neurophysiological consequences of visual cortex damage: mechanisms of recovery', in SPRAGUE, J.M. and EPSTEIN, A.N. (eds.) *Progress in Psychobiology and Physiological Psychology* Volume 8. New York, Academic Press.

SPRAGUE, R. and SLEATOR, E.K. (1977) 'Methylphenidate in hyperkinetic children, differences in dose effects on learning and social behaviour', *Science*, 198, pp. 1270–1276.

SPREEN, O. and BENTON, A.L. (1969) *Neurosensory Center Comprehensive Examination for Aphasia*, Victoria, Neuropsychology Laboratory, University of Victoria.

SPREEN, O., TUPPER, O., RISSER, A., TUOKKO, H. and EDGELL, D. (1984) *Human Developmental Neuropsychology*, Oxford, Oxford University Press.

SPRING, B. (1986) 'The effects of foods and nutrients on the behaviour of normal individuals', in WURTMAN, R.J. and WURTMAN, J.J. (eds.) *Nutrition and the Brain*, Volume 7, New York, Raven Press.

SPRINGER, S.P. and DEUTSCH, G. (1985) *Left Brain, Right Brain*, (revised ed.) San Francisco, Freeman.

SPYER, G., DE JONG, A. and BAKKER, D.J. (1987) 'Piracetam and hemispheric specific stimulation', *Paper presented to International Neuropsychology Society*, Barcelona, Spain.

SQUIRE, L.R. and ZOLA-MORGAN, S. (1988) 'Memory: brain systems and behaviour', *Trends in Neuroscience*, 11, pp. 170–175.

SQUIRES, N.K. and OLLO, C. (1986) 'Human evoked potential techniques: possible applications neuropsychology', in HANNAY, H.J. (ed.) *Experimental Techniques in Human Neuropsychology*, New York, Oxford University Press.

STAMP, T.C.B., FLANAGAN, R.J., RICHENS, A., ROUND, J.M., THOMAS, M., JACKSON, M., DURRE, P. and TWIG, C.A. (1978) 'Anticonvulsant osteomalacia', in COPP, D.H. and TOLMAGE, R.V. (eds.) *Endocrinology of Calcium Metabolism*, (International Congress Series 421) Amsterdam, Excerpta Medica.

STEGNICK, A. (1979) cited by PARDRIDGE, W.M. (1986) 'Potential effects of the dipeptide sweetener Aspartame on the brain', in WURTMAN, R.J. and WURTMAN, J.J. (eds.) *Nutrition and the Brain* Volume 7. New York, Raven Press.

STEIN, D.G. (1981) 'Functional recovery from brain damage following treatment with nerve growth factor', in VAN HOF, M.W. and MOHN, G., (eds.) *Functional Recovery from Brain Damage*, Amsterdam, Elsevier.

STEIN, D.G., ROSEN, J.J. and BUTTERS, N. (1974) *Plasticity and Recovery Function in the Central Nervous System*, London, Academic Press.

STEIN, D.G., PALATUCCI, C., KAHN, D. and LABBE, R. (1988) 'Temporal factors influence recovery of function after embryonic tissue transplants in adult rats with frontal cortex lesions', *Behavioural Neuroscience*, 102, pp. 260–267.

STEIN, L. (1978) 'Reward transmitters, catecholamines and opioid peptides,' in LIPTON, M.A. (ed.) *Psychopharmacology: a generation of progress*, New York, Raven Press.

STERNBERG, S. (1966) 'High speed scanning in human memory', *Science*, 153, pp. 652–654.

STIRLING-MEYER, J., HATA, T. and IMAI, A. (1987) 'Clinical and experimental studies of diaschisis', in WOOD, J.H. (ed.) *Cerebral Blood Flow: physiologic and clinical aspects*, New York, McGraw-Hill.

STRANACK, D. and ELLIOT, G. (undated) *Educating Children with Head Injuries*, (Booth Hall Hospital) Manchester, Manchester Education Committee.

STRANG, I., MacMILLAN, R. and JENNETT, B. (1978) 'Head injuries in accident and emergency departments at Scottish Hospitals', *Injury*, 10, pp. 154–159.

STRICH, S.J. (1956) 'Diffuse degeneration of the cerebral white matter in severe dementia following head injury', *Journal of Neurology, Neurosurgery and Psychiatry*, 19, pp. 163–185.

STRICH, S.J. (1961) 'Shearing of nerve fibres as a cause of brain damage due to head injury: a pathological study of twenty cases', *Lancet* II, pp. 443–448.

STRICKVINE-VAN REEK, P., GLAZE, D. and HRACHOVY, R.A. (1984) 'A preliminary prospective neurophysiological study of coma in children', *American Journal of Diseases in Childhood*, 138, pp. 492–495.

STROOP, J.R. (1935) 'Studies of interference in serial verbal reactions', *Journal of Experimental Psychology*, 18, pp. 643–662.

STUSS, D. and BENSON, D.F. (1986) *The Frontal Lobes*, New York, Raven Press.

SUEDFELD, P. (1979) 'The medical relevance of the hospital environment', in OSBORNE, D. (ed.) *Research in Psychology and Medicine*, London, Academic Press.

SUNDERLAND, A., HARRIS, J.E. and GLEAVE, J. (1984) 'Memory failures in everyday life following severe head injury', *Journal of Clinical and Experimental Neuropsychology*, 6, pp. 127–142.

SUTTON, R.L., WEAVER, M.S. and FEENEY, D.M. (1987) 'Drug-induced modifications of behavioural recovery following cortical trauma', *Journal of Head Trauma Rehabilitation*, 2, pp. 50–58.

SWANSON, H.L. (1987a) 'Information processing theory and learning disabilities: a commentary and future prospective', *Journal of Learning Disabilities*, 20, pp. 155–166.

SWANSON, H.L. (1987b) 'Information processing theory and learning disabilities: an overview', *Journal of Learning Disabilities*, 20, pp. 3–7.

TAITZ, L.S. (1988) 'Which children need vitamins?', *British Medical Journal*, 296, p. 1753.

TAKASHIMA, S., CHAN, F., BECKER, L.E. and ARMSTRONG, D.L. (1980) 'Morphology of the developing visual cortex of the human infant: a quantitative and qualitative Golgi study', *Journal of Neuropathology and Experimental Neurology*, 39, pp. 487–501.

TALLAL, P., CHASE, C., RUSSELL, G. and SCHMITT, R.L. (1986) 'Evaluation of the efficacy of piracetam in treating information processing, reading and writing disorders in dyslexic children', *International Journal of Psychophysiology*, 4, pp. 41–52.

TANNER, C.N., GOETZ, C.G. and KLAWANS, H.L. (1979) 'Cholinergic mechanisms in movement disorders: results of physostigmine and scopolamine administration', in BARBEAU, A., GROWDON, J.H. and WURTMAN, R.J. (ed.) *Nutrition and the Brain* Volume 5: *Choline and Lecithin in Brain Disorders*, New York, Raven Press.

TAYLOR, E. (1985) 'Drug treatment', in RUTTER, M. and HERSOV, L. (eds.) *Child and Adolescent Psychiatry: Modern Approaches* (2nd edition) London, Blackwell.

TAYLOR, E. (1986) *The Overactive Child, Clinics in Developmental Medicine No 97*, London, MacKeith Press.

TAYLOR, E., (1988) Report on an epidemiological study of childhood hyperactivity. (Unpublished.)

TAYLOR, E., SCHACHAR, R., THORLEY, G. and WEISELBERG, H.M. (1986) 'Conduct disorder and hyperactivity: I. Separation of hyperactivity and antisocial conduct in British child psychiatric patients', *British Journal of Psychiatry*, 149, pp. 760–767.

TAYLOR, H.G. (1984) 'Early brain injury and cognitive development', in ALMLI, C.R. and FINGER, S., (eds.) *Early Brain Damage*, Volume 1: *Research Orientations and Clinical Observations*, New York, Academic Press.

TELZROW, C.F. (1987) 'Management of academic and educational problems in head injury', *Journal of Learning Disabilities*, 20, pp. 536–545.

TENNANT, F.S. (1987) 'Naltrexone treatment for post-concussional syndrome', *American Journal of Psychiatry*, 144, pp. 813–814.

TEUBER, H.L. (1975) 'Recovery of functions after brain injury in man', in *Outcome of Severe Damage to the Central Nervous System*, Ciba Foundation Symposium, 34. Amsterdam, Elsevier.

THIBAULT, L.G. and GENNARELLI, T.A. (1985) 'Biomechanics and craniocerebral trauma', in BECKER, D.P. and POVLISHOCK, J.T. (eds.) *Central Nervous System Trauma Status Report*, Maryland, NIH.

TIMSIT-BERTHIER, M., MAUTANUS, H., JACQUES, M.C. and LEGROS, J.J. (1980) 'Utilite de la lysine-vasopressine dans le traitement de l'amnesie post-traumatique', *Acta Psychiatrica Belgica*, 80, pp. 728–747.

TIZARD, J. (1976) 'Nutrition, growth and development', *Psychological Medicine*, 6, pp. 1–5.

TOGLIA, J.U. (1972) 'Vestibular and medico-legal aspects of closed cranio-cervical trauma', *Scandinavian Journal of Rehabilitation Medicine*, 4, pp. 126–132.

TOGLIA, J.U. and KATINSKY, S. (1976) 'Neuro-otological aspects of closed head injury, in VINKEN, P.J. and BRUYN, G.W. (eds.) *Handbook of Clinical Neurology* Volume 23: *Injuries of the Brain and Skull*, Amsterdam, Elsevier.

TOGLIA, J.U., ROSENBERG, P.E. and RONIS, M. (1970) 'Post-traumatic dizziness: vestibular, audiological and medicolegal aspects', *Archives of Otolaryngology*, 92, pp. 485–492.

TRIMBLE, M., CORBETT, J.A. and DONALDSON, (1980) 'Folic acid and mental symptoms in children with epilepsy', *Journal of Neurology, Neurosurgery and Psychiatry*, 43, pp. 1030–1034.

TSUBOKAWA, T. (1987) 'Neurosciences for the study of coma', *Brain Injury*, 1, pp. 129–130.

TUCKER, D.M. and WILLIAMSON, P.A. (1984) 'Asymmetric neural control systems in human self-regulation', *Psychological Review*, 91, pp. 185–215.

TUOHIMAA, P. (1978) 'Vestibular disturbances after acute mild head injury', *Acta Otolaryngologica*, Supplement 359.

TWYMAN, D., YOUNG, B. and OTT, L. (1985) 'High protein enteral feedings: a means of achieving positive nitrogen balance', *Journal of Parenteral and Enteral Nutrition*, 9, pp. 679–684.

URWIN, S., COOK, J. and KELLY, K. (1988) 'Preschool language intervention: a follow-up study', *Child Care, Health and Development*, 14, pp. 127–146.

VAN DONGEN, H.R. and VISCH-BRINK, E.G. (1988) 'Naming in aphasic children: analysis of paraphasic errors', *Neuropsychologia*, 26, pp. 629–632.

VAN DONGEN, H.R., LOONEN, M.C.B. and VAN DONGEN, J.J. (1985) 'Anatomical basis for acquired fluent aphasia in children', *Annals of Neurology*, 17, pp. 306–309.

VAN HOF, M.W. (1981) 'Development and recovery from brain damage', in CONNOLLY, K.J. and PRECHTL, H.F.R. (eds.) *Maturation and Development: Biological and Psychological Perspectives, Clinics in Developmental Medicine*, No. 77/78. London, SIMP — Heinemann.

VAN HOUT, A., EVRARD, P. and LYON, G. (1985) 'On the positive semiology of acquired aphasia in children', *Developmental Medicine and Child Neurology*, 27, pp. 231–241.

VAN WOERKOM, T.C.A.M., TEELKEN, A.W. and MINDERHOUD, J.M. (1977) 'Difference in neurotransmitter metabolism in fronto-temporal lobe contusion and diffuse cerebral contusion', *Lancet*, 1, p. 812.

VAN WOERKOM, T.C.A.M., MINDERHOUD, J.M., GOTTSCHAL, P. and NOCOLI, J. (1982) 'Neurotransmitters in the treatment of patients with severe head injury', *European Neurology*, 21, pp. 227–234.

VAN WOERKOM, T.C.A.M., VAN WEERDEN, T.W. and MINDERHOUD, J.M. (1984) 'Saccadic oscillations associated with quick phases of caloric nystagmus in severe diffuse brain damage', *Clinical Neurology and Neurosurgery*, 86, pp. 21–27.

VAN ZOMEREN, A.H. (1981) *Attention after Head Injury*, Lisse, Swets Zeitlinger.

VAN ZOMEREN, A.H. and BROUWER, W.H. (1987) 'Head injury and concepts of attention, in LEVIN, H.S., GRAFMAN, J. and EISENBERG, H.M. (eds.) *Neurobehavioural Recovery from Head Injury*, New York, Oxford University Press.

VAN ZOMEREN, A.H., BROUWER, W.H. and DEELMAN, B.G. (1984) 'Attentional deficit: the riddles of selectivity speed and alertness', in BROOKS, D.N. (ed.) *Closed Head Injury: psychological, social and family consequences*, Oxford, Oxford University Press.

VARGHA-KHADEM, F., O'GORMAN, A.M. and WATTERS, G.V. (1985) 'Aphasia and handedness in relation to hemispheric side, age at injury and severity of cerebral lesion during childhood', *Brain*, 108, pp. 677–696.

VECHT, C.J., VAN WOERKOM, T.C.A.M. and TEELKEN, A.W. (1975) 'Homovanillic acid and 5-hydroxyindoleacetic acid cerebrospinal fluid levels', *Archives of Neurology*, 32, pp. 792–797.

VECHT, C.J., VAN WOERKOM, T.C.A.M., TEELKEN, A.W. and MINDERHOUD, J.M. (1976) 'On the nature of brain stem disorders in severe head injury patients: Changes in cerebral neurotransmitter metabolism', *Acta Neurochiurgica*, 32, pp. 11–21.

VERTIAINEN, E., KARJALAINEN, S. and KARJA, J. (1985) 'Vestibular disorders following head injury in children', *International Journal of Paediatric Otolaryngology*, 9, pp. 135–141.

VON WILD, K. and DOLCE, G. (1976) 'Pathophysiological aspects concerning the treatment of the apallic syndrome', *Journal of Neurology*, 213, pp. 143–148.

WAALAND, P.K. and KREUTZER, J.S. (1988) 'Family responses to childhood brain injury', *Journal of Head Trauma Rehabilitation*, 3, pp. 51–63.

WALKER, J.B., KELLEY, R.L. and RIESEN, A.H. (1975) 'Neurochemical correlates of sensory deprivation', in RIESEN, A.H. (ed.) *The Developmental Neuropsychology of Sensory Deprivation*, New York, Academic Press.

WALKER, M. (1980) *The Revised Makaton Vocabulary* (published by author).

WALL, P.D. (1977) 'The presence of ineffective synapses and the circumstances which unmask them', *Philosophical Transactions of the Royal Society of London*, Series B, 278, pp. 361–372.

WALTON, R.G. (1982) 'Lecithin and physostigmine for post-traumatic memory and cognitive deficits', *Psychosomatics*, 23, pp. 435–446.

WANNEMACHER, R.W. Jr., DUPONT, H.L. and PERAREK, R.S. (1972) 'An endogenous mediator of depression of amino acids and trace metals in serum during typhoid fever', *Journal of Infectious Diseases*, 126, pp. 77–86.

WARD, A. (1950) 'Atropine in the treatment of closed head injuries', *Journal of Neurosurgery*, 7, pp. 398–402.

WARD, J.D. and ALBERICO, A.M. (1987) 'Paediatric head injuries', *Brain Injury*, 1, pp. 21–25.

WARNOCK, H.M. (1978) *Special Educational Needs: Report of the Committee of Enquiry into the Education of Handicapped Children and Young People*, London, HMSO.

WARREN, J.M. and KOLB, B. (1978) 'Generalisations in neuropsychology', in FINGER, S. (ed.) *Recovery from Brain Damage*, New York, Plenum Press.

WEBB, M.G.T. (1981) 'A case of severe post-traumatic insomnia treated with 5-hydroxytryptophan', *Proceedings III World Congress of Biological Psychiatry*, Amsterdam, Elsevier.

WEBER, P.L. (1984) 'Sensorimotor therapy: its effects on EEG's of acute comatose patients', *Archives of Physical Medicine and Rehabilitation*, 65, pp. 457–462.

WECHSLER, D. (1974) *The Wechsler Intelligence Scale for Children — Revised* Windsor, NFER-Nelson.

WEINBERG, (1986) 'Attention deficit disorder', in FLEHMIG, I. and STERN, L. (eds.) *Child Development and Learning Behaviour*, Stuttgart, Fischer.

WEINER, E.S. (1980) 'A theoretical model of the acquisition of peer relationships of learning disabled children', *Journal of Learning Disabilities*, 13, pp. 42–48.

WEINSTEIN, G.S. and WELLS, C.E. (1981) 'Case studies in neuropsychiatry: post-traumatic psychiatric dysfunction: diagnosis and treatment', *Clinical Psychiatry*, 42, pp. 120–122.

WEINTRAUB, S. and MESULAM, M.M. (1987) 'Right cerebral dominance in spatial attention', *Archives of Neurology*, 44, pp. 61–65.

WEISKRANTZ, L. (1977) 'Trying to bridge some neuropsychology gaps between monkey and man', *British Journal of Psychology*, 68, pp. 431–435.

WELSH, M.C. and PENNINGTON, B.F. (1988) 'Assessing frontal lobe function in children: views from developmental psychology', *Developmental Neuropsychology*, 4, pp. 199–230.

WENLOCK, R.W., DISSELDUFF, M.M. and SKINNER, R.K. 1986 *The Diets of British School Children*, London, DHSS 1986.

WHARTON, B. (1978) 'Childhood', in DICKERSON, J.W.T. and LEE, H.A. (eds.) *Nutrition in the Clinical Management of Disease*, London, Arnold.

WHITTLE, I.R., JOHNSON, I.H. and BESSER, M. (1987) 'Short latency somatosensory-evoked potentials in children — part 3: findings following head injury', *Surgical Neurology*, 27, pp. 29–36.

WHURR, R. and EVANS, S. (1986) *The Children's Aphasia Screening Test*, (Published by the authors).

WHYTE, J. (1986) 'Outcome evaluation in the remediation of attention and memory deficits', *Journal of Head Trauma Rehabilitation*, 1, pp. 64–71.

WILL, B.E. (1981) 'The influence of environment on recovery after brain damage in rodents', in VAN HOF, M.W. and MOHN, G. (eds.) *Functional Recovery from Brain Damage*, Amsterdam, Elsevier.

WILL, B. E. and ECLANCHER, F. (1984) 'Early brain damage and early environment', in FINGER, S and ALMLI, C.R. (eds.) *Early Brain Damage*, Volume II: *Neurobiology and Behaviour*, New York, Academic Press.

WILL, B.E., ROSENZWEIG, M.R., BENNETT, E.L., HERBERT, M. and MORIMOTO, H. (1977) 'Relatively brief environmental enrichment aids recovery of learning capacity and alters brain measures after postweaning brain lesions in rats', *Journal of Comparative and Physiological Psychology*, 19, pp. 33–50.

WILLIAMS, D. and DENNY-BROWN, D. (1941) 'Cerebral electrical changes in experimental concussion', *Brain*, 64, pp. 223–238.

WILLIAMS, P.D., WILLIAMS, A.R. and DIAL, M.N. (1986) 'Children at risk: perinatal events, developmental delays and the effects of a developmental stimulation programme', *International Journal of Nursing Studies*, 23, pp. 21–38.

WILLS, J. (1988) 'Conflicting Statements', *Times Educational Supplement*, 12 April, pp. 18.

WILSON, B. (1981) 'A survey of behavioural treatments carried out at a rehabilitation centre for stroke and head injuries', in POWELL, G.E. (ed.) *Brain Function Therapy*, Hampshire, Gower.

WINDLEW, F., GROAT, R.A. and FOX, C.A. (1944) 'Experimental structural alterations in the brain during and after concussion', *Surgery, Gynaecology and Obstetrics*, 79, pp. 561–572.

WITTROCK, M.C. (1980) *The Brain and Psychology*, Academic Press, New York.

WITTROCK, M.C. (1986) Education and recent research on attention and knowledge acquisition in FRIEDMAN, S.L., KLIVINGTON, K.A. and PETERSON, R.W. (eds.) *The Brain, Cognition and Education*. New York, Academic Press.

WOLF, S.M. and FORSYTHE, A. (1978) 'Behaviour disturbance, phenobarbital and febrile seizures', *Paediatrics*, 61, pp. 728–730.

WOOD, R.Ll. (1987) 'Brain Injury Rehabilitation: a neurobehavioural approach', London, Croom Helm.

WOOD, R.Ll, and EAMES, P. (1981) 'An application of behaviour modification in the treatment of traumatically head-injured adults', in DAVEY, G. (ed.) *Applications of Conditioning Theory*, London, Methuen.

WOODS, B.T. (1980) 'The restricted effects of right-hemisphere lesions after age one: Wechsler test data', *Neuropsychologia*, 18, pp. 65–70.

WOODS, B.T. and CAREY, S. (1979) 'Language deficits after apparent clinical recovery from childhood aphasia', *Annals of Neurology*, 6, pp. 405–409.

WOODS, B.T. and TEUBER, H.L. (1978) 'Changing patterns in childhood aphasia', *Annals of Neurology*, 3, pp. 273–280.

WURTMAN, J.J. (1979) 'Sources of choline and lecithin in the diet', in BARBEAU, A., GROWDON, J.H. and WURTMAN, R.J. (eds.) *Nutrition and the Brain* Volume 5: *Choline and Lecithin in Brain Disorders*, New York, Raven Press.

WURTMAN, J.J. and WURTMAN, R.J. (1986) *Nutrition and the Brain* Volume 7: *Food Constituents Affecting Normal and Abnormal Behaviours*, New York, Raven Press.

WURTMAN, R.J. (1983), 'Introduction', *Journal of Psychiatric Research*, 17, pp. 103–105.

YANKO, J. (1985) 'The acute phase', in YLVISAKER, M. (ed.) *Head-injury Rehabilitation: children and adolescents*, London, Taylor and Francis.

YATES, D.W. (1988) 'Action for accident victims', *British Medical Journal*, 297, pp. 1419–1420.

YLVISAKER, M. (ed.) (1985) *Head-injury Rehabilitation: children and adolescents*, London, Taylor and Francis.

YOUNG, B., OTT, L., BEARD, D., DEMPSEY, R.J., TIBBS, P.A. and McCLAIN, C.J. (1988) 'The acute phase response of the brain-injured patient', *Journal of Neurosurgery*, 69, pp. 375–380.

YOUNG, B., OTT, L., NORTON, J., TIBBS, P., RAPP, R., McCLAIN, C. and DEMPSEY, R. (1985) 'Metabolic and nutritional sequelae in the non-steroid treated head-injury patient', *Neurosurgery*, 17, pp. 784–791.

YOUNG, B., OTT, L., RAPP, R. and NORTON, J. (1987) 'The patient with critical neurological diseases', *Critical Care Clinics*, 3, pp. 217–233.

YOUNG, S.N. (1986) 'The clinical psychopharmacology of tryptophan', in WURTMAN, R.J. and WURTMAN, J.J. (eds.) *Nutrition and the Brain*, Volume 7, New York, Raven Press.

YULE, W. (1978) 'Diagnosis: developmental neuropsychological assessment', *Advances in Biological Psychiatry*, 1, pp. 35–54.

YULE, W. (1986) 'Behavioural treatments', in TAYLOR, E. (ed.) *The Overactive Child, Clinics Developmental Medicine* No. 97, London, MacKeith Press.

YULES, R.B., KREBS, C.Q. and GAULT, F.P. (1966) 'Reticular formation control of the vestibular system', *Experimental Neurology*, 16, pp. 349–358.

ZIGLER, E. (1969) 'Developmental versus difference theories of mental retardation and the problem of motivation', *American Journal of Mental Deficiency*, 73, pp. 536–556.

ZIMMERMAN, R.A. and BILANIUK, L.T. (1981) 'Computed tomography in paediatric head trauma', *Journal of Neuroradiology*, 8, pp. 257–271.

ZUCCARELLO, M., FACCO, E., ZAMPERI, P., ZANARDI, L. and ANDRIOLI, G.C. (1985) 'Severe head injury in children: early prognosis and outcome', *Child's Nervous System*, 1, pp. 158–162.

List of Contributors

B. A. Bell
Consultant Neurosurgeon
Atkinson Morley's Hosiptal
Copse Hill
London SW20 0NE

Juliet Britton
Consultant Neuroradiologist
Atkinson Morley's Hospital
Copse Hill
London SW20 0NE

R.W.D. Clarke
Director
British Life Insurance Trust for Health
   Education
BMA House
Tavistock Square
London WC1H 9JP

John W.T. Dickerson
Formerly Professor of Human
   Nutrition
Department of Biochemistry
University of Surrey
Guildford
Surrey GU2 5XH

David A. Johnson
Clinical Psychologist
Atkinson Morley's Hospital
Copse Hill
London SW20 0NE

Denise Kingsmill
Solicitors
44 Bedford Row
London WC1R 4LL

Janet Lees
Chief Speech Therapist
Newcomen Centre
Guy's Hospital
St Thomas' Street
London SE1 9RT

Anne Maclean
Senior Dietician
St George's Hospital
Blackshaw Road
London SW17 0QT

Peter Eames
Consultant Neuropsychiatrist
Burden Neurological Hospital
Stoke Lane
Stapleton
Bristol BS16 1QT

Ruth Furlonger
ILEA Hospital Teacher
St George's Hospital
Blackshaw Road
London SW17 0QT

Lady Glenconner
14 Hillsleigh Road
Kensington
London W8

Robert Goodman
Research Fellow in Neuropsychiatry
Institute of Child Health
Great Ormond Street
London WC1N 3JH

David Hall
Consultant Paediatrician
St George's Hospital
Blackshaw Road
London SW17 0QT

H. R. M. Hayes
Child Accident Prevention Trust
28 Portland Place
London W1N 4DE

Peter Hill
Senior Lecturer in Child and Adolescent
    Psychiatry
St George's Hospital Medical School
Cranmer Terrace
London SW17 0RE

Judith Middleton
Senior Clinical Psychologist
Director, Head Injury Unit
Tadworth Court Children's Hospital
Tadworth
Surrey

Ewa Raglan
Consultant Audiological Physician and
    Neuro-otologist
St George's Hospital
Blackshaw Road
London SW17 0QT

Karen Roethig-Johnston
Research Psychologist
Department of Neuropsychology
Atkinson Morley's Hospital
Copse Hill
London SW20 0NE

Eric Taylor
Reader in Developmental
    Neuropsychiatry
Institute of Psychiatry
De Crespigny Park
Denmark Hill
London SE5 8AF

David Uttley
Consultant Neurosurgeon
Atkinson Morley's Hospital
Copse Hill
London SW20 0NE

Judith Wardle
20 Oxford Road
Littlemore
Oxford
OX4 4PE

R. H. Jackson
Child Accident Prevention Trust
28 Portland Place
London W1N 4DE

Maria A. Wyke
Senior Lecturer in Neuropsychology
Institute of Psychiatry
De Crespigny Park
Denmark Hill
London SE5 8AF

Index